ADOLESCENT PSYCHIATRY

DEVELOPMENTAL AND CLINICAL STUDIES

VOLUME 16

Annals of the American Society for Adolescent Psychiatry

ADOLESCENT PSYCHIATRY

DEVELOPMENTAL AND CLINICAL STUDIES

VOLUME 16

Edited by
SHERMAN C. FEINSTEIN
Editor in Chief

Senior Editors
AARON H. ESMAN
JOHN G. LOONEY
GEORGE H. ORVIN
JOHN L. SCHIMEL
ALLAN Z. SCHWARTZBERG
ARTHUR D. SOROSKY
MAX SUGAR

The University of Chicago Press
Chicago and London

The University of Chicago Press, Chicago 60637
The University of Chicago Press, Ltd., London

International Standard Book Number: 0-226-24062-2
Library of Congress Catalog Card Number: 70-147017

The paper used in this publication meets the minimum requirements of American National Standard for Information Sciences—Permanence of Paper for Printed Library Materials, ANSI Z39.48-1984. ∞ ™

CONTENTS

PART II. DEVELOPMENTAL ISSUES: TRANSITION TO YOUNG ADULTHOOD

JOHN G. LOONEY, Special Editor

PART V. TRAINING PRIORITIES IN ADOLESCENT PSYCHIATRY

Errata

The following are corrections of errors in the previous volume of *Adolescent Psychiatry*:

Page 33, line 1, should read "Apfel, R. J., and Fisher, S. M. 1984. *To Do No Harm: DES and the Dilemmas of Modern Medicine*. New Haven, Conn.: Yale University Press."

Pages 165–66, legends of figures 3 and 4 should be transposed.

Page 557, line 5, should read "ROBERTA J. APFEL is Assistant Professor of Psychiatry, Harvard Medical School, Boston."

PRESIDENT'S PREFACE

The loyal officers and members of the American Society for Adolescent Psychiatry (ASAP) have been proud of its growth and expansion. In recent years, the Society has developed a research fund and a research award; has presented an amicus curiae brief to the U.S. Supreme Court on capital punishment for adolescents; is a cosponsor with the American Medical Association of a three-year survey project with congressional objectives; and maintains direct liaison with the American Psychiatric Association, especially in such germane areas as public policy and subspecialization.

Our society has recently moved its offices to Washington, D.C., with David Lewis, executive director, and staff. In just the past year, we have implemented new formats for the newsletter, the brochure, and the membership directory, and, happily, a number of other exciting and stimulating projects are well on their way.

As positive as these achievements are, the original and primary goal of ASAP is and will continue to be educational. This objective is achieved through annual and regional conferences and the *Annals of the American Society for Adolescent Psychiatry*. All these represent major expenditures of devotion and energy from the authors, editors, and members of the program committees. Major themes and topics continue to examine essential core issues such as development, identity, diagnosis, and treatment, as they should, but the addition of such current topics as the neurosciences, AIDS, and domestic violence are valuable and necessary.

As president of ASAP for 1988–1989, I would like to express my enormous appreciation and offer enthusiastic congratulations to the authors, Sherman Feinstein, editor-in-chief, and the editorial group for this current volume of the *Annals*. The contents reflect ASAP's ongoing dedication to serving its membership in the pursuit of medicine's highest goals: knowledge, understanding, and the humane applications thereof for the ultimate benefit of our teenagers and their families. This volume is another great source of pride to ASAP and a welcome addition to all our libraries.

S. DION SMITH

PART I

ADOLESCENCE: GENERAL CONSIDERATIONS

EDITORS' INTRODUCTION

Peter Blos, in a presentation to the International Society for Adolescent Psychiatry, July 1987, reviews masculinity as a developmental concept. Distinct from "maleness," the early perception of sexual difference in a normal child's awareness of being a boy or girl, masculinity presents as a psychologically integrated behavioral and self-regulatory system that reaches completion only after pubertal and adolescent psychic organization has run its course. Blos further defines "gender" as the awareness of being male or female and "sex" as referring to the expressive modalities of acting and feeling male or female within the boundaries of a social and cultural definition. All this, from the vantage point of male adolescence in particular, Blos defines from sequential order (developmental or epigenetic progressions) and dynamic patterning (management of psychic and emotional needs). In this restatement of masculinity, Blos removes the Oedipus complex from its central position in the final stage of masculinity formation and recognizes as the central adolescent conflict the efforts to resolve the earlier dyadic conflict and to renounce the need for object and self-idealization. Discussions by Evan Brahm, Aaron Esman, and Vivian Rakoff help examine and clarify this major change in developmental theory.

Bertram Slaff reviews the history of child and adolescent ideas and organizations, examining, in particular, a number of conflict areas: pediatrics versus child psychiatry; medical model versus multidisciplinary team approach; general psychiatry versus child psychiatry; child psychiatry versus adolescent psychiatry; biological versus psychodynamic; credentialism versus academic openness; and centralization ver-

3

sus regional autonomy. Slaff then traces the growth of the American Society for Adolescent Psychiatry as a developmental phenomenon.

Carol C. Nadelson views adolescence from a developmental context and discusses some of the major sources of distress that parents, society, and adolescents face. Among the variations of conflict, Nadelson selects suicide, affective disorder, conduct disorder, substance abuse, and adolescent pregnancy to consider from a mental health services perspective. A discussion of financing mental health care for adolescents focuses on third-party payment from insurance, possible over-utilization of services to meet diverse adolescents' needs, special education and long-term care, as well as movement away from the medical model. The author concludes that, currently faced with major crises, adolescent psychiatrists must develop reasonable solutions in the delivery of services to adolescents and young adults.

Howard S. Baker explores the dilemmas faced by the college-bound offspring of a working-class family. Here, the response of the university environment presents a different set of developmental tasks, demanding a move out of the social class of origin. Baker approaches developmental theory from a self-psychological perspective and explores self-selfobject relationships. He documents that social class mobility must have a profound effect on both the ongoing and the developmental self-object milieu of any college student and that direct psychiatric intervention may consist of little more than understanding and encouragement. The author recommends that grasping the multiple aspects of the student's sociological environment can provide a "developmental splint" for the stressed college student.

Leo Rangell surveys adolescent development by focusing on age seventeen: a position in adolescence approaching the portal to adulthood. At seventeen the adult is getting ready to emerge: critical decisions must be made about one's future; integration and consolidation become semipermanent; and unconscious choices have become character attitudes on the spectrum of activity-passivity, object relations, sexual orientation, and identity. Rangell quotes Blos that the heir of adolescence is the self: at seventeen, he writes, the character, the emerging nature and attributes of the person, is being formed. In this unusual chapter, a synthesis of psychoanalytic perspectives are brought into focus so that the adolescent emerges as a dynamic, energetic individual on the verge of a quantum leap.

4

1 MASCULINITY: DEVELOPMENTAL ASPECTS OF ADOLESCENCE

PETER BLOS

"Masculinity" as a topic of discussion certainly deserves, at this time, a review, an update, or a revision of still too firmly held traditional formulations. Research in child and adolescent development has dislodged some of our basic assumptions that we have taken for granted, perhaps for too long. In this chapter I wish to subject to a critical scrutiny the central concept that represents the age-honored cornerstone of psychoanalytic theory dominating our thinking about masculinity.

A brief look at the literature on masculinity and femininity tells us immediately that man has been shortchanged to an astonishing degree in comparison to the endless outpourings in the effort to comprehend the enigma of woman. This is certainly true of Freud's own writings. It seemed that with the formulation of the Oedipus complex the male's sexual development and problem of masculinity was understood. It was essentially the Oedipus complex that offered the explanatory concept in relation to the sexual development of the male, normal or abnormal. I should state right here that cases of devious masculinity due to hormonal or anatomical abnormalities are excluded from this discussion.

Before we can enter the substantive part of this chapter, I suggest that we clarify the terms we use in this discourse. The term "masculinity" is obviously distinct from what we mean by "maleness," just as the term "sex" has a disparate reference from "gender." Masculinity finds its expressive definition by an endogenous system of behavior and attitudes, symbolizations, and meanings that, in their totality, are

5

characteristic and unique for any culturally coherent social structure. "Maleness," in contrast, refers to the differentiation of the anatomical sex difference in any normal child's conscious awareness of being a boy or a girl. This awareness is established early in life, whereas the operational state of "masculinity" as a psychologically integrated behavioral and self-regulatory system can reach its completion of development only after pubertal (i.e., sexual) maturation and after adolescent psychic reorganization has run its course.

The attempt to clarify terminology would be incomplete if we would fail to agree on the specific use of the two words "sex" and "gender." In my writings I have used "gender" to refer to the individual's awareness of being male or female, while I have used "sex" to refer to the expressive modalities of acting and feeling as male or female in the realm of genital sensuality and within the inclusive or exclusive boundaries of a socially and culturally codified definition. In the literature we find an irregular and often contradictory use of these terms. Consistent with my developmental reference of the terms, I speak of "gender identity" established early in life (beginning in the first year) and of "sexual identity" in its completed stage after the closure of adolescence; in fact, the attainment of sexual identity as an ego-syntonic component of the self-system determines the point of adolescent closure. We might say that, at this developmental moment, either a normal or a deviant potential within the spectrum, which lies between masculine and feminine identities, solidifies into a permanent disposition or an integrated, individual mode of personality functioning. In other words, each acquires the quality of a highly personal modality of interpersonal transaction or style, most characteristically experienced in gender-related affects and bodily expression, be these of an active or a passive nature.

Being cognizant of the fact that I write here with the focus on adolescence, I shall consequently view the issues of masculinity from the vantage point of adolescence and gauge from this perspective its protoadolescent history, its adolescent-specific contribution with reverberations into a man's adult life.

This enterprise requires that I state certain aspects of adolescent theory—and of male adolescence in particular—in order to define the theoretical position on which my contribution to the subject under discussion is based. The formulation of theory extends into two dimensions. One relates to developmental or epigenetic progressions reflecting the principle of sequential order, and the other, namely, the one of dynamic patterning, deals with the disposition and management of psychic and emotional needs. Since my adolescent research has always taken its cue from clinical observation, it seems to me appropriate to follow the same course in this presentation.

We are familiar with the psychoanalytic thesis of the Oedipus complex and the leading role assigned to it in the formation of masculinity. In essence, the successful resolution of the male Oedipus conflict, or the kind of compromise formation on which the final settlement of the male Oedipus conflict was ultimately attained, determines the uniqueness and the type of masculinity that the individual male acquires as a permanent and integral characteristic of his personality. It was only after I had practiced adolescent therapy for a long time, during which I took the centrality of the Oedipus complex as self-evident, that I came to question the psychoanalytic recapitulation theory of adolescence as the valid explanatory model of the focal adolescent developmental conflict. Voices, especially from child analysts like myself, had become increasingly more convincing in questioning the centrality assigned to the oedipal conflict in the etiology of neurotic illness in male adolescence and, consequently, doubting the exclusively defensive organization evoked by recapitulated, infantile castration anxiety at the time of sexual maturation at puberty.

The too frequent ineffectiveness of oedipal interpretations in my therapeutic work with male adolescents made me review more carefully my clinical notes. I speak here of interpretations related to the so-called typical adolescent father complex of the boy—for instance, competition with the oedipal father, patricide, state of guilt and atonement, regression to passivity, to infantile rage, and to forms of infantile self-gratification, such as masturbatory excitation or oral stimulations, inducing self-regulated mood changes.

Slowly, I came to realize that the boy's proverbial expressions of competition, oppositionalism, and defiance or, summarily speaking, his animosity toward the father or the societal father representations, such as police, law, school, and so on, have to be comprehended largely as expressions of a defensive operation against a regression to early attachment emotions in relation to the father. The etiological importance of an incomplete libidinal detachment from the early father and from his caretaking and protective presence in the little boy's life—a presence, either actual, construed, or wished for—demanded to be examined in greater detail in relation to the boy's developmental passage through adolescence. It is obvious that the physically maturing boy encounters the condition of an emotional confrontation in adolescence that repeats a trauma of the male infant when he first attempted to loosen the infantile ties of passivity to the symbiotic mother by transferring slowly and intermittently his attachment emotions to the father. Later we will consider further the similarity of the infant boy's and the adolescent boy's traumatic liberation efforts at these two crucial stages in his life, when the two denominators of male and female become irrevocably defined as sexual identity.

After I had once realized that the aggressive stance of the adolescent boy against the competitor father was only a partially correct inference and that, in addition, it had to be recognized in its unsuspected defensive function against his preoedipal libidinal father attachment, I had to take this realization one step further in terms of its consequences on the adolescent task of male psychic restructuring in its broadest sense. Implicit in the formulations just advanced is the notion that the adolescent's first heterosexual manifestations are of a defensive nature. This is to say that genuine masculinity is contingent on the adolescent libidinal severance from the dyadic father or, in other words, the removal of the defensive component from the heterosexual life of the adult male. It goes without saying that a father fixation on the dyadic stage is intimately coupled with an infantile need expressed in object idealization. Without relinquishment of infantile idealization, no individual is able to achieve the state of dependable, stable reality testing, and, therefore, he remains indefinitely at risk owing to the fact that he cannot provide for himself the necessary protection in a world that is wrought with dangers to body and mind; he requires a reliable capacity for reality testing in order to maintain an optimal and independent sense of safety. Because of these reasons, I slowly became emboldened to remove the Oedipus complex from its central position in the final stage of masculinity formation during adolescence.

Summarizing my view of the adolescent developmental task within the epigenetic schema of masculinity, I recognize as the central adolescent conflict of the boy his effort to reach an unconflicted state of masculinity via the resolution of his father complex of the dyadic period and the renunciation of the infantile need for object and self-idealization. The often noisy reverberations of the male infant's dyadic father idealization are demonstratively brought to our attention in the proverbial hero worship of peer-shared male stars in the contemporary hall of fame. With the closure of adolescence we observe a slow fading of this blind hero worship and its turn into a more idiosyncratic and critical selectivity of value and style. In my clinical judgment, these are two risk components, one infantile, one adolescent, that are central to the therapy of any adolescent boy.

Only after the dyadic libidinal attachment emotions to the father have been resolved by identification and internalization can a progression to the oedipal stage proper become viable. By the process of imitation, identification, and internalization during the toddler's life, the first decisive and irreversible cultural transmittal of sexual stereotyping occurs. The origin of an uncompromising self-evidence of the child's psychosocial typologizing, with reference to masculinity and femininity, can be traced to the transition from the male primary dyad, or other-gender dyadic tie (infant boy–mother), to the subsequent same-gender dyadic tie (infant boy–father). At this juncture are the roots of the male father complex to be found. I will return to this issue for amplification and clarification when I trace in greater detail the phases of dyadic object attachments. The only comment I will add here is to say that a progressive sense of masculinity needs to be sustained by a sense of what it is not; the latter is defined by the boy's awareness of the exclusive and the inclusive characteristics of femininity and femaleness.

The etiological importance of these preoedipal determinants in the boy's father-dependent affective life became evident to me when I realized that the diminution or resolution of the father complex in adolescent treatment was responded to with a startling decline of father-directed aggression and guilt in thought or action. The realization that the proverbial father aggression of the adolescent could be a defensive act of "turning into the opposite"—attachment into hostility—opened in my clinical work an ongoing investigation over many years into the dynamics of paternal attachment emotions during the stage of sexual maturation of the adolescent boy. The findings threw a new light on the epigenesis of masculinity.

In order to clarify this factor in the developmental complexity of masculinity, I must emphasize the originally adaptive aspect of the boy's infantile father attachment and the progressive developmental function of his infantile paternal idealization. It all has its beginning during the separation-individuation phase when the infant, under the influence of innate growth and maturation propulsion, attempts to loosen the symbiotic oneness with the mother. In this process the little boy turns to the father as a familiar other. This new, yet separate other one, the father, is to become an absolutely necessary facilitator in the separation-individuation process.

The father is not an oedipal object of fear at this stage when the parental attachment shifts from the early mother to include progressively the early father, both functioning in caretaking roles. The father presents no threat to regressive merger or to a regressive reversal of the organism's progressive ego differentiation since the new attachment object, the father, is now a vital part of the separation-individuation process and promises to secure the advance and completion of this developmental phase. Here we have to consider the fact that the father is for the infant, in Mahler's (1955) words, a so-called uncontaminated object since he had never existed as a symbiotic partner with a history of oneness or merger states. Gender identity is shared with the father and establishes a bond of sameness, inviting identification soon to be endowed with idealization. Of course, we recognize in father idealization a continuum of the merger states that the infant had experienced in the oneness with the mother and her regulating function. We notice a shift from this physical oneness and absolute security to an ideational creation of the father as the absolute protector against the regressive needs to the symbiotic past—the paradise lost.

The first move toward father idealization, with whom the little boy shares gender sameness, is closely tied to the boy's awareness of maleness, concretized in the penis, both part of object idealization and endowed with narcissistic libido. When the male infant in his effort to disengage himself from primary passivity and mother dependency turns to the father, extending his now shifting attachment emotions to the father, the new object inherits many features from the dyadic bond with the mother. Only gradually does the mother lose her role as the infant's primordial regulator or his sense of safety, security, and gratification. The pull to primary maternal dependency arouses anxiety in relation to the "reengulfing" mother (Mahler 1955). At this crucial developmental point, the father appears as a rescuer. The more desperately he is needed to ward off regression to primary passivity, the more is the rescuer idealized, not as an oedipal (triadic) but as a dyadic father. In this newly created role, the father is perceived now—at least intermittently—as more competent, more powerful, more resourceful, more dependable than the infant's first symbiotic partner, the mother. In making the distinction between the idealized dyadic and idealized triadic father, I see in the former a father greatness in which the little son shares in a significantly unambivalent relatedness, thus solidifying his earliest sense of masculinity under the benevolent guardianship of the father. This dyadic father imago can be studied in every analysis of an adult man because it represents a component of any male neurosis. In contrast, the idealized triadic or oedipal father is contained in the imago of a forbidding and vengeful, ambivalently loved, feared, admired, and degraded man.

I have concluded from my clinical adolescent observation that there are always two stages simultaneously involved in conflicted or aborted adolescence. I, therefore, stopped asking the single question, What are the oedipal or triadic dynamics in a given adolescent neurotic illness? But I ask myself in the same breath the question, What are the dyadic neurotic components in the illness?

It has become for me a categorical diagnostic requirement always to pose a dual etiological question with reference to neurotic disturbances in masculinity formation and its subsequent frailty and instability. This approach is based on my conviction that such disturbances in masculine identity formation have their dual roots in interlocking dyadic and triadic developmental derailments. Their sequential and finally irreversible resolution concludes the state of adolescence. In fact, the resolution of the dyadic father complex represents a major task of adolescence generally. The incompleteness of the transition from dyadic mother to dyadic father attachment is followed by an incapacity of the infant to share both of these early objects in pursuit of their specific and compensatory qualities. I have demonstrated the two infantile stages that are in sequence dominated by single caretaker-centered and dual caretaker-centered dyadic object relations. At the transition from one to the other we encounter the first moment of risk or the first potential break in the epigenetic progression of masculinity consolidation.

I must mention here my proposition that neither one of the two dyadic stages nor the triadic-oedipal stage of object relations arrives at a resolution—normal or abnormal—of their conflictualities in early childhood; this normative process has to be completed in adolescence. Therefore, not until adolescence is terminated can we be certain of the definite character that the masculinity of a given individual male will attain. We can expect that the study of adolescence will clarify the normative course of masculinity as well as indicate where the moments of risk lie along its developmental course during puberty. In extreme cases of effeminacy, the outcome appears already certain in early or middle childhood. In most cases the adolescent challenge—what Anna Freud has called "the second chance"—might keep sexual identity within the boundaries of gender adequacy. Residues of fragility and ambiguity in early and appropriate gender and sexual identification reappear at adolescence when the trauma of the controlling, possessive, dependency-arousing mother imago is reexperienced.

We witness this replay when the boy, because of sexual maturation, feels himself irresistibly drawn to the female with desire and fear. Should fear dominate and persist, sexual inhibition will become insurmountable; a deficient, insecure, and unstable sense of masculinity often hides behind demonstrative macho role playing. The father complex of the boy or his fixation on dyadic attachment emotions to him is drawn into the adolescent stance of pseudomasculinity. Here I refer to the adolescent boy who experiences an excruciating sense of low self-esteem and of depressive isolation due to his dependency on role playing of shared masculinity, which his idealized friend or peers in general possess in seeming abundance. This psychic pain can be averted only by being constantly heterosexually hyperactive, even though all these relationships are emotionally empty, shallow, and ephemeral. We encounter here again the infantile idealization that at adolescence congeals into a narcissistic personality disorder. This should not surprise us since these fleeting, heterosexual attachments serve a defensive purpose and are not of a genuine nature. It occurred to me that the boy's regressive pull to the dyadic father imago as his rescuer from the pubertal, highly ambivalent attraction to the female is defensively kept at bay by being excessively heterosexually active.

It is in the nature of sexual maturation that the fixation on infantile dependency attachments becomes endowed at the pubertal period with sexual, namely, genitally registered and expressed, emotions. This developmentally normal and transitory phenomenon moves adolescent heterosexuality into a new light in which we can observe it in its defensive function. We had earlier observed a similar developmental drama when the little boy encountered unsurmountable obstacles in the normal progression from the dyadic bond—other gender or same gender—to the triadic constellation of the Oedipus complex. In case the little boy, at that juncture, drifts into an effeminate libido position—either via a mother (i.e., female identification) or via a dyadic father fixation—the entire solidity and clarity of infantile gender identity becomes threatened. With the little boy's increased social awareness, his deviant masculinity, when responded to in derogatory reactions by his social surround, acquires a conflictual and ego-dystonic distinctness. When the boy's first turn away from the symbiotic mother to the dyadic father remains unrewarding, this can either be due to the unyielding strength of the infant-mother symbiotic bond or be due to the father's unresponsiveness, and it leaves the child's widening dyadic attachment and dependency needs without a participating, stage-engaged, cooperative parental partner. Such a developmental stagnation in the male infant's normal developmental progression represents the critical point at which the male child's turn into effeminacy has its decisive beginnings. Stoller and Herdt (1982) state "that the more complete and prolonged this merging (mother-infant symbiosis), and the less a father figure is present to interrupt the merging and to serve as a model for masculinity, the greater a male's femininity" (p. 33). They continue, "The most feminine of anatomically normal males—primary transsexuals—reveal these etiological elements" (p. 29). In this context I should mention a comment by Loewald (1951): "Against the threat of maternal engulfment the paternal position is not another thread of danger, but a support of powerful force" (p. 15). Following Loewald's comment we read Mahler (1955) saying that "the stable image of a father or another substitute of the mother, beyond the eighteen-months mark and even earlier, is beneficial and *perhaps a necessary prerequisite* to neutralize and to counteract the ego-characteristic over-sensibility of the toddler to the threat of a reengulfment by the mother" (p. 209, my emphasis).

While it has been an established tenet for a long time that the mother's infantilizing influence on the baby is determined by her own mothering needs—active and passive—which affirm their never relinquished emotional power at the stage of motherhood, it has been far less recognized that the father equally uses his child, especially his son, to repair his own father complex in the particular way he relates to him when called on at the dyadic stage and later, up to the closure of adolescence and beyond. Whenever a father brought his adolescent son to see me for treatment and confided in me, "I love him more than anybody in the world—he is the only one I care about," then I knew that this boy was in serious trouble. In this perspective we can say that every boy's masculinity is shaped by a three-generational confluence of infantile

attachment emotions and their resolution along overlapping developmental lines (Blos 1985).

In order to illustrate this basic concept, I shall briefly refer to the
analysis of a forty-year-old man. He had often talked about the intractability of his now four-year-old son, who refused to stay in his
own room at night but steadfastly remained a nightly visitor to his
father's bed, always bypassing the mother. The father loved this little
boy with a passion. When finally the father's own father yearning had
entered the analysis, he acknowledged the intensity of his affect with
uncontrollable sobbing, stammering, "Why did I love my father so
much; after all, I had a mother." The resolution of his father complex
in the analysis had the surprising result that the little boy listened to
his father's request and discontinued visiting his father's bed. The
father's resolution of his infantile attachment to his own father liberated
his little son from having to respond, as solicited by the father's need
for physical closeness, to his own father by substitution. With reference
to the father's masculinity, we will say briefly that he had been a
sexually inhibited youth and young man who harbored an infantile fear
of the female, which was displaced in all kinds of social and cognitive
inhibitions. These were periodically disrupted by states of anxiety,
ingratiating behavior, and deceptive imposter-like improvisations in his
adult life.

I think that developmental studies as well as clinical research have
verified Loewald's, Mahler's, and Stoller and Herdt's formulations. To
these I wish to add a typical defensive maneuver that brings the infantile
failure in the transition from the first to the second (i.e., from the
maternal to the paternal) dyadic phase of attachment emotions into a
position of correspondency with adolescence. I refer here to the fact
that the boy child's perseveration or symbiotic attachment positions
of a dyadic, male or female, partnership precludes his progression to
the oedipal level of development and thus sidesteps the confrontation
with triadic object relations and their specific conflictualities.

Conclusions

I have highlighted the developmental risk stations in diagramming
the maturational course of masculinity consolidation during the first
two decades of a boy's life. In doing so, I schematized and simplified
the etiological complexities. Each case we study in our practice reveals

a highly idiosyncratic confluence of contributing components to the general syndrome of a deviant masculinity. The ordinal position among siblings stands out in one case as a younger sister was born at a particularly sensitive time of his development, which made "being a girl" the most enviable way of being. In another case a contributory component was found in the father's absence for two-and-one-half years in the war during early childhood when the child formed the fear of the mother who supposedly had sent the father away, driving a wedge of alienation between son and father for a lifetime, associating women with danger and destruction, and remaining severely inhibited in the realm of self-assertion, confrontation, and competition. Grossly deviant masculinity is quite lucidly traceable in the history of male development, but the common disturbances of masculinity, which we observe in a vast portion of the male population without diagnosing them as deviant, require a differential diagnosis and etiological refinement in order to reveal the specificity of the developmental risk stations along the course of dyadic and triadic same- and other-gender object relations. Such clinical investigations and their theoretical conceptualization promise to be particularly helpful during the many occasions when we are called on to intervene therapeutically in the typical crises of emotional malfunction during adolescence, especially during the years of late and postadolescence and early adulthood.

REFERENCES

Blos, P. 1985. *Son and Father: Before and Beyond the Oedipus Complex*. New York: Free Press.
Loewald, H. W. 1951. Ego and reality. *International Journal of Psycho-Analysis* 32:10–18.
Mahler, M. 1955. On symbiotic child psychosis. *Psychoanalytic Study of the Child* 10:195–212.
Stoller, R. J., and Herdt, G. H. 1982. The development of masculinity: a cross-cultural contribution. *Journal of the American Psychoanalytic Association* 30:29–59.

EVAN BRAHM

One of the privileges of being a discussant is that one is afforded the opportunity to review the presenter's contributions in depth and, as a result, to develop a deeper appreciation of them. I have enjoyed the opportunity to read and reread many of Dr. Blos's formidable contributions and to wrestle with the considerable challenges that he has put before us for over four-and-a-half decades.

The presentation by Dr. Blos follows from his recent book *Son and Father* (1985). In this work, he has placed increased emphasis on the early relationship of the infant and young male child with his father, which he has called the isogender dyadic relationship. In emphasizing the importance of the early father-son relationship in the development of masculinity, Dr. Blos has stated his disagreement with the mainstream psychoanalytic view that the successful resolution of the triadic Oedipus conflict or, alternately, the kind of compromise formation obtained primarily determines the type of masculinity acquired. He cites Loewald and Mahler as other analysts who, more than thirty years ago, raised the importance of the early relationship with the father, although neither they nor others to whom he also refers so clearly detailed the importance of the early dyadic relationship to the development of masculinity. While Dr. Blos describes the progression from the primary dyadic relationship with the mother, to that with the father, to the oedipal relationship, he states that it is the task of adolescence to resolve all three. His emphasis is on drawing our attention to the importance of the early dyadic relationship with the father and its resurgence in adolescence when its final resolution can take place. This theoretical position emanates from his extensive clinical experience. The emphasis that he places on the importance of the early father-son relationship for the development of masculinity is one with which I agree. My own analytic work with adolescents and adults, although quite modest in comparison to that of Dr. Blos, supports his emphasis.

His description of the early dyadic relationship with the father is one of attachment, in which the father is progressively included in caretaking roles and promises to secure the advance and completion of the early developmental phase of merger and regulation. Dr. Blos provides us with a portrayal of a shared gender identity and of sameness leading to identification and idealization. He describes a "shift from this *physical* oneness and absolute security to an *ideational* creation of the father as the absolute protector against the regressive needs to the symbiotic past" (p. 10, emphasis mine). His clinical description of a warm, loving, caretaking relationship is well described in this paper and, I believe, is amply supported by clinical evidence. I found his elucidation of the concept of a shift from a sense of a physical experience of attachment to the development of an ideational experience of protection to be a wonderful way of capturing the role of the early father in the infant's development from an archaic state based on the experience of his physical needs being met to the early development of a capacity for rudimentary conceptualization in which idealization becomes possible. There may be similarities with Kohut's (1971) formulation of two poles of the self and their corresponding lines of development—a grandiose self dependent on the experience of mirroring and an idealized parental imago, which requires an experience of a selfobject on whose strength the infant can count—ultimately leading to the development of a capacity for idealization.

Dr. Blos views the loosening of the male infant's tie to his mother by slowly and intermittently transferring his attachment emotions to his father as traumatic. Based on this, he postulates an emotional confrontation in adolescence that repeats this infantile trauma. I would like to raise some questions regarding his view of both stages.

In optimal infantile development, does the male inevitably experience a trauma when he forms an attachment to his father? Might there instead be the inborn potential in infants to form several early attachments, allowing for different secure feelings of caretaking from parents of each gender? In *Son and Father*, Dr. Blos stated that, if the father was "perceived and used differently [from the mother], then a healthy expansion and enrichment of the child's incipient personality becomes discernible'' (1985, p. 25). I understand him to mean that both parents have different constitutional dispositions that facilitate different developmental aspects for the infant and young child. While the shift from the dyadic attachment to one parent to dyadic attachments to two may be traumatic for some, or even many, young children, we can ask whether this is due to developmental necessity or whether, when it occurs, it is due to developmental difficulties, such as those resulting when a mother has a need to engulf her child or a father who, because of his own unresolved issues, does not make himself adequately available to his son or forms an excessively merged relationship. Any of these would not be optimal to the young boy's developmental needs and would lend greater likelihood to his experiencing difficulties in adolescence with the pressures brought to bear by the pubertal thrust of sexuality.

As a brief aside, while Dr. Blos's paper and my discussion focus on the boy's experience of dyadic attachments to his mother and to his father, we can wonder about the extent to which the boy is constitutionally predisposed to experience maternal and paternal attachments and his capacity to experience this unfolding epigenetic schema even when he has only one parent for all or part of his childhood and adolescence.

Dr. Blos has challenged the traditional psychoanalytic view that adolescent aggression against the father or the societal father representations is a defensive manifestation of unresolved, triadic oedipal conflicts. He has persuasively suggested that better clinical results ensue when attention is paid to the dyadic father relationship, a view that, as I have already said, I find supported by the clinical evidence in his publications and in my own work. Dr. Blos further suggests that both the adolescent's aggressive and his sexual behavior can be seen as defensive functions against the regressive pull of his preoedipal, libidinal father attachment.

From my analytic experience with some adolescent males, I wonder whether this issue can be pursued further. Does it result from the resolution of the dyadic relationship with the father as an inevitable aspect of adolescent development, or is this the manifestation, albeit common or even virtually ubiquitous, of inadequacies in paternal attachment, possibly more pronounced when the boy experienced an extra need for his father to compensate for deficiencies resulting from his relationship with his mother?

Dr. Blos describes how both parents may impose their own unresolved needs on their child and presents us with an illustration from the analysis of a forty-year-old man of how as a result of his own unresolved infantile attachment, manifesting as a need for closeness to his own father, by substitution, he solicited his four-year-old son to come to his bed nightly. His son's behavior ceased when Dr. Blos was able to help his analysand to resolve his infantile attachment. However, we can wonder what kind of adolescent difficulties this four-year-old boy might have experienced had his father not been able to resolve his difficulties. Dr. Blos tells us that "every boy's masculinity is shaped by a three-generational confluence of infantile attachment emotions and their resolution along overlapping developmental lines" (pp. 13–14).

This had led me to wonder whether it would be useful to expand on the view, as I have understood him, that normal adolescent development involves a defense against the unresolved dyadic bond with the father. It seems to me that the nature and extent of the male adolescent's aggressive and sexual difficulties, while stemming from his intrapsychic state, are often heavily influenced by his experience of the insufficient provision of an attachment relationship with his father in early childhood. This is further complicated when he continues to experience similar difficulties in his current relationship with his father during adolescence, whether these result from his distortions or whether his father continues to manifest unresolved difficulties similar to those that he had when the adolescent was an infant and toddler. Whatever difficulties the four-year-old son of Dr. Blos's analysand in fact will experience in attempting to resolve his dyadic relationship to this father in his adolescence, we can speculate that the nature of his difficulties would be significantly greater had his father's unresolved infantile attachment persisted through his adolescence and young adulthood. In addition to whatever difficulties the adolescent male experiences in his relationship with his father, he must also cope with his internalized experience of his mother in childhood and his ongoing adolescent experience of her.

From this vantage point, I would like to inquire further into Dr. Blos's view that much of adolescent aggression is a defense against the regressive pull of unresolved dyadic attachment to the father and that it could be a defensive act of "turning into the opposite"—attachment into hostility. Clinically, the advent of aggression in adolescence is clearly quite common. I would like to suggest that at least some of this may be anger, ranging from mild protest in some to rage in others, against the experience of inadequacy in the infantile and childhood paternal dyadic bond as well as angry affect accompanying the emerging need to sort out his adolescent voyage via a process of deidealization, whether perceived through a dawning realization in conscious awareness or experienced only in confused, poorly understood affect and behavior.

What I am raising for consideration is the extent to which the trauma described by Dr. Blos in the transferring of infantile attachment emotions from mother to father and the repetition of this trauma in adolescence represents optimal developmental potential or is influenced by inadequate parental experiences. It may be useful to inquire into the optimal development of masculinity with a view to the boy's experience of his infantile attachment to his mother, and subsequently to his father, and then, at adolescence, to consider how this might unfold with parents who are relatively unencumbered by their own unresolved developmental issues.

I am in accord with Dr. Blos that infant research together with clinical observations have facilitated an opportunity for us as clinicians to reconsider our traditional views, and I am optimistic that the ongoing interchange between developmental psychologists and clinical researchers will assist us in our task of continuing to question our metapsychological and clinical theories and assist us in our struggle to understand our patients better.

REFERENCES

Blos, P. 1985. *Son and Father: Before and Beyond the Oedipus Complex.* New York: Free Press.
Kohut, H. 1971. *The Analysis of the Self.* New York: International Universities Press.

AARON H. ESMAN

It is always a pleasure and a privilege to share a platform with Dr. Peter Blos. It is a pleasure because it affords an occasion for a reunion with one who has been teacher, colleague, and friend for more years than either of us would like to acknowledge. It is a privilege because it permits an intellectual dialogue with one of the masters of the field, one of those rare few who have enlarged our knowledge of a major aspect of human growth and behavior. Today Dr. Blos has indeed enriched our grasp of the central theme of this meeting, a theme to which he has devoted himself for some time now, deepening his and our understanding as he pursues his work.

Dr. Blos's reformulation of our conception of male adolescent development has, as its cornerstone, a reassessment of the central role of the Oedipus complex and the identifications with the father established at that time, largely as a defensive maneuver. He emphasizes the crucial importance of the preoedipal tie to the father both as a primary identificatory component of the sense of maleness and of masculine role patterns and as a determinant of central aspects of male adolescent behavior—in particular, its rebelliousness and negativism and its assertive machismo. He advises us of the necessity to deal with this preoedipal tie and its ramifications in our therapeutic work with such patients and, in particular, to recognize its manifestations in the transference, especially the tendency alternately to idealize and devalue the therapist as the young man struggles with his early idealization of the father and the necessity to undergo a normative process of disillusionment and reality testing in the course of establishing a new, more mature mode of relation with father and father figures in his life.

It has long been clear to observers and therapists of children and adolescents that the father assumes a crucial role in his son's life long before the conflictual struggles of the oedipal phase make their intrapsychic appearance. Father as early object of imitation and idealization and father as aid and support in the process of disidentification with mother during separation and individuation have long been recognized, in large part as a result of Dr. Blos's teaching. Recent infant observation studies have indicated that discrimination between mother and father—especially the sounds of their voices—can be observed in early infancy, suggesting that differential relatedness can begin almost ab initio. This differentiation is in turn abetted by the very different patterns of handling, motor stimulation, and address adopted by fathers with their sons as opposed to their daughters and as opposed to the ways mothers do these things. Thus, it is clear now that, virtually from the beginning of life, the intrinsic biological disposition to maleness is fostered by the interactional events between boys and their fathers, the fantasies both parents nourish about their little one's future course of life, and sociocultural expectations and role patterns, all of which shape first the basic gender identity and then the sexual role behaviors of the developing boy.

We know from the researches of such workers as Zuger (1984) and Green (1987) that, in a distressing number of cases, the failure to assume a masculine identity by early latency may definitively foreclose the possibility of doing so, that the "sissy boy" or male cross dresser of five or six has a very high probability of becoming an overt effeminate homosexual in adolescence.

Blos's work has highlighted the preoedipal, preconflictual pattern of identification and idealization and the adolescent struggle to break free. I should like to address myself to another aspect of the development of masculinity and the preparations for adolescence—the course of events that occurs during that increasingly neglected phase, the period of so-called latency. As Freud pointed out, it is during this period, when, ideally at least, the storms of the oedipal struggle have waned in intensity, that the child becomes educable. In traditional cultures and in an earlier, less complicated time than ours, this has meant for the boy child a period of apprenticeship with his father or father surrogate, during which the lore of the society and the technology of the specific tasks he is destined by birth to pursue are imparted to him. In the process, he learns what it means to be a man in his culture. He learns, that is, the forms, modes of relationship, and skills that make up the traits of masculinity in his world.

In such cultures, the arrival of puberty is commonly marked by rites of passage that often take the form of a symbolic rebirth, an emergence from the world of women and children into full membership into the male order. Unlike the adolescent process that Dr. Blos describes, in which the boy breaks from the preoedipal attachment to the father to assume his autonomous place in the world, the boy in a traditional culture intensifies his ties to the world of the father, breaking away from his preoedipal attachment to the mother and thus assuming masculine sexual prerogatives and social status.

In this connection, Stoller and Herdt (1985) report the fascinating situation of homosexual development in a man reared in a New Guinea culture characterized by unlimited, culturally sanctioned fellatio among prepubertal boys and older youths. Despite this practice, eagerly engaged in by all concerned, adult male homosexuality is virtually unknown. The case cited was deviant in his developmental experience in that he was regarded as a bastard and reared without a father or father surrogate by a mother who was bitter against men and reared him in isolation. Unlike "normal" men in his culture, he continued his interest in and excitement about fellatio with young boys until his adult life and had no interest in sexual activity with women.

In this culture, boys remain with their mothers until late latency; fathers are distant, engaged in hunting, warriorhood, and ritual. At the first initiation, which occurs between seven and ten, the boys are abruptly separated from their mothers and begin their indoctrination into the world of men, actively—and at times brutally—encouraged to identify with their father's male roles. It is at this time that the boy begins to suck older boys' penises, in order to accumulate the semen that will make him a man. At puberty, he changes roles and becomes the one whose penis is sucked by younger boys. Finally, in late teens or at about twenty, he marries and becomes actively, aggressively, and exclusively heterosexual. Here, clearly, there appears to be no break from the relationship with the father in adolescence; the homoerotic behavior of late childhood and youth is culturally normative and experienced as an aspect of acquiring masculine identity, of becoming like the father and assuming his social role.

The point of this digression into anthropology is to underscore the importance of the boy's latency age nonconflictual relationship with his father in his education toward masculinity, even in industrialized cultures. I would suggest that a significant contributor to the difficulty some boys have in acquiring a conflict-free sense of masculinity in our time is the declining role of just such a relationship in their lives, in this era of long-distance commuting, single-parent families, and sporadic father-son contacts marked in many cases by ignorance on the boy's part of his father's actual occupational pursuits. As Malmquist (1978) has pointed out, most published studies of paternal influence have shown that "boys from father-dominant homes display more sexual preference according to the masculine sexual standard and are more identified with fathers than are boys from mother-dominant families" (p. 214). It is the intensification of the oedipal and preoedipal tie to the mother that makes adolescence so turbulent in father-absent situations—the need aggressively to break away from both the sexual and the dependent attachments that have not been adequately mitigated by a close connection with the father, one that might prepare the boy adequately for his masculine role. Thus the importance of pop-culture male idols and of the male peer culture in presenting to the boy models—however dubious they may at times be—of what masculinity means in the contemporary world.

Conclusions

My purpose in these remarks is in no way to deny or even to minimize the importance of the epigenetic and dynamic issues advanced by Dr. Blos in his elucidation of the development of the sense of masculinity in the male adolescent. His clinical evidence and the constructions he derives from it are solid and persuasive, and those of us who have followed the evolution of this work have already been illuminated by it. I intend merely to propose that the process is a gradual and progressive one that accrues identificatory elements through all phases of childhood and to emphasize the critical role of latency-phase factors that Dr. Blos has, for what I assume are purposes of argumentation, elected to ignore.

In the crises of our time, I find major sociocultural contributions to the increasing malaise of our male adolescents and the need many of them find to assume exaggerated caricatured masculine postures in order to sustain the tenuous stability of their masculine identities. The seed of these developmental distortions I see both in early childhood and in the latency stage as the precipitate of the failures in fathering that are increasingly evident in these times. It is this lack that many of our male adolescent patients seek to replenish in the treatment situation, and it is this longing from which they defensively recoil, insofar as it threatens their shaky sense of autonomy, heterosexual identity, and masculine pride: thus the acting out, the devaluation of the therapist, and the premature terminations that so often mark the course of treatment for these youths.

REFERENCES

Green, R. 1987. *The "Sissy Boy" Syndrome and the Development of Homosexuality.* New Haven, Conn.: Yale University Press.
Malmquist, C. 1978. *Handbook of Adolescence.* New York: Aronson.
Stoller, R., and Herdt, G. 1985. Theories of origins of male homosexuality. *Archives of General Psychiatry* 42:399–404.
Zuger, B. 1984. Early effeminate behavior in boys. *Journal of Nervous and Mental Diseases* 172:90–97.

4   DISCUSSION OF PETER BLOS'S CHAPTER

VIVIAN M. RAKOFF

As one would expect, Dr. Blos has given us an elegant, intellectually consistent, clinically perceptive, and wise overview of the development and consolidation of "masculinity" during adolescence. There is a richness and precision in his overall schema that makes comment difficult; in particular, it makes reservations and criticism seem fragmentary. Dr. Blos's description of the move from an early infantile dyadic relationship through a triadic child, mother, father, developmental phase and the later dyadic phase is a map firmly based on Freud's description of the development of the oedipal stage and its resolution. Although Dr. Blos specifically distances himself from the classical oedipal formulation, he too asserts that the process of achieving masculinity is one of creating a necessary distance from the mother to an eventual realistic perception of the father and a degree of identification with him. His view is supported not only by his own clinical vignettes but also in certain aspects by the empirical studies of Green (1987), Money and Russo (1979), and others and—as Dr. Blos indicates—by Stoller and Herdt's (1985) anthropological description of the development of "masculinity" in the Sambia tribe of New Guinea. These support the notion that close bonding, excessive affectionate relationships with the mother, and a distant or less involved father constitute an essential threat to heterosexual masculinity, with its concomitant developmental possibilities of bisexuality and homosexuality in adolescence and adulthood.

However, for all its elegance and completeness, the explanation leaves us with a mystery, a mystery that Freud (1905) himself stated in these terms: "It may be questioned whether the various accidental influences would be sufficient to explain the acquisition of inversion without the co-operation of something in the subject himself" (pp. 140–141). Green (1987), after his essential acceptance of this schema, writes with a kind of worried modesty that, even after one has accepted the general short-hand picture of the need to escape close bonding with the mother and the development of attachment/distance from the father, there appears to be another factor.

I am, of course, evoking the time-worn problem of nature versus nurture, and (if I may take a brief moment on this topic given the pressure of time) I am forced to make my remarks in aphoristic form. Nature and nurture are in a fundamental sense neither opposed nor discontinuing. It is part of our human nature to be nurtured in a human family, as it is part of our nature to be nurtured in varying human families. Given the varieties of human personality and possible config-urations of the family within a given society and across varying cul-tures, there should be an expectation of varying kinds of masculinity and varieties of sexuality as normative human possibilities. Further-more, if Freud's statement that there must be some contributing com-ponent in the individual is given serious weight, then the responses of a particular mother to a particular boy have to be carefully examined. Green (1987) approaches this in his case records of "sissy boys" who are perceived as "very beautiful." This may not be an idiosyncratic perception of the mother. They may indeed be "easier to love and to cuddle." They bring to the mother-child bonding and rearing process their particular characteristics; they are not passive, doll-like manne-quins but active participants who evoke specific responses from the mother by the cues they emit. Thus, the reciprocal choreography of close bonding makes the relationship of the mother to a potentially "effeminate" son a subtle dyadic interplay, one that is not entirely the expression of the mother's nurturing patterns.

I also want to question Dr. Blos's implication, which I may have misunderstood, that adolescence is indeed, in Anna Freud's terms, a "second chance." Green's (1987) fifteen-year histories of effeminate males support the idea of an essentially continuous process in which early "effeminacy" shows itself in adolescence and adulthood in a high proportion: two-thirds of his sample of effeminate boys developed a homosexual or bisexual sexual orientation in adolescence. Similarly, Stoller and Herdt (1985) suggest that the almost brutal masculinity of the Sambias is determined from infancy and childhood, so that the absence of any known homosexuality (excepting for one egregious example) in their rough society cannot be ascribed to an adolescent conflict or task having been resolved.

The implications of my comments are as follows. I am aware that I may have misunderstood some of Dr. Blos's intentions. He too after all is constrained by a very short time to deal with a complex issue. However, the title of his chapter contains a significant assumption, an assumption that I have questioned in my written manuscript by putting the word "masculinity" between quotes since it appears that Dr. Blos in his precise formulation has given us a convincing diagram of the development of heterosexual masculinity. There is an implication that other forms of sexual orientation of the male sex are not masculine. Of course there may be a "commonsense" validity underlying this assumption, but since, as I have suggested, the human possibility exists for a great variety of mother/child, father/child interactions, and if these interactions are indeed as formative as Dr. Blos's argument suggests, then the possibility, indeed the probability, of a variety of male human sexual behavior is "normative."

The society of the Sambias described by Stoller and Herdt, which, at least in their account, contains almost no variations on adolescent heterosexual masculinity, appears to achieve this purpose by an imposed separation of the sexes; by a distrust on the part of the males of all things feminine; by a brutal subjugation of latency-age boys; and by a superstitious overvaluing of sperm (young boys being inducted into adulthood are forced to perform ritual fellatio on their seniors). The Sambias believe that sperm is not generated in each male but has to be passed from generation to generation through fellatio. This is manifestly a radical distortion of the potentialities of human variety through an imposed and rigorous formula. If then the implicit assumption of Dr. Blos's paper is that the kind of masculinity he describes is the only proper kind and since he cites Stoller and Herdt's (1985) paper in support of his thesis, is he, even by remote implication, suggesting that a formula of male child-rearing similar to that of the remote Sambias should be imposed to produce only heterosexual males in our society?

I realize that my argument is hyperbolic and a kind of a reductio ad absurdum, but it is made to emphasize that a consequence of our society's tolerance of varieties of expression of personality and identity may be varieties of interrelationships and varieties of sexual orientation.

There are also significant consequences for the treatment of adolescents and, indeed, adults in Dr. Blos's paper. Since sexual orientation, however it is established, appears to be largely achieved—although it may not be expressed until later—in early childhood, and since it appears to be the consequence of something akin to what the ethologists refer to as "imprinting," it becomes an almost unalterable component of the individual's personality and behavior. It is to a large degree beyond choice and most elaborate forms of psychotherapy and/or behavior modification—if the therapeutic aim is to change sexual orientation.

The therapeutic task then should probably not be directed at change but at understanding. In one Dutch series of 120 homosexual men who sought therapy to change their behavior, there was only one successful case (W. Sengers, "Homosexuality as a Complaint" [1969], cited in van Naersen). While one is aware of the anecdotal reports of success in changing sexual orientation, essentially the matrix of sexual identity and behavior may at best be modified—and, I suggest, modified only within the available repertoire of sexual responsiveness the patient possesses before coming into treatment. Bisexuality and other forms of sexuality other than a fully expressed heterosexual orientation appear to lie on a continuum, and therapeutic work may best be served by carefully discovering the position of an individual patient along that continuum. In addition, there will need to be exploration of the societal influences rather than the individual need that may have brought the patient into treatment. Should the therapist share the implicit assumption that a valid masculinity is to be expressed only as a fully heterosexual sexual orientation, then the uncertain, troubled adolescent will undoubtedly be given invalidating messages rather than the support and education he requires.

A few other matters. Dr. Blos's epigenetic journey toward adolescent masculinity is derived almost entirely from a conflict model, and, as far as it goes, it is self-consistent and convincing. I suggest that there are other epigenetic models that may be of use in understanding how adolescent sexual orientation may be developed. In particular, Erikson's model of stage-specific tasks may free us from the theoretical exigencies of a solely conflict instinct/defense model. Achieving secure identity is the prime task of adolescence, and it is a precursor of the later stage-specific task of authenticity. Secure identity must incorporate the authentic sexual needs of the adolescent as opposed to the imposed societal (and I should say in many instances therapeutically imposed) notions of an acceptable sexuality. In addition, the epigenesis of selfhood demands from the therapist an empathic compassion for socially variant forms of sexuality. Furthermore, Blos's statement that the achievement of a secure sexual identity marks the end of adolescence and an affirmation of adult masculinity fails to take into account the factors of work and taking one's place in the historical/political aspects of society, as components of an adult masculine identity. Blos's focus appears to be exclusively erotic, and, while in other writings he extrapolates the erotic into other modalities of function, his model, as it stands, does not encompass the multivariate experiences and duties beyond the erotic, which any society—with variations—may perceive as masculine.

Dr. Blos draws our attention to the valuable role the father plays in helping the boy, and later the adolescent, achieve adult masculinity. To extrapolate the point somewhat, the father in most societies is the bridge from the domain of intimacy, emotional bonding, sexuality—the locus of our "unclothed" experience—to the public culture of duty, the performance principle, the life of political mankind—our "clothed" experiences. In his transitional role-giving capacity, he models and guides the child-to-become-adolescent toward the protean forms of masculinity demanded in any complex society.

REFERENCES

Freud, S. 1905. Three essays on sexuality. *Standard Edition* 7:140–141. London: Hogarth, 1953.
Green, R. 1987. *The "Sissy Boy Syndrome" and the Development of Homosexuality.* New Haven, Conn.: Yale University Press.
Money, J., and Russo, A. 1979. Homosexual outcome of discordant gender identity roles: longitudinal follow-up. *Journal of Pediatric Psychology* 4:29–41.
Stoller, R. J., and Herdt, G. H. 1985. The development of masculinity: a cross-cultural contribution. In R. J. Stoller, ed. *Presentations of Gender.* New Haven, Conn.: Yale University Press.
van Naersen, P. T. O. Theories on homosexuality among professional therapists. *Journal of Homosexuality* 13:145–155.

5 HISTORY OF CHILD AND ADOLESCENT PSYCHIATRY IDEAS AND ORGANIZATIONS IN THE UNITED STATES: A TWENTIETH-CENTURY REVIEW

BERTRAM SLAFF

Child and adolescent psychiatry as a subspecialty begins with William Healy (1869–1963) in 1909. A group of philanthropically minded individuals in Chicago had proposed a five-year study of Illinois delinquents that would, according to Jane Addams, one of the sponsors, "get at the root of the exact causes that make children go wrong" (Jones 1987, p. 18). Financial support was offered, and, on the recommendations of Adolf Meyer and William James, a forty-year-old neurologist, William Healy, was asked to head their research project at the Juvenile Psychopathic Institute, later to be known as the Institute for Juvenile Research (Gardner 1972).

Gardner wrote that Healy had emigrated to this country from England at age nine. For economic reasons, he had dropped out of grammar school at age thirteen and had gone to work as an office boy in a bank. During the next ten years, while working at the bank, he became so successfully self-educated that he was accepted as a student at Harvard University, where he entered the William James faculty-student circle. Afterward, he went to medical school, becoming, successively, a general practitioner, a gynecologist, and, finally, a neurologist, when he was tapped for the new study.

Healy stated in 1960, "As a fair-minded researcher, I don't think I had any idea of what I would find out. I didn't have any preconceived theories. I had never studied children before that, in that sense. . . .

All I hoped to accomplish was to find out what needed to be done by way of treatment" (quoted in Gardner 1972).

Healy was charged to work with the Juvenile Court of Chicago, providing the court with a detailed scientific record on each subject, and was also to collect data about the medical, psychological, and social background of frequent offenders in an effort to determine the causes of juvenile delinquency. In 1915, *The Individual Delinquent* was published. In this work, Healy introduced a psychodynamic perspective, demonstrating the role of disturbing social and developmental events in bringing about delinquent behavior. Each child's actions had a meaningful history, and only through studying this background could one hope to understand and to help. Healy included psychoanalysis in his 1915 list of "working methods" and made use of a psychologist and a social worker in this collaborative effort in studying the emotional problems of children, introducing Southard's term "clinic team" to describe this activity.

Healy was disappointed at the lack of adequate facilities for the treatment of delinquents in Chicago. In 1917, he and his collaborator, Dr. Augusta Bronner, a psychologist, opened the clinic known as the Judge Baker Foundation (later the Judge Baker Guidance Center) in Boston after receiving assurances of improved opportunities for the treatment of delinquents there. He continued to be active in the Boston area until his death at the age of ninety-four.

Some earlier events must be noted. In 1904, G. Stanley Hall had published *Adolescence*. The same year, Freud's *The Psychopathology of Everyday Life* had appeared; in 1905, he had given his statement of psychosexual development in the *Three Essays on the Theory of Sexuality*. Freud himself was to lecture in America in 1909.

In 1905, Binet and Simon in France developed tests to measure intelligence. Noshpitz (1979) reported that a specific norm was developed for each increment of age. Intelligence thus became an invariant; once measured, it would theoretically be firm and lifelong. This instrument became universally accepted as the first modern psychological test. Intelligence was regarded as having many aspects. It was, therefore, to be studied by means of asking the child to accomplish a variety of different tasks. Multiple dimensions of cognitive functioning, verbal and nonverbal, were measured simultaneously. Each measurement was quantifiably scored. This approach has been basic to subsequent psychometric testing.

Goddard made these tests available at the Vineland Training School in New Jersey in 1910. These tests are currently under challenge as being vulnerable to the effects of racism, elitism, and cultural bias.

In 1909, Clifford Beers founded the National Committee for Mental Hygiene. Its slogan was "the prevention of insanity and delinquency," and it emphasized preventive work with children (Curran 1978).

At Yale, another dimension of child psychology was opening up. The existing Psychoeducation Clinic in 1911 acquired a new director, Arnold Gesell. Renamed the Yale Clinic of Child Development, it provided many valuable studies of the fine details of the unfolding of the human being (Noshpitz 1979).

In 1918, the Commonwealth Fund was established with the goal of furthering medical knowledge; its interests came to include delinquency. The National Committee for Mental Hygiene and the Commonwealth Fund proposed, in 1922, that eight test clinics be established in various cities with five-year support to be given by the Fund; afterward, these clinics were to be supported locally. The term "child guidance clinic" was chosen.

These eight clinics were established successfully and gained community support; many additional clinics were subsequently founded. They provided child psychiatrists with an institutional base for their activities. Diagnosis took up most of their energies, but they also did some pioneer treatment. The "team approach" prevailed. Generally, the psychiatrist treated the child, the social worker took a history and worked with the parents, and the psychologist did testing. The clinics discovered that, in addition to their basic tasks, they had to function as child advocates, work with community groups, and liaison with other agencies that dealt with children.

Delinquency had been the prime object of study, but, in the 1920s, attention began to be paid to children whose behavior was disruptive at home or at school but who had not come to the attention of the law.

This was a period of increasing acceptance of psychoanalytic theory. In this era, before the development of ego psychology, the key concepts were libido, transference, and insight. In 1928, Anna Freud published her *Introduction to the Technique of Child Analysis*. Melanie Klein's *The Psychoanalysis of Children* followed in 1932.

In 1923, Karl Menninger wrote to twenty-six psychiatrists, stating, "In spite of the rapidly increasing prestige of neuropsychiatry and the behavioristic or psychological attitude toward conduct disorder, there

33

exists no centralizing organization of the representatives of the neuropsychiatric or medical view of crime." This led ultimately to the formation of the American Orthopsychiatric Association (AOA) (Lowrey 1948, p. 190). Originally, active membership was limited to psychiatrists, with associate membership made available to others engaged in the study and treatment of behavior disorders. Later Ph.D. psychologists and then social workers were admitted to membership. The 1926 program included the statement, "The American Orthopsychiatric Association has as its purpose the centralizing of the techniques, objectives, and aspirations of psychiatrists, psychologists, and social workers, whose primary interests lie in the problems of human behavior, particularly conduct disorders of the antisocial types, providing a common meeting ground for students of these problems, and fostering scientific research in this field."

Major figures in the establishment of the AOA included Herman Adler, David Levy, Arnold Jacoby, Lawson Lowrey, George Stevenson, and William Healy. Healy was elected first president. "Ortho" became the central meeting place for the professionals of the child guidance clinics.

Seven specific conflict parameters come to the fore at various times: (1) pediatrics versus child psychiatry, (2) medical model versus interdisciplinary team approach, (3) general psychiatry versus child psychiatry, (4) child psychiatry versus adolescent psychiatry, (5) organic (biological) versus psychological (psychodynamic), (6) strong credentialism versus relative openness, and (7) centralized national organization versus regional autonomy. The last two relate particularly to the contrasts between the American Academy of Child Psychiatry (renamed the American Academy of Child and Adolescent Psychiatry [AACAP] in 1987) and the American Society for Adolescent Psychiatry (ASAP).

In 1926, Piaget published *The Language and Thought of the Child*. In this and many succeeding works, Piaget was able to show the development of cognitive structures in an orderly and predictable developmental sequence. He described the sensorimotor stage until about eighteen months, the preoperational stage until five to six years, the stage of concrete operations from about six to eleven, and, finally, the potential for abstract operational thought of the adolescent.

The first pediatric-psychiatric service was opened in 1930, when Leo Kanner joined the Harriet Lane Pediatric Clinic at the Johns Hopkins University. He was asked by the Josiah Macy Foundation to study the "rank and file of patients in the pediatric clinics for the formulation of psychiatric problems." The purpose of the study was to help pediatricians learn how to cope with such issues (Noshpitz 1979, p. 88). Kanner developed the first specialized facility for the study, diagnosis, and treatment of seriously disturbed children and their parents.

In 1930, the *Journal of the American Orthopsychiatric Association* was founded. It was a period of some considerable wrangling between pediatricians and child psychiatrists; they differed on whose responsibility it was to care for the infant, and they had other differences as well. Joseph Brenneman, a distinguished pediatrician, read a paper in 1931, later published in the *American Journal of Diseases of Children* (1931), called "The Menace of Psychiatry." Noshpitz (1979) recalls that he took out after IQ tests; the need for child psychiatrists to have pediatric training; the dangers of parent education, especially in respect to behaviorism; the dubious effect of public acceptance of norms with the resultant labeling of all variety as pathological; and the overorganization of children's lives in the service of health. He found the term and the idea "Oedipus complex" to be nauseating. He asserted that sex played a very minor part in early child life. He closed by suggesting that the psychiatrists should investigate the current psychiatric movement as a psychiatric problem.

In 1931, amphetamine, a substance with a remarkable capacity to stimulate the central nervous system, was synthesized.

Howard Potter studied children housed in institutions for the retarded and reported the finding that many of these were psychotic. His work in 1933 gave an early picture of childhood schizophrenia.

In 1934, the American Board of Psychiatry and Neurology came into being.

In 1935, Leo Kanner issued the first English textbook on the topic, *Child Psychiatry*. In 1938, he began to study a curious group of children whom he was presently to call autistic.

In 1937, an adolescent psychiatric ward was opened at Bellevue Hospital in New York City, under the direction of Frank Curran (Curran 1978).

In 1938, Lauretta Bender, director of the Child Psychiatric Ward (founded in 1923) at New York's Bellevue Hospital, published her *Visual-Motor Gestalt Test and Its Clinical Use*.

Stella Chess (1988), writing on the last half-century of child and adolescent psychiatry, notes that fifty years ago these were truly in their infancy periods as scientific disciplines. A pessimistic constitutional-hereditary point of view was being increasingly challenged and discredited. Freud and Pavlov had demonstrated how much of behavior formerly labeled as preformed and predetermined actually arose out of the child's life experiences. Psychodynamic-psychoanalytic ideas based on Freud's work took hold in child psychiatry. Behaviorism, based on Pavlov's studies of conditioning, became an important influence among clinical and experimental psychologists. Child psychiatry was isolated from other scientific disciplines to which it should have been closely linked: developmental and social psychology, pediatrics, and the neurosciences.

The 1940s saw an interesting development in the realm of delinquency. An early seminal concept emerged that was to make child psychiatry especially alive to the power of family factors in the genesis of emotional disorders. Articles appeared describing the unconscious fostering by parents of child acting-out behavior, formulations later to be couched in terms of "superego lacunae" (Johnson 1949).

David Levy (1937) wrote on primary affect hunger. Rene Spitz (1945, 1946) described hospitalism and anaclitic depression. He reported on the effect of separation and object loss in the second half of the first year of life. John Bowlby (1946) considered the affectionless character as someone whose disturbance is directly attributable to maternal deprivation. He later (Bowlby 1951) became known for his work on attachment. These are the early manifestations of the new field of infant psychiatry. The World Association for Infant Psychiatry and Allied Disciplines was formed in Lisbon in 1980.

Frederick Allen published *Psychotherapy with Children* in 1942. In the previous twenty years, "A methodology had emerged in which one engaged in play with an emphasis on establishing a good relationship with a child. Some counseling with parents was the rule, including advice giving and an attempt to change sources of overstimulation or other forms of mismanagement. This combination of parent work and relationship was the basic modality of the approach. A certain amount of interpretation was also employed, depending on the amount of analytic training or consultation available" (Noshpitz 1979, p. 129).

Kanner (1944) had described a special group of children characterized by loss of speech, lack of human contact, an obsessive preoccupation with repetitious sameness, and cold distant parents. He suggested a psychological origin for autism on the basis of the emotional climate within which these children were reared. This ushered in a new era in the study of childhood psychosis and a tremendous controversy about nature, nurture, genetics, and whether parents should be blamed (or blame themselves) for the serious psychiatric illnesses of their children.

Stella Chess (1988) observed that by the 1940s the constitutional-hereditary view of the infant as a homunculus had been thoroughly discredited. Now, the neonate was seen as a tabula rasa, a blank slate on which the environment would inscribe its influence until the adult personality was etched to completion. The first few years of life were considered crucial. With this premise, it was no surprise that child psychiatrists began to place the blame for a child's disturbed behavior on the parents, especially the mother. Concepts such as the "schizo-phrenogenic mother," the "double bind" theory put forward by the anthropologist Gregory Bateson, and the "hostile, rejecting mother" began to dominate child psychiatrists' thinking and practice. This *mal de mère* ideology (Chess 1964) caused untold guilt and anxiety to in-numerable mothers. Some decades later, after this phase had declined, Kanner was to tell a meeting of parents of autistic children, "I exon-erate you."

In the 1940s, Fritz Redl and S. R. Slavson were active in doing group work. Group psychotherapy has been defined as a process in which therapeutic forces are deployed in a setting in which several patients meet with one or more therapists. The patients are brought together for the purpose of helping each other change in the direction of "normal development." Intrapsychic, interpersonal, transactional, and group psychodynamic frameworks are involved (Kraft 1979).

In 1946, Fritz Redl organized a research-oriented residential treat-ment center, which accepted a number of "hyperaggressive" boys. This was in the tradition of the work August Aichhorn had done in Vienna in 1918, which had led to the publication of *Wayward Youth* (1925). From this research, *Children Who Hate* and *Controls from Within* were published by Fritz Redl and David Wineman. They were included in *The Aggressive Child* (1957).

In 1946, the Group for the Advancement of Psychiatry (GAP) was formed, building alongside the more conservative American Psychiatric Association. William Menninger was a guiding spirit. Its membership of approximately 185 psychiatrists has been organized in the form of a number of working committees, including the Committee on Child Psychiatry and the Committee on Adolescence. These committees direct their efforts toward the study of various aspects of psychiatry and toward the application of this knowledge to the fields of mental health and human relations. Collaboration with specialists in other disciplines has been one of GAP's working principles.

In 1948, fifty-four child guidance clinics came together and created the American Association of Psychiatric Clinics for Children (AAPCC), under Frederick Allen's leadership. This was to be the first standard-setting body for child psychiatric services and for the training of child psychiatrists. These clinics manifested the multidisciplinary "team approach" and were not necessarily under medical supervision. Accreditation by this organization became one of the proudest forms of recognition an agency or an individual could receive (Curran 1978).

The National Institute for Mental Health was set up in 1949 under Robert Felix. It would be the principal federal agency concerned with improvement of the mental health of Americans. Daniel Blain has called the years 1945–60 the "magic years" of American psychiatry. During this period, mental illness and mental retardation were recognized as major mental health problems. Large public investment was made in training, research, and service programs. Perhaps, inevitably, along with these went the expectation of instant relief (Noshpitz 1979).

In 1949, the American Psychiatric Association (APA) authorized the formation of the first APA Committee on Child Psychiatry. Noshpitz observed that from the onset child psychiatrists have worked within "team" contexts. What would have most likely been the child psychiatrist's professional organization, the AOA, had very quickly taken on a multidisciplinary "team" character. The new standard-setting association of clinics, the AAPCC, was also multidisciplinary. Eventually, some professors of psychiatry began to object. Why should nonpsychiatrists be setting standards for psychiatrists (even if they were only child psychiatrists)? Within the APA, similar concerns were expressed. Was child psychiatry a separate discipline, or was it some kind of hybrid, fated forever to carry other professions along in its train?

That the general psychiatry–child psychiatry conflict parameter still exists is suggested by a cartoon that appeared in the spring 1988 *AACAP Newsletter*. It shows an individual labeled "Psychiatry Department," wearing a crown with the title "Chairman," saying, "Of course I think we should have a Child Psychiatrist in the Department. After all, someone has to pick out the toys for the waiting room."

In 1949, Frederick Allen was chairman of the APA committee that recommended board certification for child psychiatrists after examination. The APA's Committee on Child Psychiatry approved this recommendation and sent it on to the APA council, where it died. For the next nine years, this proposal was resubmitted and rejected (Curran 1978).

During the 1950s, behavioral therapy emerged. Dynamic therapy was subjected to direct attack. Eysenck (1952) critiqued existing psychotherapeutic technology and found it ineffective.

In 1951, at an AOA meeting in Cincinnati, a group of child psychiatrists led by George Gardner met to consider the desirability of forming a child psychiatry organization ("The History of the American Academy of Child Psychiatry" 1962). In 1953, the American Academy of Child Psychiatry (AACP) formally came into existence, with George Gardner as president. Membership was to be by invitation. To be eligible for fellow membership, an individual had to be a member of the APA; had to be certified by the American Board of Psychiatry and Neurology or be board eligible; had to have had at least two years of training in child psychiatry; had to have practiced child psychiatry for a total of at least five years following completion of his training period; had to be able to demonstrate a chief professional interest and activity in the field of child psychiatry; and had to have made an "outstandingly significant" contribution to any one of—or combination of—the following activities: (1) therapy with children and adolescents; (2) teaching of child psychiatry; (3) training of physicians for the eventual practice of child psychiatry; (4) research relative to problems in child psychiatry; (5) the administration of a child psychiatric clinic or of significant child psychiatric programs at the local, state, or national level.

Invitation to associate membership in the AACP was to be extended to those physicians not eligible for fellow membership who had made outstanding contributions to the field of child psychiatry. Associate members were not to have the power to vote or to hold office in the AACP.

It should be noted that the AACP was set up as an "academy" in the classic sense of that term. It was an organization made up of the recognized leaders in the field who proclaimed the goal of setting and maintaining the highest standards. At that time, the AACP did not have the goal of being an organization that included the rank and file of child psychiatrists in the nation.

Family therapy was a major development in the 1950s. Noshpitz (1979, p. 168) remarks, "Systems theory was applied and the concept of the family system, or the family as a system, became commonplace. All this presently moved in the direction of a view of family therapy, which regarded the child as a function of family interaction. The child's psychopathology was accordingly viewed as a product or an expression of intrafamilial forces. Ultimately this would beget a good deal of controversy with child psychiatrists who looked in vain in these formulations for any explicit discussion of child development, or for an account of the interaction of the child's psychic structures with the family vectors that were being described."

Margaret Mahler (1952, 1975) was a great contributor to the understanding of childhood psychosis. She began to correlate the behavior of her patients with the developmental events in their early lives. She studied the ego aspects of early personality unfolding and conceptualized this in terms of a series of stages of infantile progress. First, there was an autistic stage, lasting through the first two months. From then to about nine months, she postulated a stage of infantile fusion with the caretaker, known as symbiosis. This, in turn, was followed by a series of stages of separation and individuation, with the child achieving separate functioning in the presence and emotional availability of the mother. The psychic fusion she saw as symbiosis, and, in contrast to Kanner's autistic children, who had never achieved fusion, she defined a different group of psychotic children as "symbiotic." These were children who had indeed gone beyond autism and accomplished the psychic fusion but had then failed in their work of separation-individuation. Successful separation-individuation was thought to be reached by about age three, culminating in the attainment of stable object constancy and a sense of autonomy.

In 1953, it became known that chlorpromazine affected the symptoms of psychosis. Organicists vied with psychodynamicists in the diagnostic and therapeutic spheres of interest. The successful use of these drugs reinforced the search for alternatives to hospitalization.

In December 1957, the Council of the APA capitulated and accepted that child psychiatrists be certified after a specialized training curriculum. In 1959, the American Board of Psychiatry and Neurology set up a Committee on Certification in Child Psychiatry. Training standards were formulated, and examinations for candidates for certification were established. (In 1987, there was a name change to the Committee on

Certification in Child and Adolescent Psychiatry.) The subspecialty of child psychiatry had been established. The AAPCC was thus relieved of the responsibility of setting standards for child psychiatry training.

In 1957, Congress passed a law providing for medical care for the children and spouses of members of the uniformed forces, known as "CHAMPUS."

In 1958, the Society for Adolescent Psychiatry (SAP), under the leadership of James Masterson, was founded in New York City. General psychiatrists who were interested and active in treating adolescents as well as child psychiatrists were welcomed into SAP.

In 1960, the New York Council on Child Psychiatry was formed, under the direction of Exie Welsch. Membership was open to physicians, qualified for membership in the APA, who were interested in child psychiatry.

A preliminary report of the Joint Commission on Mental Illness and Health was prepared in 1960 and came out ringingly against the large mental hospitals where adults had been "warehoused" for so many years. In their place, it held out the model of community services that would reach everyone at a site near home and without regard for ability to pay. The report left out consideration of the needs of children and adolescents.

Early child psychiatry evolved in the freestanding community service units, the child guidance clinics. Now, many were growing as subunits of departments of general psychiatry. Before the decade was over, however, in many an academic setting, battle lines would be drawn between the parent department of psychiatry and the younger child psychiatry division. By 1979, child psychiatry had become, in large measure, an academic discipline.

The growth of psychiatric units attached to general hospitals went on apace. In many institutions, adolescent patients were housed on the adult units and treated by general psychiatry residents under the supervision of a cadre of adolescent preceptors. Inevitably, there was some rivalry between this group and the child psychiatry supervisors.

The 1960s was an era of the development of group psychotherapy, encounter groups, drug treatment methodologies, and the use of supervised paraprofessionals. There was great interest in the new community mental health centers.

In 1963, a conference on career training in child psychiatry was sponsored by the APA and the Association of American Medical Colleges (not including the AAPCC). This expressed the gradual movement to bring child psychiatry closer to its sources within medicine.

In 1965, Congress provided for a first Joint Commission on the Mental Health of Children to be organized by Reginald Lourie. The same year, Project Headstart was launched; Julius Richmond had suggested a preschool program to include parent counseling, health care, and comprehensive child development. Also in 1965, the American Association for Child Psychoanalysis was formed.

In 1967, the four societies for adolescent psychiatry in New York, Philadelphia, Chicago, and Southern California confederated to form the ASAP, with William A. Schonfeld as president. To the question, "Another Society! Why?" Sherman Feinstein and Bertram Slaff responded (1971, p. 12):

The essential function of an adolescent psychiatry society is to provide a forum for the encouragement and discussion of the psychiatric needs of youth. Teenagers are treated by child psychiatrists and adult psychiatrists, as well as by those who limit their work to this age group. Therapists' conceptualizations and approaches vary greatly, depending on their training opportunities and experiences. The forum approach encourages communication in a specific area among psychiatrists of diverse backgrounds.

The purpose of the Society is not to create a subspecialty but rather to stimulate interest in this phase of life. Adolescent maturational tasks may be secondary only to early developmental issues and as such may have a profound impact; they give the growing individual a second chance to negotiate healthy character defenses.

An adolescent psychiatry society does not compete with or duplicate the groups formed by child psychiatrists. In organizational terms adolescent psychiatry societies should cooperate with child psychiatry groups, with the former encouraging the participation of interested members from adult psychiatry. Child psychiatrists see their functions as covering early development through the resolution of adolescence while many adult psychiatrists work with patients from the assumption of adolescence through its transformations into the adult years of life. This leaves many years of overlap and mutuality of interest.

42

It will be noted that powerful contrasts existed between the beginning conceptions of the AACP and the ASAP. The stringent requirements for membership in the AACP have been mentioned. The ASAP merely required eligibility for membership in the APA and an interest in adolescence. The AACP was a strong central organization; the ASAP was a confederation of local societies, each of which had considerable autonomy. Members of local societies automatically became members of the ASAP. Membership in local child psychiatry groups was and is separate from membership in the AACP. (In 1988, about two-thirds of the members of the New York Council on Child Psychiatry also are members of the AACAP.) The AACP was structured to represent the highest standards of the profession; the ASAP was developed to meet the manpower emergency in adolescent psychiatry (Slaff 1970).

Clarice Kestenbaum (1987, pp. 2–5) has reviewed the child psychiatry training experience in the mid-1960s. "Child psychiatry in 1964 was a relatively new field. Certification had existed for a mere five years. There were no formal standards for residency training—each program specialized in what the professor knew best. . . . Training was catch-as-catch-can. . . . Despite the value of therapeutic eclecticism, however, lack of a central integrating developmental theory began to cause problems."

Kestenbaum has considered the research efforts of the 1930s and 1940s as investigating the belief that early experience determines adult behavior. In the 1950s and 1960s, research activity was devoted to the study of mothering as a set of attitudes. In the 1970s, researchers began to study the role of the child hitherto left out, his particular constitutional makeup and his particular effect on his caretaker. The mother-child fit, the transactional model, became an important research strategy. Serious attention was paid to inborn predisposition to particular temperamental traits, character formation, and neurosis. Research in the 1980s has continued to delve into questions of fetal development, intrauterine influences, and the genetic basis of behavior, personality, and character formation.

The late 1960s was the era of increasing social disorganization, related to the Vietnam conflict and the assassinations of Martin Luther King, Jr., and Robert Kennedy; student revolts at Columbia, Harvard, and many other universities were manifestations of this crisis.

A major transformation occurred in 1969 within the AACP. Sidney Berman (1970, pp. 197–198), then president, described the issue:

It should be noted that between 1963 and 1967 the roster of the Academy increased from 245 to 264 members. In 1967 the Committee on Regional Planning compiled a national directory of child psychiatrists with basic training qualifications, and these numbered 835. Council faced this critical question, asking how the Academy could meet the needs of young child psychiatrists, colleagues whom we have trained and with whom we practice, and yet justify, by its membership roll call, the concept of an Academy. [This] . . . culminated in the decision by the members to make the Academy truly the representative voice for child psychiatry nationally. The Committee on By-Laws, in keeping with the mandate of the members, drafted changes in the by-laws to broaden the base for membership. This included admission by application. The members overwhelmingly approved these changes by a vote of 176 to 11 and so closed this chapter on the thorny issue of membership by invitation which we had struggled over for years. We who shared academic pursuits of excellence with our colleagues in the Academy were awakened by a powerful ground swell of reality.

The present requirements for active members are that they be physicians who (1) "shall have been certified in child and adolescent psychiatry by the American Board of Psychiatry and Neurology or have completed two years of training in a child and adolescent psychiatry training program accredited by the Accreditation Council on Graduate Medical Education, and have completed general psychiatry training; or have had child psychoanalytic training and have been certified as such by the psychoanalytic institute in which child psychoanalytic training was received; (2) shall demonstrate, through documentation, that this major professional interest and activity is in the field of child and adolescent psychiatry" (American Academy of Child and Adolescent Psychiatry, *By-Laws* [1988], p. 5).

As part of the new openness, the AACP welcomed local child psychiatry groups into its Assembly of Regional Organizations. In 1988, AACAP had 4,000 members, and there were forty-two regional child psychiatry organizations. Scientific meetings take place each autumn.

In 1968, the final report of the Joint Commission on the Mental Health of Children was published. Its major effect lay in the introduction of the term "advocacy." This notion asserted that within the meshwork of American society children were being neglected, that their mental health was in jeopardy, and that their problems were not receiving adequate responses.

White House Conferences on Children and Youth had been held in 1909, 1920, 1930, 1940, 1950, and 1960. In 1970, the administration could hardly avoid maintaining this tradition. An ominous note was sounded when Stephen Hess, the national chairman of the White House conference, told the delegates of the Council of National Organizations for Children and Youth (of which I was a member because of my then presidency of the ASAP) that the report of the Joint Commission on the Mental Health of Children, on which many child and adolescent psychiatrists had worked arduously at the government's request, would not ("repeat, would not") be admitted to the agenda of the White House conference—this "on the highest authority."

In 1970, the AAPCC, no longer responsible for training in the field of child psychiatry, changed its name to the American Association of Psychiatric Services for Children (AAPSC). It would serve its 157 member clinics as a clearing house for child mental health information, provide mental health consultation to agencies and organizations, serve as a source of public information, and act as an advocate for child mental health.

In 1971, the first ASAP-sponsored annual volume, *Adolescent Psychiatry,* was published, under the editorship of Sherman C. Feinstein, Peter L. Giovacchini, and Arthur A. Miller. By 1988, fifteen volumes have been issued.

In 1988, the ASAP celebrated its twenty-first birthday. A historical review mentioned the invitation in 1967 by Robert Stubblefield, chairman of the Committee on Certification in Child Psychiatry, to the ASAP to make recommendations regarding the "timing, amount and nature of the training experiences for general psychiatrists and for child psychiatrists in work with adolescents." An ASAP position paper was prepared. In 1969, an ASAP Conference on Training in Adolescent Psychiatry met at the University of Chicago under Daniel Offer's leadership. This led to the publication of the 1971 volume *Teaching and Learning Adolescent Psychiatry,* edited by Daniel Offer and James Masterson.

In 1971, the ASAP participated in the First Panamerican Congress on Adolescent Psychiatry in Buenos Aires, Argentina. This led to the formation of the Panamerican Forum for the Study of Adolescence, which was charged with planning biennial conferences on this topic for the Americas.

In 1972, the Long Range Planning Committee recommended "consideration that ASAP's present position as a loose confederation of an increasing number of constituent societies be reviewed critically. To facilitate the effectiveness of the organization on a national level it may be necessary to make ASAP the primary group, with concurrent membership in the local societies" (*American Society for Adolescent Psychiatry Newsletter* [August 1972], p. 5).

The same year, it was reported that a continuing education program for the ASAP was feasible and desirable.

In 1973, the ASAP was invited to send its president to appear on the podium with other representatives of national organizations at the following APA convocation.

Membership "at-large" was instituted in 1974 to permit individuals who did not live in areas with societies or with the potential for forming societies to join the ASAP.

In 1977, policy was set on interregional meetings, which were to be balanced geographically.

A new category, fellowship, for selected members was established in 1978.

Areas of activity included the Mental Health Law Project, the Juvenile Justice Standards Project, Guidelines on Pharmacotherapy of Institutionalized Adolescents, and Education of the Handicapped.

The first of a series of teaching institutes took place in 1980.

Preliminary meetings toward the formation of the International Society for Adolescent Psychiatry were held at the International Association of Child and Adolescent Psychiatry and Allied Professions meeting in Dublin in 1982.

An enhanced role was sought for Lois Flaherty and her Training Standards Committee, especially in developing a model curriculum for adolescent psychiatry.

Richard Sarles met the challenge of securing accreditation for the ASAP in the continuing medical education arena.

An ASAP archive was begun with the taping of John Schimel's conversation with Isaac Bashevis Singer.

In 1983, the Council of Delegates approved the recommendation that a Future Directions Task Force be established to study the structure, future, and operations of the ASAP. The task force, chaired by Richard Marohn, presented its report in 1986 with its recommendations, many of which are now being implemented.

An ASAP Research Fund has been established.

The Organizing Conference of the International Society for Adolescent Psychiatry met in Paris in 1985. Sherman C. Feinstein, an ASAP past president and longtime senior editor of *Adolescent Psychiatry,* was elected president.

In 1987, the ASAP filed an amicus curiae with the Supreme Court in *Thompson v. Oklahoma,* supporting the argument that the execution of an individual who was under age eighteen at the time he or she committed a capital offense was cruel and unusual punishment in violation of the Eighth Amendment. Recently, the Supreme Court sustained this position.

In 1988, the ASAP has twenty-eight chapters and 1,427 members. Of the members, 521 also belong to the AACAP.

Scientific meetings are held twice yearly. Annually, an individual is selected to receive the Distinguished Service Award, subsequently termed the William A. Schonfeld Award, named after the ASAP's late first president. Awardees have included Peter Blos, William Schonfeld, Irene Josselyn, Dana Farnsworth, Rudolf Ekstein, E. James Anthony, Fritz Redl, Phyllis Greenacre, Melvin Sabshin, Moses Laufer, Robert Coles, Hilde Bruch, Heinz Kohut, George Tarjan, Selma Fraiberg, Otto Kernberg, Margaret Mahler, Bruno Bettelheim, Daniel Offer, John Bowlby, Jerry Lewis, and Vivian Rakoff.

The ASAP serves as an essential bridge between child psychiatrists who naturally concern themselves with adolescents and general psychiatrists who also treat adolescents, in a continuing effort to satisfy the enormous need for adolescent psychiatric services.

Jerry Wiener (1988, p. 9) has stated in his 1987 presidential address to the AACAP:

Who knows how much closer to the melting heat of the mental health sun this Icarus of Child Psychiatry might have flown, borne aloft as it were by wondrous but waxen wings, had not some French physicians made the serendipitous observation that chlorpromazine affected the symptoms of psychosis. And so was ushered in the biological revolution and a consequent struggle for the mind and soul of psychiatry in general and of child and adolescent psychiatry in particular. First one and then more slowly the other returned to their roots and identifications in medical traditions and medical models in a giant grinding of gears referred to as the "remedicalization" of psychiatry. Of course, as we became re-medicalized we found ourselves in the same boat with medicine in general, bobbing and floating in the ever-increasing turbulence created by the currents of increasing competition, cost-containment, prospective payment, and expectations for kinds of documentation we were ill prepared to provide.

Wiener listed major gains in the recent decades: the growth of biologically based theories for the etiology, pathogenesis, and treatment of infantile autism, schizophrenia beginning in childhood or adolescence, Tourette's syndrome, and obsessive-compulsive disorder; the recognition of depression as a distinct disorder in children and youths; improvements in DSM-III and DSM-III-R; improved assessment instruments; the movement of almost all training into hospital and academic-based medical centers; an increasing commitment to raise training standards; and a significant expansion of a scientifically sophisticated research establishment.

The "bad news" has to do with cost containment and cost reductions. "Cost containment takes many forms, most of them burdensome and time consuming, including precertification, peer and nonpeer review, gatekeeping, prospective payments, capitations and managed health care. Unfortunately, there yet is no evidence that this time and effort in any way affect quality or accessibility of health care, except perhaps adversely. . . . We are now in a consumer-oriented marketplace environment in which the values and methods of the marketplace are much more a part of our professional lives. . . . Competition will increase" (p. 9).

Wiener includes in the "good news" that child and adolescent psychiatry will remain the single greatest shortage specialty for the rest of this century, that it will increasingly establish itself as an important integrative academic discipline, that training will progressively become more rigorous, and that the commitment exists to the progressive expansion of a scientific data base.

Stella Chess (1988) concluded her study of the last fifty years of the development of child and adolescent psychiatry with observations that long-term longitudinal studies report the unpredictability of later functioning from early life experiences and behavior. "There are so many factors that influence an individual's life at all stages of development and so many unpredictable maturational changes that emerge, that any formulation, concentrating primarily on the first few years of life is bound to be inadequate. . . . The emotionally traumatized child is not doomed, the parents' early mistakes are not irrevocable, and our preventative and therapeutic intervention can make a difference at all age-periods" (p. 4). A multifactorial approach is called for that takes into account the interaction of biological, psychological, and sociocultural influences at all age-stage levels of functioning.

Conclusions

From the simple to the complex is the developmental pattern of child and adolescent psychiatry as presented in this history. The challenge presented to William Healy in 1909, at the beginning of child and adolescent psychiatry as a professional discipline, was to "get at the root of the exact causes that make children go wrong." Almost eighty years later, the search for furthering understanding continues on many fronts, with recognition that the "exact causes" may be a reductionist concept, inappropriate to the complexities of each individual.

As our field has advanced, many "certainties" have faded. As our knowledge has increased, so has our awareness of how much is unknown. Child and adolescent psychiatry has moved from the courts and the child guidance clinics into the medical-psychiatric mainstream. Former conflict parameters such as organic (biological) versus psychological (psychodynamic) must be replaced by syntheses that regularly seek to integrate newer findings. It has been an exciting time.

NOTE

I would like to acknowledge the contribution of Joseph D. Noshpitz to this historical survey. He made available to me his extensive "History of Childhood and Child Psychiatry in the 20th Century" (Noshpitz 1979), which had to be eliminated from the four-volume *Basic Handbook of Child Psychiatry* (New York: Basic, 1979) because of lack of space, even though the editor-in-chief was Joseph D. Noshpitz.

REFERENCES

Aichhorn, A. 1925. *Wayward Youth*. New York: Viking.

Allen, F. 1942. *Psychotherapy with Children*.New York: Norton.

Bender, L. 1938. *A Visual-Motor Gestalt Test and Its Clinical Use*. Monograph no. 2. New York: American Orthopsychiatric Association.

Berman, S. 1970. Epilogue and a new beginning. *Journal of the American Academy of Child Psychiatry* 9:193–201.

Bowlby, J. 1946. *Forty-four Juvenile Thieves, Their Characters and Home Life*. London: Bailliere Tindall & Cox.

Bowlby, J. 1951. Maternal care and mental health. *Bulletin of the World Health Organization* 3:355–534.

Brenneman, J. 1931. The menace of psychiatry. *American Journal of Diseases of Children* 42:396–402.

Chess, S. 1964. Mal de mère. *American Journal of Orthopsychiatry* 34:613–614.

Chess, S. 1988. Child and adolescent psychiatry come of age: a fifty year perspective. *Journal of the American Academy of Child and Adolescent Psychiatry* 27:1–7.

Curran, F. 1978. Child psychiatry, USA, 1928–1978: one man's perspective. Paper presented to the New York Council on Child Psychiatry, May 18.

Eysenck, M. 1952. The effects of psychotherapy: an evaluation. *Journal of Consulting Psychology* 16:319–324.

Feinstein, S., and Slaff, B. 1971. Another society! Why? *American Society for Adolescent Psychiatry Newsletter* (April), p. 12.

Freud, A. 1928. *Introduction to the Technique of Child Analysis*. New York and Washington, D.C.: Nervous and Mental Disease Publishing Co.

Freud, S. 1904. The psychopathology of everyday life. In A. Brill, ed. *The Basic Writings of Sigmund Freud*. New York: Random House.

Freud, S. 1905. Three essays on the theory of sexuality. *Standard Edition* 7:125–243. London: Hogarth, 1953.

Gardner, G. 1972. William Healy, 1869–1963. *Journal of the American Academy of Child Psychiatry* 11:1–29.

Hall, G. S. 1904. *Adolescence*. New York: Appleton.

Healy, W. 1915. *The Individual Delinquent*. Boston: Little, Brown.

The history of the American Academy of Child Psychiatry. 1962. *Journal of the American Academy of Child Psychiatry* 1:196–202.

Johnson, A. 1949. Sanctions for superego lacunae of adolescents. In K. Eissler, ed. *Searchlights on Delinquency.* New York: International Universities Press.

Jones, K. 1987. "Straightening the twig": the professionalization of American child psychiatry. New Brunswick, N.J.: Rutgers University, Department of History. Typescript.

Kanner, L. 1935. *Child Psychiatry.* Springfield, Ill.: Thomas.

Kanner, L. 1944. Early infantile autism. *Journal of Pediatrics* 25:211–217.

Kestenbaum, C. 1987. Child psychiatry today—a view from the bridge. Paper presented to the New York Council on Child and Adolescent Psychiatry, October 1.

Klein, M. 1932. *The Psychoanalysis of Children.* New York: Norton.

Kraft, I. 1979. Group therapy. In J. D. Noshpitz, ed. *Basic Handbook of Child Psychiatry,* vol. 3. New York: Basic.

Levy, D. 1937. Primary affect hunger. *American Journal of Psychiatry* 94:643.

Lowrey, L. 1948. The birth of orthopsychiatry. In *Orthopsychiatry, 1923–1948, Retrospect and Prospect.* Menasha, Wis.: Banta.

Mahler, M. 1952. On child psychosis and schizophrenia: autistic and symbiotic infantile psychoses. *Psychoanalytic Study of the Child* 7:286–305.

Mahler, M.; Pine, F.; and Bergmann, A. 1975. *The Psychological Birth of the Human Infant.* New York: Basic.

Noshpitz, J. 1979. History of childhood and child psychiatry in the 20th century. Washington, D.C.: George Washington University School of Medicine. Typescript.

Offer, D., and Masterson, J. 1971. *Teaching and Learning Adolescent Psychiatry.* Springfield, Ill.: Thomas.

Piaget, J. 1926. *The Language and Thought of the Child.* New York: Harcourt, Brace.

Potter, H. 1933. Schizophrenia in children. *American Journal of Psychiatry* 89:1253–1270.

Redl, F., and Wineman, D. 1957. *The Aggressive Child.* Glencoe, Ill.: Free Press.

Slaff, B. 1970. The manpower emergency in adolescent psychiatry. *Psychiatric Opinion* 7:25–28.

Spitz, R. 1945. Hospitalism. *Psychoanalytic Study of the Child* 1:53–74.

Spitz, R. 1946. Anaclitic depression. *Psychoanalytic Study of the Child* 2:313–342.

Wiener, J. 1988. The future of child and adolescent psychiatry: if not now, when? *Journal of the American Academy of Child and Adolescent Psychiatry* 27:8–10.

6 TEENAGERS IN DISTRESS

CAROL C. NADELSON

When we discuss teenagers in distress, we immediately flash to television reports of "epidemics of suicide," rampant drug abuse, pregnancy, newspaper headlines screaming crisis, and increasing societal anxiety about the plight of our young people.

In the twenty-year period between 1960 and 1980, we have learned that deaths of sixteen- and seventeen-year-olds in vehicular accidents increased more than 40 percent, homicides by over 230 percent, and suicides by 140 percent. Drug use among white twelve- to seventeen-year-olds increased by almost 140 percent and alcohol use 56 percent. The delinquency rate of ten- to seventeen-year-olds rose by over 130 percent, and the birth rate of unmarried white women fifteen to nineteen rose by more than 140 percent. Welfare spending for teenagers has continued to rise, as has teenage unemployment. At the same time, SAT scores for high school seniors dropped 11 percent on the verbal portion and 6 percent in mathematics. In the six years since these data were collected, there has been no evidence that any of these alarming figures have turned around.

Let me put our current dilemma in another perspective and suggest that we are not and have not been alone in our concern. Aristotle said,

> The young are in character prone to desire and ready to carry any desire they may have formed into action . . . they are changeful, too, and fickle in their desires, which are as transitory as they are vehement; for their wishes are keen without being permanent, like a sick man's fit of hunger and thirst. They are passionate, irascible,

apt to be carried away by their impulses . . . if the young commit
fault, it is always on the side of excess and exaggeration . . . for
they carry everything too far, whether it be love or hatred or
anything else.

Still another opinion was voiced by Shakespeare in *The Winter's
Tale*. He said, "I would there were no age between ten and three-and-
twenty, or that youth would sleep out the rest; for there is nothing in
the between but getting wenches with child, wronging the ancientry,
stealing, fighting."

Although many cultural anthropologists suggest that there is marked
intercultural variability in teenage norms and behavior, challenging the
view of the inevitability of turmoil, it is likely that we are looking at
the picture from different perspectives. It may indeed be that there is
enormous cultural variability, and perhaps the experiences of Shakespeare and Aristotle are closer to us today. On the other hand, it may
be that the large majority of adolescents do experience relatively little
turmoil but that those who are in crisis are capable of creating massive
chaos. Since adolescents are no longer small children, they no longer
commit innocent, childish sins; suicide, drug abuse, alcoholism, pregnancy, and delinquency are forever.

Physiologically, since adolescence begins when sexual maturity is
attained, it does not occur at a fixed time. In fact, the age has changed
substantially over the last century. Scandinavian records suggest, for
example, that in 1850 the average Norwegian girl reached sexual maturity after the age of seventeen and a half, and the figure has steadily
moved downward. The implications are important since developmental
processes are set in different biologic environments and are thus potentially affected in different ways.

Adolescent development is a complex series of physical and emotional changes, and reactions to the changes range widely and are
mutually interactional. Puberty confronts the adolescent with immut-
able physiological changes that have multiple implications, are difficult
to understand, and cannot be controlled. The adolescent experiences
changes in feelings, mood, and behavior, as Aristotle told us, that are
unpredictable and perplexing. Inconsistency and ambivalence are the
hallmarks of this march toward adulthood and the development of a
stable self-image, a sexual identity, and a concept of self as an individual
and as a responsible adult in society. These processes do not proceed

in a fixed, orderly sequence, but they evolve in varying ways at varying rates.

Inherent in the development of an identity and self-image, which has enormous cultural variation, are the formulation of life goals and commitments, the development of a capacity to tolerate delay, and a mastery over instinctual needs for action. With this there is the development of a more consistent system of morality, which includes flexibility and empathy.

As Shakespeare reminded us, we cannot close our eyes, but we must tolerate the anxiety and uncertainty that both parents and children experience. There is no turning back. A new parental identity must also emerge as parents return to their childless days or take on a new role in society. At times, parental reactions parallel those of their children, and the adolescent may lose the reassurance and support of parental authority and stability. In this process, parents, society, and adolescents are often pitted against each other in a struggle toward mutual definition, tolerance, and responsibility.

Suicide

Having set out a developmental context, let me pick from among the major sources of distress in adolescents the issues that have been most compelling and have caused the greatest concern. First, the tragedy of teenage suicide. It is estimated that about 25,000 suicides take place in the United States each year, and approximately ten times as many suicide attempts are made. Five thousand of the suicides are adolescents, and 12 percent of the suicide attempts are made by adolescents. It is estimated that 10 percent of those who attempt suicide later go on to commit suicide (Caine 1978).

As with adults, most of the attempts are made by girls. While the ratio of completed suicides is three to two, male to female, this grim statistic is changing, and an increasing number of teenage girls are successfully committing suicide. Suicide is the second leading cause of death in adolescence, followed closely by accidents, many of which may also be seen as suicidal equivalents.

Why do young people commit suicide or make attempts? The causes are complex and involve psychological, biologic, and sociocultural factors. While not all young people who attempt or commit suicide have an underlying psychiatric disorder, depression and chemical dependence are major risk factors for suicide. Those young people who demonstrate antisocial or impulsive behavior, such as truancy, stealing, confrontations with the law, and running away from home, and are more impulsive and aggressive are also at increased risk for suicide.

Thus, an important preventive strategy is the early detection and treatment of a variety of mental disorders, including affective illness, conduct disorders, and chemical dependency. A family history of suicide increases the risk eight times. Explanations for this are complex and include identification with the family member who has committed suicide and genetic and other biologic factors. Reduced levels of the neurotransmitter serotonin may be associated with increased aggression in violent suicide attempts and completions, increasing the risk of completed suicide twenty times.

Of the psychosocial risk factors, the loss of a loved person, multiple moves and stresses, chronic illness, being the victim of child abuse, being a runaway, having an unwanted pregnancy, and having experienced recent humiliation in front of family or friends that injured self-esteem are important.

A recent study (Salk, Lipsit, Sturnan, and Reilly 1985) has suggested that there are perinatal risk factors related to later adolescent suicide; respiratory distress for more than one hour at birth, no antenatal care before twenty weeks of pregnancy, and chronic disease of the mother during pregnancy may affect risk in adolescence. Although the methodology of the studies has been criticized, the data point to important areas for future investigation and attention.

So-called suicide clusters appear to be occurring at increasing rates among adolescents. The term refers to the phenomenon of one suicide appearing to trigger others in a group, school, or community. These suggest the major role that peer pressure plays, particularly in those who are suggestible.

What are the warning signs? They include (1) depressed mood; (2) change in sleep and appetite patterns (increased or decreased); (3) decline in school performance, which may be secondary to decreased concentration ability and/or increased oppositionalism, both of which can be manifestations for depressive syndrome; (4) increased withdrawal from family and friends; (5) loss of interest and pleasure in previously enjoyable activities; (6) preoccupation with themes of death, such as reading books on death and dying; (7) increased irritability and behavior problems; (8) statements like, "I wish I were dead," which may appear manipulative but may also indicate poor coping skills and impulsive self-destructive risk taking; (9) giving away important possessions; (10) use of drugs and alcohol, which can represent self-destructive wishes as well as the adolescent's attempt to medicate his depression (unfortunately, drugs and alcohol may serve to affect reasoning ability and decrease inhibitions, helping to make a potentially suicidal adolescent truly suicidal); (11) history of previous suicide attempt (studies note that 40 percent of attempters had one or more previous attempts); (12) history of abuse and neglect; (13) history of learning disabilities associated with a sense of failure and frustration; and (14) frequent somatic complaints.

From the perspective of the mental health professional evaluating suicidal tendencies, the following must be considered. (1) What does the adolescent feel suicide would accomplish? (2) What was the method, including the extent of lethality, and why was that method chosen or considered? For example, if the plan was to overdose, then the question is, On what pills, how many, and whose were they? This can help with understanding the meaning of the attempt. (3) How long has the person been thinking about suicide; for example, is it an impulsive act or planned? (4) Has suicide ever been tried before? How close has the patient come to doing it? (5) What are the person's fantasy reactions of others to his or her death? (6) Is a psychiatric illness present, especially depression or psychosis? (7) What kind of interaction does the adolescent have with his or her family, and what areas of conflict can be identified? (8) How is the adolescent functioning at school, at work, and in his or her peer group?

Adolescent suicide can be prevented. The risk factors can be addressed. Intervention is necessary, but the specifics must be determined after careful evaluation.

Affective Illness

Confusion and myth about the nature and prevalence of "adolescent turmoil" have perhaps contributed to the lack of clarity about how to determine what is psychopathology. The appearance particularly of bipolar illness and major depressive disorders during adolescence must be recognized and addressed.

It has been noted (Ryan and Puig-Antich 1986, p. 422) that "one unwarranted use of explanatory paradigms before the full extent of the phenomenology is assessed'' may confuse the picture regarding prevalence and incidence and even make etiology difficult to assess. There are no good estimates of the prevalence of affective illness among adolescents in the general population. In their Isle of Wight follow-up study, Rutter, Maughan, Mortimore, and Ouston (1979) found that, among 2,000 fourteen- to fifteen-year-olds, thirty-five (1.7 percent) had a major depressive disorder. The incidence figures in child psychiatric services vary a great deal, as expected from referral patterns and diagnostic practices. A conservative estimate for the incidence from new adolescent cases of affective illness presenting to the child psychiatric services in a general hospital was 15 percent of adolescent intakes (Kupferman and Stewart 1979; Pearce 1978).

Since the majority of affective symptoms are experienced subjectively, the development of assessment techniques has been critical to any advances in nosology, psychobiology, and treatment. DSM-III has provided a useful diagnostic framework, and recent evidence suggests that, although the frequency of some symptoms vary with age and are related to developmental patterns, their nature does not vary. In fact, until recently the diagnosis of bipolar disorder was rarely made in adolescents, but emerging evidence has made it clear that a substantial proportion of those with unipolar diagnosis do have bipolar illness. This obviously makes a difference in the course of the illness and its treatment.

The danger of suicide in adolescents with bipolar illness is high. Carlson and Strober (1978) reported that over 80 percent of their sample had suicidal ruminations and that over 35 percent committed suicidal acts, which was significantly greater than 15 percent of adult bipolars who had committed suicidal acts. Successful suicide accounts for 2.4 percent of all deaths in the first half of adolescence and for 8 percent in the second half (Shaffer 1985).

In general, the view that depressive clinical pictures in these age groups are transient is inaccurate (Ryan and Puig-Antich 1986). The course is often chronic, persistent, and recurrent with associated psychosocial defects. It is important to emphasize that among the important risk factors is family history of affective illness. Adults with onset of depression before age twenty have been shown to be even more likely to come from families with this disorder than those with later onset depressive illness (Weissman, Leckman, Merikangas, Gammon, and Prusoff 1984b). In looking at these data, however, it is important to emphasize that they are preliminary, that morbidity risks in these family studies are also raised for other psychiatric disorders, alcoholism (Puig-Antich, in press; Strober 1984), anxiety disorders (Puig-Antich, in press; Weissman, Leckman, Merikangas, Gammon, and Prusoff 1984a), and conduct disorders (Puig-Antich 1982; Weissman et al. 1984a) and that there is evidence that there may be an increased prevalence of depression (Weissman et al. 1984a) and suicide (Shaffer 1985) among young people today.

Although psychosocial variables have been cited as risk factors, there is little evidence that marital status of the parent, size of the sibship, socioeconomic status, parental separation, divorce or marital functioning, or familial constellation or structure play much of a role in the causation of depressive disorders in children. In only one study (Weissman et al. 1984a) has parental divorce been shown to have an effect, albeit minor. Since the diagnosis and treatment of these disorders is not, at this time, definitive either, biologic interventions clearly are effective, but considerable diagnostic and therapeutic research will be necessary to provide more efficacious approaches.

Another group of disorders that have become more clearly elucidated recently are conduct disorders. Current DSM-III criteria are the presence, for at least six months, in patients under age eighteen of a repetitive and persistent pattern of conduct in which the basic rights of others are violated. A high incidence of psychomotor epilepsy (Lewis 1976), history of injuries especially to head and face, and psychotic, especially paranoid, symptomatology (Lewis and Shanok 1977) have been reported in adolescents with conduct disorders. Schizophrenia is the most common discharge diagnosis in hospitalized adolescents previously diagnosed as having conduct disorder (Lewis 1985). The major factor leading to diagnosis of conduct disorder appears to be violence, with no other significant symptomatic differences from other psychiatrically hospitalized adolescents.

Because of the potential for making this diagnosis and failing to investigate symptoms appropriately to rule out potentially treatable neuropsychiatric disorders, Lewis (1985) has advocated that the diagnosis be limited to patients showing no sign of neurological dysfunction or mental retardation and no history of non-drug-induced psychotic symptoms or violent behavior.

Early investigations of etiology focused primarily on psychogenic and social determinants, including intrapsychic conflict, family disorganization, and learned behavior. More recent research has suggested an association between attention deficit disorder and delinquency (Lewis 1985), and it has focused on the important role of temperament (Thomas, Chess, and Birch 1968). Family studies also suggest the possibility of genetic factors (Guze 1976), and, as noted, the possible rate of neurological dysfunction has been emphasized (Cantwell 1978).

Clearly, since there are many diagnostic questions, no single etiologic theory appears to explain the clinical presentation. It is likely that this is a group of heterogeneous disorders with multiple etiologies. In any event, the prognosis is generally poor, unless a specific etiology is identified, for example, bipolar disorder in which 20 percent of bipolar adolescents have a history of prepubertal onset that at the time was diagnosed as attention-deficit disorder or conduct disorder (Ryan and Puig-Antich 1986). About half the children and adolescents with conduct disorders become antisocial adults.

The treatment available for conduct disorders is far from definitive, and, since spontaneous remission is unlikely, it is clear that research is essential to delineate effective therapeutic strategies. A variety of approaches has been attempted, including the full range of the treatment armamentarium, with discouraging results except in specific situations. Behavior modification, for example, makes youngsters more manageable in residential programs but does not affect overall behavior, recidivism, or the number and severity of offenses following discharge (Shamsie 1982). Those reports of efficacy of psychotherapy do select cases that appear to be amenable to this approach, for example, those with neurotic conflict (Adams 1961; Aichhorn 1935; Persons 1967; Rutter 1975). Likewise, it is important to identify biologically treatable psychopathology such as depression (Puig-Antich 1982).

Lewis (1985, p. 1759) indicated that "the failure of special types of programs to address individual differences and meet individual needs probably accounts in great measure for the lack of success of any single treatment modality . . . that the very best therapeutic and educational programs will fail if they do not recognize and treat appropriately psychotic symptoms, severe depression, attentional disorders, seizures, and other psychosocial vulnerabilities that interfere with a child's ability to take advantage of even the finest programs." Even patients receiving benefit from somatic therapies require combined intensive multimodality psychosocial treatments, usually in residential settings.

Arguing against the notion that residential programs are useless (based on the frequency of loss of gains on discharge), Lewis sees such youngsters as having continued needs for social and psychological assistance beyond that available from their families and calls for availability of ongoing treatment in the form of hospital, residential, community, and group-living programs, special schooling, medication, and psychotherapy, alone or in combination, depending on the nature and seriousness of the disorder and the stability of the home environment.

Other studies (e.g., Offer, Marohn, and Ostrov 1979) suggest that hospital treatment programs be aimed either at converting true neurotic acting out into treatable neurotic symptomatology or at providing external structure sufficient to compensate for internal psychological deficits and, in either case, to develop in the adolescent the capacity for self-observation and introspection. Thus, a number of studies continue to emphasize the importance of intensive long-term hospitalization and an in-depth, comprehensive approach to these adolescents.

Substance Abuse

Another major crisis for adolescents is substance abuse. There are conflicting reports regarding the prevalence of these problems, and some even suggest that drug use has decreased or at least leveled off in teenagers. Drug use must be distinguished from abuse.

The prevalence of drug use in adolescents differs markedly for different drugs. The more socially accepted drugs are most widely used. The proportion of adolescents and young adults who have experimented with drugs has increased dramatically over the past two decades. Between 1962 and 1979, experimentation with marijuana increased from less than 5 percent to almost 70 percent, and cocaine use increased from zero to almost 25 percent of adolescents. A recent New York State study of adolescents found that 99 percent used alcohol, 72 percent marijuana, 25 percent psychedelics, 30 percent cocaine, and 3 percent heroin (Henreden 1986). Henreden also reported that, if the subjects had not experimented with these drugs by age twenty, they were unlikely to do so. Patterns of drug use were similar for men and women. Although there are reported higher rates for men in all drugs, except minor tranquilizers and stimulants, there has been some recent suggestion that sex differences are disappearing. Use of alcohol and cigarettes generally precedes marijuana use, and half those who try marijuana in their teen years progress to stronger drugs (Lettieri and Ludford 1981).

Even among very young adolescents the picture is troubling; 40 percent of New York State twelve-year-olds reported using alcohol (Barnes 1984). Some say that alcohol is currently the drug of choice among teenagers, and 10–20 percent of adolescents are said to be problem drinkers. The arrest rate for intoxication for those under eighteen has escalated dramatically over the past few years. What do we know about etiology? Age, sex, peer and parental values, cultural factors, individual personality characteristics, and psychopathogy as well as genetic and biologic factors all play a role.

Adolescents are more likely to use alcohol and marijuana if their parents use them. With regard to other drug use, a permissive parental attitude appears to be more important than actual parental drug use. Adolescents who use drugs are significantly more likely to have one or both parents who used them as adolescents. Peer influences are especially important in marijuana use. There is some recent evidence suggesting that biologic risk factors are important. Twin studies of adopted children who were not raised with their biologic parents indicate that the sons of alcoholics may be four times as likely to be alcoholics as the sons of nonalcoholics (Henreden 1986).

The influence of cultural values and attitudes has been shown through longitudinal studies of drug-abusing adolescents. These studies suggest that those who abuse drugs early continue to do so through their young adulthood. Further, drug-abusing women are more likely to have had pregnancies when they were teenagers, and drug-abusing men were more likely to be exempted from military service (Henreden 1986). The rate of criminality is twice as high among those who are drug abusers, although not with marijuana use.

Some use alcohol or drugs as an attempt at self-treatment for conflicts around self-esteem, sexuality, and dependence. The single most important personal dimension linked with drug abuse is lack of traditional values, including rebelliousness, resistance to authority, high need for autonomy, and social (but not personal) alienation. Sensation-seeking behavior and drug use is also correlated. Although most studies find weak correlations between psychopathology, including lower self-esteem and drug use, there is some suggestion that depression may be an important variable.

Adolescent Pregnancy

Recent reports about adolescent pregnancy have been alarming. We are told that we have the highest rate among Western nations and that we have steadily moved up in the last two decades. It is estimated that more than half the population of fifteen- to nineteen-year-olds in the United States and a fifth of the thirteen- to fourteen-year-olds are sexually active. Of the over 10 million adolescent women aged fifteen to nineteen in the United States, one in ten becomes pregnant—almost 2 million each year. The rate in 1982 was 185 pregnancies per 1,000 black and ninety-six per 1,000 white fifteen- to nineteen-year-olds (Moore, Simms, and Belsey 1986). Of these, almost 30 percent have live births, and more than 20 percent that we know of have abortions. For those fourteen and under, there were almost 30,000 pregnancies, half of which ended in abortion and one-third in live births.

Even more alarming is the fact that, although an increasing proportion of adolescents are sexually active, the percentage of those using effective means of contraception has not risen as rapidly; thus, large numbers of teenagers are at risk for pregnancy.

Tension between those who advocate preventive programs in schools and communities and those who favor approaches that primarily advocate family responsibility may have resulted in a lack of clear definition of responsibility and inadequate attention to prevention. The fear that providing information would stimulate sexual activity among teenagers has repeatedly been shown to be erroneous. In fact, those communities that have lowered their pregnancy rate have active educational programs and provide access to contraception. A recent article reported a substantial reduction in teenage pregnancy after these programs were instituted. They generally advise sexually active teenagers how to obtain and use contraceptives and prenatal care and how to get back into school and avoid having more babies. At one school there was a day-care center, it was noted, as a "grim reminder" to other students that "parenthood is no picnic."

The reasons for pregnancy are multiple. In some adolescents it may be linked with psychopathology, depression, anxiety, low self-esteem, and a range of developmental conflicts, but this is clearly not true in the majority of cases. Family crisis and loss are risk factors, and a large number of pregnant teenagers report alcohol and drug abuse and physical and sexual abuse. There is also considerable peer pressure and a sense of hopelessness about the future, which are important factors.

The consequences of pregnancy for the teenager herself as well as for her child can be monumental. Not only are there medical problems, including obstetrical complications, because prenatal care tends to begin late, in part related to denial of pregnancy. But there are greater risks. An infant born to a teenager is three times more likely to die in the first year of life than a baby born to a woman between twenty and twenty-nine years of age (*AMA News* [January 17, 1986]). Although all the reasons are not clear, nutritional habits among teenagers are generally poor, and substance abuse is a major problem.

A "syndrome of failure" is perpetuated in many teenagers who deprive themselves of the chance to escape poverty. They do not return to school, and they are more likely to be unemployed, be on welfare, and have subsequent pregnancies. Although a recent longitudinal study suggests that the long-term outcome is less negative than we have previously thought, it cannot be seen as positive (Furstenberg 1986).

The consequences for the children of these teenagers are influenced by the presence of extended family networks and ties and other support systems. The frequency with which teenage fathers are absent provides an unreal environment for children and presents models for adult men that may contribute to the perpetuation of the problem.

Mental Health Services

Let me turn now to the problem of access to mental health services for those needing them. What happens to the families who must care for the teenagers in crisis? What resources can they draw on?

The problems of financing mental health care for adolescents are particularly complex because, in addition to the specific health care issues, parental involvement and educational requirements must be considered. Since most treatment involves family members, educational resources, and even living arrangements, the cost and complexities increase. Most adolescents in the United States are financed for health care via insurance, usually their parents', and receive similar benefit packages from most major insurance plans. Public services do supplement these benefits, but the amounts are quite variable.

One question, recently raised, is whether adolescents have been overutilizing psychiatric resources to meet other needs. This concern is registered because of the increase in treatment of adolescents in long-term care facilities. Whether this represents a reallocation because of underutilization in the past or a new "crisis" is not clear.

In 1978, the President's Commission on Mental Health estimated that 15 percent of children and adolescents were in need of psychiatric services for disorders, including major affective illness and alcohol and substance abuse. These conditions often require long-term and expensive care, especially if adequate community services are not provided.

The current prospective payment system appears to be even more inadequate in its predictions for adolescents than for adults. A recent report from the University of California, Los Angeles, Neuropsychiatric Institute indicated that costs for psychotic children and adults are not comparable.

Most reimbursement for psychiatric treatment includes evaluation, inpatient hospitalization, outpatient visits, and partial hospitalization, including family work—but collaboration with teachers, schools, and other consultations often cannot be directly reimbursed. Moreover, with lifetime limits on treatment, the idea of using up benefits for the future early in life creates substantial problems. It has been suggested that this, coupled with the stigma of mental illness, leads people to wait rather than utilize services. This may result in delays until "crises" are even greater.

Parents whose benefits provide cafeteria-type programs are more likely to choose more extensive pediatric services or dental care before considering coverage for mental illness. The Employee's Assistance Society of North America has indicated that approximately 40 percent of employees seek assistance for emotional problems of their children or families. As noted, since most adolescents are covered through their parents' policies, employers will probably seek to find ways to identify high-risk families early. This could cause substantial problems in the future.

Likewise, organized-care settings are another place where family members are seen. Children and adolescents represent up to 25 percent of health maintenance organization (HMO) members, and a psychosocial diagnosis has been reported in between 5 and 15 percent of children seen in HMOs, with another 8–10 percent having psychosomatic diagnoses. The range of services provided is generally not consonant with the nature or complexity of those needed by children and adolescents.

While social security insurance provides income and care for needy families and Medicaid programs are available, the options and coverage vary. The CHAMPUS program (Civilian Health and Medical Program of the United States) provides medical benefits to individuals who are dependents. In 1984, it provided inpatient psychiatric care and payments of approximately $130 million, 64 percent for patients under age nineteen. In the past, unrestricted use was possible, but more recently there have been changes. For example, an inpatient limit was set at sixty days and fifty outpatient visits per year for both children and adults. Waiver policies exist but are limited to patients showing significant risk to self or danger to others. CHAMPUS has also paid for residential treatment, which is costly, and recently it has been curtailed to those children who are severely emotionally ill. This treatment is not covered by the sixty-day limitation. CHAMPUS has not reimbursed for partial hospitalization, a recommendation made frequently by child psychiatrists. It is clear that there are enormous difficulties in developing reimbursement mechanisms for alternative programs.

The Alcohol, Drug Abuse, and Mental Health Administration (ADAMHA) Block Grant program mandated, in 1984, that at least 10 percent of the mental health share of services be for seriously disturbed children and adolescents or for other unserved or underserved populations. Again, this may be only the tip of the iceberg. Among the major problems in allocating resources are some of the jurisdictional problems and responsibilities for emotionally ill and handicapped children and adolescents. In some states, the responsibilities may be in departments of education and, in others, in departments of health or mental health. Depending on jurisdiction, health insurance companies may consider these services to be health or psychosocial—but not medical services, in the traditional sense; thus, they may not cover them.

The situation is further complicated by state education codes that often require the provision of appropriate educational services for all "handicapped" children. The problem then becomes how to differentiate who is responsible for what type of care and service. Excluding the comprehensive long-term care of the mentally ill and disabled from insurance coverage is possible if education and housing are seen to be part of the package, and these are considered government responsibilities. Institutions that serve emotionally disturbed adolescents often contribute to the confusion by representing themselves in chameleon-like fashion. They can be called schools or medical facilities depending on the political or economic circumstances. While it is clear that definitions must be firmer, the problem may be in the conceptualization of insurance itself.

An additional problem relates to diagnosis. DSM-III has added clarity with regard to adults more than to children and adolescents. The nomenclature is not so precise or specific, and the danger of stigmatization results in attempts to avoid premature labeling. Vague terms are often used, increasing third-party payers' suspicion and enhancing the long-term planning problems.

This is further complicated by the movement away from medical models for treatment while still using them for funding. The varieties of therapists employed without clear definition of roles and functions do not make the task simpler. Even more of a problem is the increasing use of group insurance. In order to provide good rates, long-term, costly care could spell disaster. Group members would prefer reduction of benefits, particularly for problems they do not see themselves as encountering; thus, the services adolescents need are more likely to be eliminated, especially as "cafeteria" policies become more popular.

Conclusions

In all, then, we are currently faced with major crises in mental health care availability and delivery for adolescents, with clearly escalating problems and inadequate mechanisms for coping, either programmatically or fiscally. It is incumbent on us to come up with reasonable solutions and not to wait for them to be imposed on us.

REFERENCES

Adams, E. 1961. *Effectiveness of Interview Therapy with Older Youth Authority Wards: An Interim Evaluation of the PICO Project.* Research Report no. 20. Sacramento, Calif.: California Youth Authority.

Aichhorn, A. 1935. *Wayward Youth.* New York: Viking.

Barnes, G. 1984. *Alcohol Use among Secondary School Students in New York State.* Buffalo, N.Y.: State of New York Division of Alcoholism and Alcohol Abuse, Research Institute on Alcoholism.

Caine, E. 1978. Two contemporary tragedies: adolescent suicide/ adolescent alcoholism. *Journal of the National Association of Private Psychiatric Hospitals* 3(Spring): 4–11.

Cantwell, D. P. 1978. Hyperactivity and antisocial behavior. *Journal of the American Academy of Child Psychiatry* 17:252–262.

Carlson, G. A., and Strober, M. 1978. Manic-depressive illness in early adolescence: a study of clinical and diagnostic characteristics in six cases. *Journal of the American Academy of Child Psychiatry* 17:138–153.

Furstenberg, F. 1986. Study: '60's teen mothers made gains. *AMA News* (April 11).

Guze, S. B. 1976. *Criminality and Psychiatric Disorders*. New York: Oxford University Press.

Henreden, R. L. 1986. Adolescent alcoholism and substance abuse. *APA Annual Review* 5:468–479.

Kupferman, S., and Stewart, M. A. 1979. The diagnosis of depression in children. *Journal of Affective Disorders* 1:213–217.

Lettieri, D. J., and Ludford, J. P. 1981. *Drug Abuse and the American Adolescent*. National Institute of Drug Abuse Research Monograph no. 38/Research Analysis and Utilization Systems Review Report. Rockville, Md.: U.S. Department of Health and Human Services.

Lewis, D. D. 1976. Delinquency, psychomotor epileptic symptoms and paranoid ideation: a triad. *American Journal of Psychiatry* 133:1395–1398.

Lewis, D. D. 1985. Conduct disorders and juvenile delinquency. In B. Saddock and H. Kaplan, eds. *Comprehensive Textbook of Psychiatry/IV*. Baltimore: Williams & Wilkins.

Lewis, D. D., and Shanok, S. 1977. Medical histories of delinquent and nondelinquent children: an epidemiological study. *American Journal of Psychiatry* 134:1020–1025.

Moore, J.; Simms, K.; and Belsey, C. 1986. *Choice and Circumstance: Racial Differences in Adolescent Sexuality and Fertility*. New Brunswick, N.J.: Transaction.

Offer, D.; Marohn, R. C.; and Ostrov, E. 1979. *The Psychological World of the Juvenile Delinquent*. New York: Basic.

Pearce, J. 1978. The recognition of depressive disorder in children. *Journal of the Royal Society of Medicine* 71:494–500.

Persons, R. 1967. Relationship between psychotherapy with institutionalized boys and subsequent community adjustment. *Journal of Consulting Psychology* 31:137–141.

Puig-Antich, J. 1982. Major depression and conduct disorder in pre-puberty. *Journal of the American Academy of Child Psychiatry* 22(1): 29–39.

Puig-Antich, J. In press. Effects of age and puberty on psychobiological markers of depressive illness. In M. Rutter, C. Izard, and P. Read, eds. *Development of Affect*. New York: Guilford.

Rutter, M. B. 1975. *Helping Troubled Children*. New York: Plenum.

Rutter, M. B.; Maughan, B.; Mortimore, P.; and Ouston, J. 1979. *Fifteen Thousand Hours: Secondary Schools and Their Effects on Children*. Cambridge, Mass.: Harvard University Press.

Ryan, N. D., and Puig-Antich, J. 1986. Affective illness in adolescence. *APA Annual Review* 5:420–450.

Salk, L.; Lipsit, L. P.; Sturnan, W. Q.; and Reilly, B. 1985. Relationship of maternal and perinatal conditions to eventual adolescent suicide. *Lancet* 1(8429): 624–627.

Shaffer, D. 1985. Depression, mania and suicidal acts. In M. Rutter and L. Hersov, eds. *Child and Adolescent Psychiatry: Modern Approaches*. London: Blackwell.

Shamsie, S. 1982. Antisocial adolescents: our treatments do not work—where do we go from here? In S. Chess and A. Thomas, eds. *Annual Progress in Child Psychiatry and Child Development*. New York: Brunner/Mazel.

Strober, M. 1984. Familial aspects of depressive disorder in early adolescence. In E. B. Weller and R. A. Weller, eds. *Current Perspectives on Major Depressive Disorders in Children*. Washington, D.C.: American Psychiatric Press.

Thomas, A.; Chess, S.; and Birch, H. C. 1968. *Temperament and Behavior Disorders in Children*. New York: New York University Press.

Weissman, M. M.; Leckman, J. F.; Merikangas, K. R.; Gammon, G. D.; and Prusoff, B. A. 1984a. Depression and anxiety disorders in parents and children. *Archives of General Psychiatry* 41:845–853.

Weissman, M. M.; Leckman, J. F.; Merikangas, K. R.; Gammon, G. D.; and Prusoff, B. A. 1984b. Onset of major depression in adulthood. *Archives of General Psychiatry* 41:1136–1143.

7   IF ROCKY GOES TO COLLEGE: DILEMMAS
OF WORKING-CLASS COLLEGE STUDENTS

HOWARD S. BAKER

The movie *Rocky* portrayed many of the dilemmas of American working-class life with considerable sensitivity. We saw the often intense pain inflicted by financial limitation, a narrowed worldview, and almost constant narcissistic injury. Rocky repeatedly says, "I don't want to be just another bum on the block." In the increasingly absurd sequels, we can observe with equal clarity the desperate efforts at narcissistic repair that Stallone seeks. We are privy to an unchecked excess of macho defenses that might work under some circumstances despite their primitive grandiosity.

What if Rocky went to college instead of going back into the ring? In that circumstance, he, of course, would have brought with him his narcissistic vulnerability and his tendency toward grandiosity, but the response of the university environment would have presented a very different set of developmental tasks. While the scenario of Rocky in a university may seem unlikely, many young men and women from the same background do, in fact, attend college.

Because of their class, they may have some advantages—they often, for example, know the meaning and value of hard work. Unlike their middle- and upper-middle-class peers, however, they will almost certainly begin a process of changing social class. There are many ways that this shift will complicate the lives of these students, burdening them with impediments to both academic success and psychological development. These added challenges will, moreover, continue once they graduate and enter the business and adult social worlds.

Although upward social mobility has been a traditional goal of American culture, people who climb well up the class ladder often experience this move as a deviation out of and away from what was familiar and dear. Relationships at home that have been vital to psychological health and necessary for continued emotional development may be seriously disrupted. Relationships at school may be difficult to establish. This isolation may complicate or cause psychiatric symptomatology.

This chapter summarizes clinical experience with approximately 300 college students from blue-collar backgrounds. Some grew up within blocks of where *Rocky* was actually filmed. Many have shown great strength, others have barely succeeded, and some have collapsed under the pressure imposed by demands of their education. For some, families have provided exceptional support and encouragement, but others have been sabotaged both covertly and overtly. All have placed themselves in a foreign environment that has moved them out of their social class of origin, sometimes catapulting them from the bottom of the lower-middle class to the top of the upper-middle class with dramatic speed. This shift, while at least arguably positive, undoubtedly stressed both their personal, psychological development and the stability of their family and social networks. There was a price to pay for social advancement. It was often great and more than some could bear.

Despite receiving little recent attention, understanding social class issues is important when treating these people. There are, furthermore, implications in working with the many patients who have made less pronounced socioeconomic gains. The purpose of this study, therefore, is to describe complicating elements of upward social mobility and to offer some treatment recommendations.

For purposes of clarity, only people that come from Caucasian, unquestionably blue-collar backgrounds are considered. They are first-, second-, or third-generation ethnic Americans with family roots in Europe—principally Italy, Poland, and Ireland. The parents hold laboring or semiskilled jobs. The religious preference is most frequently Roman Catholic, and they live in working-class neighborhoods in the Philadelphia area that often have a distinct ethnic character. They are members of the first generation to attend college.

The following generalizations are, of course, just that—generalizations. People from all groups vary substantially, and we all are, to use Sullivan's term, more simply human than otherwise. What follows applies to many if not most of them, but it does not apply to all. Social class, moreover, is but one factor shaping the lives and symptoms of these patients. While it can never be separated sensibly from other variables, it is, nevertheless, pervasive, coloring nearly all aspects of intrapsychic, intellectual, family, and social functioning.

A Self Psychological, Developmental Perspective

Recent contributions in developmental theory have created a richer perspective for understanding the effect of social status. The work of Erikson (1950), Levinson (1978), Mahler, Pine, and Bergman (1975), Offer and Sabshin (1984), Stern (1985), Vaillant (1977), and others is consistent and leaves little room to challenge the assumption that psychological development must continue throughout the life cycle. Stern (1985) and the self psychologists (Kohut 1971, 1977, 1984; for a summary, see Baker and Baker 1987) have stressed that psychological development is fundamentally imbedded in relationships and that it cannot proceed optimally without sufficient empathic responsiveness within those relationships. Kohut labeled the essential relationships "self-selfobject relationships," and he insisted that they were necessary from birth to death.

The success a person has in traversing developmental challenges will, to a great extent, depend on the phase-appropriate, empathic responsiveness of the selfobject milieu. Throughout life, intrapsychic capacities for trust, individuation, self-esteem regulation, tension regulation, and so forth must be reworked. Successful developmental reworking or arrests and regressions will be determined by a complex interaction of internal and environmental factors. Biological and previously established psychological capacities and vulnerabilities will interdigitate with relative empathic successes and failures on the part of those aspects of the ongoing environment that must meet the individual's selfobject needs. The vicissitudes of these factors will determine the course of the individual's life.

Self psychology also stresses some psychological themes that are different, although not necessarily in conflict with other developmentalist approaches. A Kohutian perspective on young adult development certainly would address biological drives and the inevitable associated conflicts, but it would not make them the core organizing focus of the personality. Instead, the central themes are establishing a cohesive experience of self that is able to express core ambitions and goals effectively and vigorously and avoiding the internal experiences of fragmentation and depleted depression. To accomplish these two goals, individuals must have established endopsychic structures that will be sufficient to maintain self-cohesion and vigor with only phase-appropriate responsiveness on the part of self-selfobject milieu. That is to say, as healthy people grow, they develop increasingly effective structures that enable them to manage stress while depending on self-selfobject relationships less absolutely and more flexibly. This intrapsychic development enables them to shift their selfobject needs from archaic to mature levels, so that the average, expectable environment will be satisfactory.

Kohut used the term "selfobject" to describe the intrapsychic experience of using someone or something outside the self either to maintain a sense of vigorous self-cohesion or to avoid fragmentation or depleted depression. He divided selfobject needs into three categories: mirroring, idealizing, and alter ego (or twinship). In essence, mirroring deals with self-esteem regulation, feeling an entitled sense of ambition, and the ability to enjoy one's activities. Idealizing is concerned with the ability to regulate tension and affect, channeling and regulating the drives, and the development of meaningful goals and ideals. Alter ego deals with the feeling of connectedness to others in a collegial way and the development of talents into usable skills.

The way people use selfobjects to obtain sustenance may be clarified by a familiar example. Imagine an actress giving a performance. If the audience is appreciative, their response functions as a mirror that reflects back to her that her performance was good. She is able to use the audience as a mirroring selfobject that will enhance and consolidate her sense of self-esteem. If applause is modest, less than she anticipates, the audience cannot be used as a mirroring selfobject. If the response is one of derision, the experience will be traumatic narcissistic injury and many precipitate some degree of self-fragmentation.

Self psychology holds that the essential self-sustaining functions mentioned are met through some fluctuating balance of intrapsychic and interactive nurturance. The average, expectable environment will normally be sufficient to meet the needs of a reasonably healthy person. Although nearly all interactions may meet selfobject needs, the extent to which a particular interaction is salient depends on several factors. (1) Is the environment valued? Our actress may value a New York theater critic's response more than that of an entire small-town audience. (2) Is the interaction considered important? Our actress may demand applause when she comes on stage but may not expect to be recognized on the street. (3) How mature is the person? Has he or she been able to develop reasonably effective intrapsychic structures to sustain the self? Is our actress, for example, confident of her abilities and internally certain of her self-worth? If her intrapsychic capacity to regulate self-esteem is severely limited, each person in any audience—or even strangers on the street—may precipitate narcissistic injury. (4) How much stress is the person enduring? If our actress has just been left by her husband or if she is having trouble getting work, she will probably be more needy of a positive audience response.

Relating the same four questions to students from working-class backgrounds, several things are obvious. These students show all levels of maturity, but younger students are, of course, rarely completely mature. Whatever their grade, some of the subjects had serious intrapsychic vulnerabilities, and others were quite strong. Relationships both at home and in school were important and valued, but it was often virtually impossible to reconcile the conflicting demands of home and school. The opinions of professors and popular classmates were extremely difficult to dismiss. College is a major stressor for all students, but it is probably greater for those with limited social and educational backgrounds. In summary, school, family, friends, and dates were all needed to function as selfobjects. Interactions with them were not readily dismissed. Many working-class students did not, however, receive responses that helped sustain self-esteem or provided needed calming. Some found situations and relationships that actively interfered with maintaining a cohesive and vigorous sense of self. At times, they were even traumatized when they needed help most. Others merely encountered disinterest or emotional distance. In either case, they could not use the university or many new or old relationships as selfobjects to meet legitimate selfobject needs. This complicated or even entirely derailed psychological development, occasionally precipitating emotional collapse and psychiatric symptomatology.

Interactions across Class Barriers in the University

If the theory is correct, social mobility must have a profound effect on both the ongoing and the developmental selfobject milieu of any college student. When blue-collar youths go to college, they are entering a new, unusual environment; in America, college is the most frequent pathway to a change in status. Jencks, Bartlett, Corcoran, Crouse, Eaglesfield, Jackson, McClelland, Mueser, Olneck, Schwartz, Ward, and Williams (1976) state this succinctly: "The highest grade of school or college . . . completed is the best single predictor of . . . eventual occupational status" (p. 223). Success in college is, therefore, particularly necessary if one hopes to share in the American dream of upward mobility and improved economic standards.

Most colleges begin this process immediately by providing an overwhelmingly upper-middle-class milieu. Certainly, the faculty and administrators fall into that category, and the student body comes predominantly from middle- and upper-middle-class backgrounds. The university setting, however, is unusual in that there is much direct contact between classes. It is neither trivial nor accidental that in other circumstances we tend to live and socialize with people from our own class. Although most of us work with people from all classes, it is generally true that these relationships are well structured and that when the class difference is greater the interpersonal intimacy is more limited or even ritualized. We often become uncomfortable when in the company of others who are unlike ourselves. While contact with others who are different is interesting, it is like salt—a little bit is generally enough. Although this discomfort operates in both directions across class barriers, it may be easier for people who look down the ladder to dismiss interactions as unimportant.

In each interaction between people, there is a potential selfobject mirroring function—each person inevitably reads the other as a commentator about self-worth. If the interaction is positive, it is helpful. If it is negative and minimal and the people involved are secure, the mirroring aspect of the interchange may be dismissed as irrelevant. But, if the contact is greater, the others generally valued, and the people themselves not secure, it is harder to dismiss a negative response.

Imagine an interaction between two college seniors that I shall call Charles and Stan. Although those are not their names, they are real people—not caricatures. Charles, because of many family trips to Europe, knew the Paris metro before he spent his junior year there. He pieced together much about European history visiting the castles, palaces, and battlefields. His intellectual parents discussed the significance of the places they visited. Before he was twelve, he knew the difference between Gothic and Romanesque architecture, that the castles were built throughout the countryside because the threat of war was constant, and that the church played an important role in preserving learning. He is handsome, works out regularly to keep in good physical condition, and is a fine athlete. His clothes fit well and are chosen to show casual good taste. His physicist father and teacher mother both love their work. He is not a patient.

Stan's family does not own a car. They have had a only handful of family vacations, leaving Philadelphia for the nearby Pocono Mountains or the New Jersey shore. He has never been more than 200 miles from home, never flown in an airplane, never really thought about European history, and certainly never discussed it at home. His inexpensive clothes cannot fit his moderately overweight body well, and he might wear plaid shorts with a striped shirt. His idea of a fine restaurant is a franchised seafood chain, and he has eaten there only twice. He has been to only a handful of movies, no legitimate theater, and only a very few rock concerts. The money to go just is not available. He speaks with a clearly discernible working-class accent and makes regular grammatical errors. His father hates his job in a factory and complains about it continuously, and his mother does not work and has no established job skills.

These two men may sound exceptional, but, at the Ivy League university that Charles attends, he is by no means unusual. In fact, unlike many of his classmates, he did not go to boarding school, his parents are not really wealthy, nor are they listed in the social register. There are hundreds of people with backgrounds similar to Stan's at his vocationally oriented university.

How might these two men experience each other if they were in the same history class? Charles might feel uncomfortable, sensing his privilege and feeling constrained in discussing what has, for him, been his regular experience. Stan would probably feel inferior immediately, unsure of himself. Even if both had equal IQs, the material would be more difficult for Stan to grasp because of the limits of his experience. He might, moreover, react by either excessively embracing or rejecting upper-class American values. Charles and Stan probably would not like each other and would avoid each other outside the classroom. Neither could use the interaction to provide a positive mirroring experience.

Stan labeled history as irrelevant claptrap and dismissed people like Charles as stuck-up snobs. He chose to withdraw from exploring large areas of cultural and intellectual life—leaving gaps that will almost certainly never be filled and that might make themselves known in future interactions. Avoiding contact with people like Charles means that Stan will not learn how to conduct himself in the private club environment where much high-level business is transacted. When a new cluster of small shops that can be found in any suburban mall opened near his campus, Stan dismissed the complex as filled with "weird" or "faggot" places. In other words, Stan does not know how to interact in a middle/upper-middle-class milieu, and, if his current attitudes continue, he may never learn. But, if he does enter that environment, interactions will be unfamiliar and stressful, and this may limit his progression up the corporate ladder.

He has chosen, instead, to try to obtain a secure (but less challenging) accounting job in a large corporation rather than one in a better-paying, more prestigious accounting firm. He is probably correct in his belief that this will decrease the amount of contact he will have with those he considers "snobs." He wants to live near his friends (only a few of whom have gone to college) and his parents (although he hates his alcoholic father). Naturally, he wants a more economically comfortable life than his parents had, but he has chosen to minimize shifting his social status despite the consequences this may have for his income.

For many students, similar decisions in no way reflect either psychopathology or developmental arrest. Rather, such decisions may simply be wise and healthy, meaning something like, "I don't like the stress of that other life, and I would prefer to remain close to my roots. I think any other decision would risk unwanted distance between me and my family and friends, and I can make enough money to meet my needs."

Family, Peer, and Social Interactions

Rubin (1976), Sennett and Cobb (1972), and Sexton and Sexton (1971) have provided reviews of working-class life, and they all conclude that blue-collar families live in what Rubin calls "worlds of pain." Much of their anguish centers around their jobs. Although they may provide valued social contacts, the work is generally repetitive, boring, and even dangerous. It is unlikely that either the money or the nature of the work itself will provide many hourly workers with enhanced self-esteem. Rather, those authors are unanimous in their insistence that many aspects of work provide endless insult. There is a pervasive sense of powerlessness that is at best faintly disguised by defensive, macho bravado (the Rocky solution).

The family structure is hierarchical, with the father as at least the titular head, the person to whom all must show what is called "respect." But this often means almost abject obedience and avoiding anything that might either challenge the illusion of his position on top of the pecking order or threaten his precarious self-esteem.

The parents generally do not read regularly; if they do, it is only parts of the newspaper. There are few, if any, books in the home. Both financial and loyalty considerations ensure that they rarely venture out of their neighborhoods unless such excursions are necessary. Without a car, it is obviously necessary to shop at a local store, which will surely be geared to a lower-income market and taste. These people certainly do not dine in expensive restaurants, attend orchestra concerts or theater, or visit art museums. People from higher classes are considered outsiders, are not trusted, and are generally labeled snobs. For most, the religious preference is Roman Catholic, and the families are often very large.

While men are burdened with the need to prove their macho power and must avoid anything hinting of effete intellectualism (which may be considered evidence of homosexuality), the lot of women is no better. These women have been expected to remain in a relationship to their husbands and authority males that is at least overtly subordinate. Although current economic realities are having an effect (women are working and attending college), hidden doubts persist about the wisdom of a higher education for women. It is often thought that what limited funds are available should, after all, be spent on the male children, who will eventually become primary breadwinners.

Nonstudents generally marry at an early age, often within the teens. Even in the parents' generation, marriage was frequently precipitated by pregnancy. Many wives still hope for little more than a husband who has a stable job and does not drink or beat them. Some of the men are equally satisfied if the sex is regular and pregnancies infrequent.

While these comments about working-class family life may seem stereotyped and bigoted, they provide a pattern that accurately describes many in this circumscribed group. The comments do not, however, note these people's particular strengths. Often they know how to work and genuinely know how to work hard, possess valuable "street smarts," are often quite self-reliant, and are able to fight hard to get what they want. Although they do not expect Mom and Dad to "fix it all," many parents will make tremendous sacrifices for the benefit of family members and friends. The positive side of a narrow worldview may well be intense loyalty and support for those who conform. Students from this background tend to be cooperative, hard working, and respectful. In general, I find them nice, decent people who sincerely try to make things work instead of behaving in a way that might be considered entitled, self-centered, and, frankly, offensive.

Despite their strengths, a multitude of factors combine to humiliate them regularly. Even jokes deliver insult—we do, after all, tell Polish, not Swiss, jokes. When regularly disparaged, people routinely follow one of two basic paths: denial that the insult matters, accompanied by deprecation and devaluation of outsiders, or efforts to compensate through grandiose or perfectionistic defenses. Either path, of course, complicates the life of both the family and the member who changes status.

University and college students in particular often seem a threat, even the enemy, to many blue-collar people, but this is also "the way out" for their children. Parents must greet the experience with considerable ambivalence and trepidation. Will the children they love become different, their "betters," or even strangers? Who will they marry: one of the outsiders with different values and a foreign worldview?

When someone from a working-class background goes to college, he or she is likely to provoke competitive feelings in family members or life-long friends. This is particularly so if the other person is narcissistically vulnerable. For example, one student was offered a promotion at his cooperative education job that would give him an hourly wage higher than that of his father. His mother insisted that he reject the promotion, stating clearly that his father "won't be able to handle it." Another father greeted the news that his son was accepted to a prestigious college with, "We'll see how long you last there." The boy flunked out and transferred to an easier school, where he continued to pursue premedical studies. His father's response to that was, "When you get to be a big doctor, don't come driving around here in your Cadillac." Other fathers worry that their children will become one of the bosses that they and their friends all hate.

Obviously, much of the issue here is the fathers' narcissistic vulnerability, not their social status. But these men are often humiliated by the circumstances of their class, and this imposes substantial impediments to the development of well-consolidated self-esteem. The simple fact that their child attends college creates a competitive situation not present in the children of college-educated parents. Suddenly, life becomes replete with potential for assaults on the father's self-esteem. This surely diminishes the ability of many fathers emotionally to support their children's education.

It can be equally problematic if the child is a narcissistic extension of the parents. When the college education proves the parents' worth, it may deny much of the child's unique individuality. School may come to be a burden, an activity unrelated to the development of the "true self" (Winnicott 1965), a loathsome effort of the "false self" to meet parents' needs. Not infrequently, both narcissistic competition and narcissistic extension operate simultaneously.

These attitudes extend beyond parents to siblings, other relatives, and friends, all of whom may be threatened and overtly or covertly sabotage the student. For example, one student experienced such repeated and intense attacks as a snob and a phoney big shot that he and an uncle both lost control and got into a serious fistfight at a family wedding. Needless to say, he came to avoid family gatherings, but he felt guilty about this decision, and his parents were extremely (and not quietly) upset by it.

In many working-class high schools, the dropout rate before graduation is well over 50 percent. As noted, pregnancy is often involved, and the teenagers are forced into premature marriage and must take jobs with little future. Those who do not attend college are often locked into limited opportunities. There will be a stark difference between their lives and those of a friend, brother, or sister who graduates from college and marries another graduate. Income disparity alone may create tension. The dropout will not be able to afford many vacations skiing in Europe. What should be given for Christmas, a generous gift or something in the price range that your sibling can afford? But the differences are more pervasive than those of economics. There may be an entirely different set of interests and style of life. The mirror that siblings provide each other can become increasingly distasteful. They may become strangers, making obligatory family gatherings increasingly uncomfortable. Siblings will tell the entire family that they are doing "good enough," that college educations are an unnecessary waste of time. They may repeatedly question why the parents are wasting money on a brother's or sister's tuition, and so on.

Although mothers can be competitive with children, clinical data suggest that they are more commonly worried that they will lose the contact with children they both value and need. For example, one mother idolized her brilliant son: he was particularly important to her because of the empty nature of her relationship with her husband. She soon realized that she no longer understood what her son was interested in. With increasing difficulty, she encouraged only those aspects of his education that were practical and discouraged the more culturally oriented classes that were of particular interest to him. He loved music and wanted to attend concerts given by the Philadelphia Orchestra, but she absurdly insisted that the danger of street crime between the concert hall and the parking lot was too great, so he never went. She found tasks that needed to be done at home just when there was an exam. He would get angry; she would become hurt and withdrawn; he would feel guilty and eventually do the work rather than study. The bottom line was, of course, poor grades.

Comparing a laborer father or a checkout clerk mother to a professor may precipitate a traumatic deidealization of a previously idealized parent. This can be a calamity for both generations. A son may do an about face, suddenly valuing nothing about his father. This deprives the father of a mirroring selfobject that could help maintain the older man's self-esteem. The son is deprived of an idealized source of strength and calming. This happened to an architecture student when his carpenter father, thinking he would need management skills he did not possess, refused to take an independent contracting job. Suddenly, the son could admire nothing about his father and became obsessed with homosexual fantasies. The prior idealization was undoubtedly poorly consolidated or even defensive in nature, and the dynamics were not simple. An important element, however, was the collapse of the idealization that precipitated a sexualized longing for a self-selfobject relationship to replace the functions previously provided by the father.

Not only family relationships are disrupted when a student starts a climb up the class ladder. Peers demand time, and socialization in these neighborhoods consists of "hanging on the corner" or drinking in neighborhood bars. Conversation is generally limited to gossip, drinking stories, drugs, sports, and sex for the young men and boys, clothes, and babies for young women. Studying also takes time and pulls the student away from friends, whose response varies from uncomprehending support to overt sabotage. As part of a class assignment, one young man made his first—and last—visit to the art museum with his girlfriend. That behavior was labeled as clear evidence of homosexual tendencies, and the student himself could not believe that his friends were only (or even principally) joking.

Peer and family problems, of course, apply to women. Marie was the ninth of eleven children and the only one in her immediate or extended family to attend college. Nor did the spouses of her older siblings attend college. A few admired her perseverance, but most clearly expressed that she was wasting her time. Her parents complained bitterly about the tuition payments, that she was not helping sufficiently with family finances or housework, and so forth. At family parties, aunts and uncles continued to comment on how she had grown, as if she were six. One aunt assembled an album with pictures of all the cousins—except Marie, the deviant. She graduated shortly after a sister married, and the sister was given a big wedding. At the formal graduation, her parents claimed great pride and pleasure, but the celebration consisted of a few drinks in a local tavern, and Marie had to organize and pay for her own graduation party.

Large families are common in the working classes, and coming from a family the size of Marie's can present some particular problems as well as providing many joys. There is little room for privacy, so finding quiet for study can be a challenge. There are obvious financial difficulties. Perhaps most important, in many families there is little possibility for individualized responsiveness, and normative thinking and behavior are necessary for daily functioning. Efficiency is a necessity; things work most smoothly if everyone has similar tastes, interests, and values. Imagine the potential for conflict if different members could enjoy or even tolerate only either hard rock, disco, standards, or classical music—particularly if there are twelve people living in a seven-room row home.

Although hard data are difficult to obtain, it seems that the educational and social system of blue-collar students routinely urges conformity instead of diversity. In *Women's Ways of Knowing*, Belenky, Clinchy, Goldberger, and Tarule (1986) present the concept of "received" knowledge, referring to taking information in as it is presented by an all-knowing source. It is presented back without change, with an absence of the feeling of having created the knowledge. There are correct answers and incorrect answers, and the authority knows which is which and does not want to be challenged. Received knowledge may be best in the powerless circumstances of an assembly-line job, in which there often appears to be no use for, expectation of, or even tolerance for innovative thinking.

This attitude is continued into the primary and secondary schools as well. University faculty, particularly those with experience teaching at a variety of schools, routinely notice that many students from blue-collar backgrounds have not been trained to question information, that they just do not ask the difficult questions. Operating from a Marxist perspective, sociologists Bowles and Gintis (1976) do not find this observation surprising. In *Schooling in Capitalist America,* they write that the United States has three basic types of education. One is geared toward creative thinking and is taught principally in private and good suburban high schools. At the other end of the spectrum are schools for the lower classes, which stress rote learning. The third group falls between the other two. These authors believe that the goal of the American educational system is to maintain the status quo while providing the illusion of equality of opportunity. One may easily disagree with their explanations about the reasons, but it is difficult to contradict the data marshaled by them and others (e.g., Jencks, Smith, Ackland, Bane, Cohen, Gintis, Heyns, and Michelson 1972) that upward mobility is extraordinarily difficult and that the educational system fails to facilitate that shift as it should.

Students themselves are well aware of these differences and often blame their poor preparation on dogmatic teachers, but the attitude is more pervasive, extending throughout the family and the culture. Since Weber (1958) described the Protestant ethic, many have wondered if it is essentially discouraged in a predominantly Roman Catholic environment. Rosen (1965), for example, notes the importance that others have attributed to a theology that is given by the priests (and ultimately by the pope), is not open to question, and stresses obedience. Interestingly, many parochial schools use uniforms, which, despite their advantages, consolidate a leveling uniformity.

Although much of this may be changing in today's schools (perhaps because of the shortage of nuns and priests), if the school excessively stresses received knowledge, the mirroring it provides for its students may have seemed like, "I know the correct answers. Your ideas are correct only when they match mine, and ideas generated within you are not valuable." Certainly, many teachers try to avoid that position and try to listen carefully to their students' ideas—something not easily done when classes are too big. But when there is a tendency at home, a tendency at work, and a tendency at school not to question authority, the overlapping tendencies leave little opportunity for mirroring experiences that lead students to respect and value the originality of their own thinking, to believe that they create useful, new ideas.

Whatever the cause may be, it is clear that the total environmental pattern generally known to these students has valued and established intellectual patterns that are not well suited to academic work. Their first task may be to learn to think more flexibly. Moreover, even the quality of the knowledge that has been received is typically inadequate. Perhaps because of the current emphasis on the failure of the ghetto school, we regularly ignore that the schools in white, working-class areas are not good either. Since only a minority of students are college bound, it is often necessary to gear the curriculum to levels well below the national norm—and few would argue that the national norm is genuinely satisfactory.

These students often enter college with academic limitations that tend to make for negative mirroring experiences in the classroom. When academic material becomes more complex, a limited fund of knowledge or a rigid cognitive style becomes an increasing handicap. For example, although received knowledge may be satisfactory for learning basic skills or in introductory levels of technological subjects, it is generally only a stepping stone and not sufficient in advanced physics or liberal arts subjects. Interestingly, lower levels of management rely primarily on technical skills and ask that the orders of superiors be carried out without much questioning, whereas upper management must cope with new material and should deal with it innovatively. It is not surprising, then, that most lower management comes from technical or business backgrounds while a high percentage of upper management pursued liberal arts majors in college. Even the cognitive style encouraged in the working classes holds people close to that class.

Working-class students have some other academic problems that are relatively straightforward. They generally must live at home to save money, so they often must spend hours commuting to and from school when classmates are studying or relaxing. Families cannot offer the help with schoolwork that others can get from the person down the hall in the dormitory or from an older sorority sister. Nor are fraternity exam files open to them. Parents may know how to work hard, easily painting the house for hours without a break. That is, however, the way that they may think their children should study calculus—study breaks are mere laziness.

While the home environment is unable to provide much help in some areas, these students find the university environment quite uncomfortable. Thinking back to Charles and Stan, obviously Stan would tend to form friendships with other commuting students. But these people often live in divergent parts of the city and need to be home for dinner (which is often as early as five o'clock). Staying late to study together can be difficult or impossible—particularly if they must travel by public transportation, which can be dangerous after the rush hour. They avoid most campus organizations since they bring them into direct contact and competition with the very students they fear most. All this means decreased study and social opportunities.

I described Stan, who reacted to his many problems by remaining in school but preserved a primary loyalty to his community of origin. Others drop out, finding the tension too great to bear. Still others try to join the establishment, and many fall anywhere on the spectrum between the extremes. Mike was a student from a Polish-American, Roman Catholic family who tried to out-WASP the WASPs. He began his career at a nationally recognized university in the suburbs that primarily educates the children of well-to-do Catholics. Living at home, he had to commute an hour and a half on public transportation from his row home through some of our country's most magnificent suburbs. He was filled with envy and a desire to live there. Misled by a high class rank at his mediocre high school, he was stunned to realize that his preparation was entirely inadequate. An ROTC scholarship enabled him to attend that college, but it placed major time demands on him. Several factors ensured his academic failure: too little time for study, poorly established academic skills, the moderately difficult curriculum, and—most important—the hours lost to fantasies of grandiose repair of real and imagined daily narcissistic injuries. His poor grades humiliated him, but he was able to transfer to another university. Although his new school was probably more academically demanding, it held as part of its mission educating students from working-class backgrounds.

Mike entered the second university determined to get straight A's. My best estimate of his intellectual gifts was that they were only modestly above average, so this would have been a difficult task indeed. Again, failure was ensured, and his narcissistic grandiosity intensified. His longing to be perfect extended to his understanding of social position as well. He chose to pursue crew as a sport. His ability enabled him to join (but not be really accepted into) one of the city's prestigious rowing clubs. His dress was determined by the most careful study of "preppie" taste. Grammatical errors and unwanted accents would, however, occasionally leap from his mouth like a frog at a debutante ball.

I often wondered how he got any real studying done when so many hours were spent rowing and lost in grandiose fantasy. Many hours of psychotherapy, many dropped courses, and two extra years of college later, he graduated with more realistic assessments of his capabilities and a better-developed capacity to use his talents and skills. I hear from him occasionally; he is living with an apparently charming woman, works effectively, and plans to attend an appropriate law school in the fall.

We both agreed that his success was the result of his ability to use our relationship to help him regulate his self-esteem. He established, in other words, a useful mirroring transference. We repeatedly examined both the inevitable disruptions of our relationship and the myriad of narcissistic assaults provoked by his perfectionism. This enabled him to establish a more realistic and internally based sense of self-esteem. Little attention was focused on oedipal conflicts. I understood his psychopathology as based principally on deficits in self-structure rather than as a narcissistic defense against conflict.

Discussion

Because of finances and many other limitations outlined, Rocky, or his academically talented neighbors, would have to negotiate perilous shoals in their journey through college. They would begin a major upward shift in social position. No particular difficulty is fatal for these students, but, with obstacles coming one on another, many are indeed stressed. Some of the challenges that result from this shift are basically sociological in scope. Although we are well advised to take note of them, direct psychiatric intervention may consist of little more than understanding and encouragement. There are, however, important developmental and intrapsychic factors that are directly affected by movement up the class hierarchy.

Recent contributions of self psychology are particularly helpful in efforts to understand how social mobility complicates the intrapsychic task of maintaining a cohesive, vigorous self, one with well-established ambitions and clear and attainable goals. The shift itself often creates disruptions in essential self-selfobject relationships that have previously sustained these people. Likewise, mobility imposes particular difficulties in establishing psychologically necessary contacts in the new environment. Maintaining or developing self-selfobject relationships may become so difficult that talented individuals will be forced to or simply choose to remain in or near their class of origin. Those who do not, who substantially change social status, may feel like someone with one foot on the boat and the other on the dock. This is a precarious position from which to negotiate the stresses of college.

Perhaps a majority will find that their friends and family provide self-selfobject relationships sufficient to meet their developmental needs. These relationships will yield a solidity and reliability that will more than compensate for any lack in sophistication. But others are left weakened and will survive only if they find special self-selfobject relationships within the university community that provide a developmental splint (Doctors 1987). This will enable both restorative and ongoing personal development. If a sufficiently empathic relationship can be established, and with a bit of luck, they may mature and succeed brilliantly.

Effective treatment of these students requires continuous, careful attention to the disruptions in self-selfobject relationships that may be imposed by their developing social mobility. Sometimes it will be a background issue; other times it will represent the central focus of treatment. I have never found it irrelevant.

When they graduate, moreover, these students will continue to face similar burdens—though without the assistance of the university environment. They, too, may also need a developmental splint, and many will need to find it in a psychotherapeutic relationship.

Kohut (1984) has recommended that treatment will be facilitated by establishing selfobject transferences. Accomplishing this with these students may require some alteration in therapeutic technique. While it is important to help anyone realize that they are understood from their own particular perspective, this obtains particular salience in the blue-collar population. These patients generally see psychiatrists as members of the other social group, the representative of the bosses and the country club set. Initially, we are not trusted. Moreover, their home environment has never encouraged seeking psychiatric help: "Shrinks are for crazy people, and I'm not crazy."

It seems wise, therefore, to take any steps that encourage accessibility if they do not unnecessarily complicate the therapeutic stance. Baum and Felzer (1964) and Gould (1967) found a more accessible, open, and flexible approach helpful in their work with nonstudent, lower socioeconomic status patients. Heitler (1976) stressed the importance of preparatory techniques in dealing with similar patients, noting that they do not have the same understanding of the therapeutic process that middle-class patients do. These patients need to see psychiatrists as normal, and it is often useful for them and their parents actually to see an apparently normal psychiatrist at freshman orientation meetings. They also need to know that we really understand the factual dilemmas that they face because of their backgrounds. It helps if we know specifics of their ethnic heritages.

Many face a painful realization that family members and friends are, in truth, undercutting their progress in college. These people, who had been so important in the past, may be experienced as actively destructive. When that happens, students often need both emotional support and confirmation that their perceptions are not crazy.

In general, it is the nontherapeutic environment that provides collegians their most salient self-selfobject relationships. Selecting the right type of university is, therefore, especially important. Many people, particularly those with intrapsychic vulnerabilities and/or ambivalent family systems, will be wise to select schools that have student bodies with large numbers of people from their own class, where they can find a larger network of genuine peers. Vocationally oriented universities may offer some particular benefits by providing clear goals. In that environment, "street smarts" may give them an advantage over more sheltered, middle-class students. Parents may be more supportive when there is the clear end point of a specific job. Because working-class people often tend to distrust people who do nothing practical, they may even see earning money by thinking as a "con job." Real work is done with the hands and yields a product (Sennett and Cobb 1972). Engineering and accounting may rely principally on thinking, but most people believe that a real product is made and think they know what the job consists of. Consequently, parents may be more supportive when their child is pursuing a definable major.

For some, however, the correct choice may be an Ivy League or other prestigious school. Although it is important that all universities establish special facilities to support working-class students, it is essential at these schools. In fact, government programs are available to help schools accomplish this goal, and most universities have established organizations in place. Social support, tutoring, and encouragement are provided. This is often a very valuable adjunct to treatment, but it may be necessary to persuade these students to use available facilities. Psychiatrists can generally find out about them through the dean of students' office.

Therapists' attitudes and countertransferences are, of course, vital in any psychotherapeutic endeavor. Again, working-class students may have special problems because most therapists have established beliefs about people from the lower classes, who are often seen as more sexual, more impulsive, more authority bound, less intelligent, and so on. We may prefer to treat people from backgrounds similar to our own, feeling more important if our patients seem more important. The son of the chief executive officer of a large corporation may appeal to us more than the daughter of the person who cleans the president's office. The more prestigious physicians do, after all, care for the more prestigious patients. It is obvious that we all share most of these attitudes to some degree, and it is certainly true that they will negatively affect our work more if we deny them or are unaware of them.

Siassi and Messer (1976) have pointed to another attitudinal danger. Obvious social problems may lead us to ignore intrapsychic difficulties. The self psychological perspective is, at its deepest level, an intrapsychic one. I have tried to show that the intrapsychic tasks of continued development have been complicated by interpersonal problems imposed, in part, by social class. We must remain principally concerned with our patients' psyches, but intrapsychic development needs continued consolidation from a supportive, empathic environment during a college student's education. Without this support, expression of the nuclear program of the self or even maintaining cohesion and vigor are more difficult—or may even be impossible.

Sometimes these students will decide to continue their education, distancing themselves from family and old friends. At other times they will withdraw from school to reestablish themselves in the neighbor-hood. The successful ones will figure out some way to balance all the conflicting demands effectively. Sometimes they may need support to continue their education, but it is all too easy for therapists to support that decision and unconsciously sabotage the option to quit. That may reflect our values and needs, not theirs.

Conclusions

A satisfactory grasp of the multiple aspects of the person's socio-logical environment and a careful awareness of their and our own class prejudices will help us provide a needed developmental splint—and help facilitate the efforts of those patients to find hidden support in other aspects of their lives. Then they will be able to reduce the im-pediments they and others place in the way of their progress.

REFERENCES

Baker, H., and Baker, M. 1977. Heinz Kohut's self psychology: an overview. *American Journal of Psychiatry* 144:1–9.

Baum, O., and Felzer, S. 1964. Activity in initial interviews with lower-class patients. *Archives of General Psychiatry* 10:345–353.

Belenky, M.; Clinchy, B.; Goldberger, N.; and Tarule, J. 1986. *Women's Ways of Knowing*. New York: Basic.

Bowles, S., and Gintis, H. 1976. *Schooling in Capitalist America*. New York: Basic.

Doctors, S. 1987. The developmental splint: meanings and functions of symptoms in adolescence. Paper presented to the tenth annual Conference on the Psychology of the Self, Chicago, October 25.

Erikson, E. 1950. *Childhood and Society*. New York: Norton.

Gould, R. 1967. Dr. Strangeclass; or, how I stopped worrying about the theory and began treating the blue-collar worker. *American Journal of Orthopsychiatry* 37:78–86.

Heitler, J. 1976. Preparatory techniques in initiating expressive psy-chotherapy with lower-class, unsophisticated patients. *Psychological Bulletin* 83:339–352.

Jencks, C.; Bartlett, S.; Corcoran, M.; Crouse, J.; Eaglesfield, D.; Jackson, G.; McClelland, K.; Mueser, P.; Olneck, M.; Schwartz, J.;

Ward, S.; and Williams, J. 1976. *Who Gets Ahead? The Determinants of Economic Success in America.* New York: Basic.

Jencks, C.; Smith, M.; Ackland, H.; Bane, M. J.; Cohen, D.; Gintis, H.; Heyns, B.; and Michelson, S. 1972. *Inequality: A Reassessment of the Effect of Family and Schooling in America.* New York: Basic.

Kohut, H. 1971. *The Analysis of the Self.* New York: International Universities Press.

Kohut, H. 1977. *The Restoration of the Self.* New York: International Universities Press.

Kohut, H. 1984. *How Does Analysis Cure?* Chicago: University of Chicago Press.

Levinson, D. 1978. *The Seasons of Man's Life.* New York: Knopf.

Mahler, M.; Pine, F.; and Bergman, A. 1975. *The Psychological Birth of the Human Infant.* New York: Basic.

Offer, D., and Sabshin, M. 1984. *Normality and the Life Cycle.* New York: Basic.

Rosen, B. 1965. Race, ethnicity, and the achievement syndromes. In M. Kornrich, ed. *Underachievement.* Springfield, Ill. Thomas.

Rubin, L. 1976. *Worlds of Pain.* New York: Basic.

Sennett, R., and Cobb, J. 1972. *The Hidden Injuries of Class.* New York: Knopf.

Sexton, P., and Sexton, B. 1971. *Blue Collars and Hard-Hats.* New York: Random House.

Siassi, I., and Messer, S. 1976. Psychotherapy with patients from lower socioeconomic groups. *American Journal of Psychotherapy* 30:29–40.

Stern, D. 1985. *The Interpersonal World of the Infant.* New York: Basic.

Vaillant, G. 1977. *Adaptation to Life.* Boston: Little, Brown.

Weber, M. 1958. *The Protestant Ethic and the Spirit of Capitalism.* New York: Scribner's.

Winnicott, D. W. 1965. *The Maturational Process and the Facilitating Environment.* New York: International Universities Press.

8   SEVENTEEN: A DEVELOPMENTAL VIEW

LEO RANGELL

In surveying the psychological conflicts of adolescence, I am choosing to write not on a phase, or a stage, or an age group, but on a year. I am focusing on age seventeen, a year of life that I see not as at but approaching the portal to adulthood. It is a time close to the end of the gestation period for the emerging of the adult.

Partial structures, psychic and somatic, and their derivative traits and characteristics are beginning to assume definitive form and to be united into a cohesive whole. I do not say final whole because finality does not occur until the end of life. Physically, one can begin to see the shape and look of the face and body of an adult. The same is true of the psychological as of the somatic. Beginning to be reliably visible is also the self, the character, the emerging nature, and attributes of the person. To a large extent, the die is being cast for the central nature of the total specific and unique individual being formed.

In the seventeenth year, we can see this process leading to the adult well on its way, an agglutination of partial and incomplete developments shaping into a more formed and static structure. At seventeen, the adult is getting ready to emerge and be born. His final characteristics are beginning to take shape in preparation for the event of the adult coming out. In the comparable seventh or eighth month of intrauterine pregnancy, we cannot see the same happening as visually, although with the fluoroscopes and sonograms of today that is indeed beginning to be the case. But, in outer as compared to intrauterine life, we are in a position to have a better view. This chapter is meant to help train us look at what is before us.

It is surprising that in psychoanalysis, which, as a paradigm, is dedicated to seeing the past in the present, which sees life as a series of successive unfoldings and constantly exposes repetitive cycles, we have not thought before that the first succession of developmental phases—oral, anal, phallic, preoedipal, and oedipal, latency to puberty—can be and typically is repeated immediately afterward in the adolescent years, while the first epigenetic unfolding is still fresh. As such, adolescence can be recognized as a recapitulation of the earlier tasks and achievements. From thirteen to twenty, the next phase of the evolving maturation traverses at this next succession of stages the same sequences as it did the first time. Oral taking in from the environment, anal independent self-sufficiency, phallic, vaginal, genital exchanges with objects, now as a more total sexual and aggressive entity, evolve in accordance with a combination of constitutional givens, maturational characteristics, and experiential inputs implanted and developed from the first sequential developmental series from birth to puberty.

Since Erikson (1950), the unfolding of the epigenetic stages of later life are being seen more concretely but not yet so visibly and consciously during this earlier transitional period. Every aspect is recapitulated, drive pressures, old and new, a steady expansion of ego development, superego characteristics that take more definitive forms, the same and different from before, all leading to separation-individuation again, only much more so, and changed object relations from a combination of all these. But, unlike the drama, suddenness, and violence of the original birth and the burst of physical changes at the birth of the adolescent, the birth of the adult slips in more quietly. It is my impression that it is easily overlooked. Perhaps this is because it means so much now. There is less turning back and fewer changes ahead, at least major ones.

Just as progression culminates in a new whole at puberty after the first unfolding sequence, so does the whole adult, albeit a young adult, emerge after the adolescent second sequence. The initial phasic yet continuous development has repeated itself in a new concentric layer, with the original forms either consolidating their structures and characteristics or acquiring new contents and shapes as progressive development continues. The next nodal point, of the appearance of a significantly new level of person, finds the physical and the psychological not unexpectedly integrated or at least parallel and interrelated. Perhaps it is no accident but in accordance with man's phylogenetically developing sense of time and cognition that the changes and new developmental forms of the first third of life correspond numerically to the mathematical division into decades. Childhood, the teens, and the twenties could have come to be divided by the tens in accordance with the observed and experienced changes in the cycle of life.

Mahler's (Mahler, Pine, and Bergman 1975) felicitous phrase "the psychological birth of the infant"—between symbiosis and individuation during the first year of life—introduces more than the specific insight this points to. Birth need no longer be confined to the body but can be applied to psychological achievements as well. But it also leads to a general principle, which can be reflected on with profit, that birth need no longer be limited to the moment of physical separation of the fetus from the protective environment inside the mother's body. Life after birth is indeed a succession of births as well as deaths or passings of stages and organizations.

If we distance ourselves from conventional but imprecise generalizations, we see at once that, just as life begins not at birth but at conception, so is birth not limited to that most dramatic moment when the newborn traverses the border between the intrauterine and the external environment. Birth as inception occurs at conception. Maturation, formerly limited to the organic, and development, to the psychological, a distinction introduced by Hartmann (1939), actually occur to both physiological and psychological elements. And both are to be taken into account not only in studying the original libidinal and ego phases but in understanding all stages of the life cycle. Late adolescence, on which I will focus, is no exception.

A number of distinctions of concepts and terms, often merged or confused or at least not clearly separated, need to be differentiated. Congenital is not the same as constitutional. Congenital characteristics, that is, those present at birth, are already a product of constitution and environment and contain somatic and psychological potentials. The earliest intrauterine environment is determined by both somatic and psychological aspects of the maternal surround. The newly "born" is already a combination of the constitutional and acquired. With Hartmann's (1939, 1950) ego-id matrix, innate ego apparatuses, and possible ego energies, Rapaport's (1953) inborn discharge channels, the innate releaser mechanisms of Tinbergen (1951), Lorenz (1950), and other ethologists, although birth does occur later, there are already, as with somatic factors, psychological *anlagen* and potentials present prebirth as well. Affect attunement (Stern 1983), object synchrony, mutuality (Erikson 1950), active reciprocity (Winnicott 1957), all observed by infant observers from birth on, and Freud's (1896; Breuer and Freud 1893–1895) descriptions of affects as deriving phylogenetically from inherited hysterical attacks make the distinction between psychic and somatic an academic question and the acrimonious debate between nature and nurture outmoded. Constitutional and acquired, psychic and somatic, are united and reciprocal in each pair. Both distinctions and continuities are necessary to encompass the data of development scientifically. Borders and overlapping are each operative and important, not only in studies of infancy and childhood, but in the derivative understanding they cast throughout life.

It is from this as a background that I wish to turn to the subject I have chosen to focus on in this chapter. I have for many years had nascent, and not so latent, thoughts about the arrival not just at late adolescence but at the more specific and precise age of seventeen and the particular dynamics operative at that moment in life. From my exposure to clinical and theoretical psychoanalysis for over four decades, as well as from observations made more quietly in life, I have long felt that this critical and formative developmental period has a nodal significance that has not commanded a sufficient intensity of attention.

Psychoanalysis, following Freud, has pinpointed the oedipal period to age four to six, studying, discussing, and constantly rethinking its apical position. Secondarily, perhaps even reactively, attention shifted to what was first called the pregenital years; when genital was discovered to antedate the oedipal (Galenson and Roiphe 1974; Roiphe 1968; Roiphe and Galenson 1972), it was called preoedipal instead. From this, concentrated attention moved on to mother-child and finally to the earliest mother-infant relationships. Prodigious literature eventuated for each. This present centering on the passage from adolescence to adulthood does not detract from any of these. My experience in confronting psychoanalytic issues has always been that turning to an unfamiliar or at least underattended area has usually been met by a defense of the familiar or preceding areas of interest and attention. This is not necessary here. Everything gained previously still stands. But new veins, as Ferenczi (1930) put it, can be found in old mines, which need constantly to be explored.

Eleven to twelve initiates puberty quite visibly with surface changes and glandular action. The adolescent that follows has been openly prepared for. The intergenerational activity that ensues is intense, tense, determined, but usually good natured. The problems come on, many and concentrated, and with wide oscillations. The patience of all is tested and honed. Characteristics are demonstrated across the spectrum of actions and affects, good and bad, acceptable, horrid, predictable, surprising, steady, changeable, chaotic. This is the most action-oriented period of parent-child relations. I will pass through this rapidly to come to the age I have selected for this presentation.

The year is the junior year in high school, the year before the final year and the moving on to bigger things. This is known to students and faculty—I have only recently seen it officially noted and described as such in an educational brochure—as the most decisive year in a young person's course of life. Decisions are made after the junior year; the grades in the last year do not count. But all that has preceded leads now to a series of crucial choices at many crossroads. Until now, life has mainly provided what was needed; progress has been passively received. The young person applies or does not apply to college. Each chooses his social, occupational, and geographic directions, usually with surface knowledge appearing to choose but deeper unconscious elements directing.

Where will he go to college? Does one go at all, near the family, or away from them? What goals will he reach for, who will his friends be, and his loves, and how will he relate to them? These choices, made with all levels of the psyche participating, from which later occurrences will derive that will be attributed to chance, will determine the more enduring states, chronically over time, in love and work. If this strikes one as a young and tender age to be given such decisive importance, I think of the fact that, just as in a horizontal sense, conscious decisions—I am speaking of the major ones—are preceded by long preparatory unconscious formative stages, the same obtains in a longitudinal, developmental sense, that crucial and active periods of decision are similarly prepared and shaped by preliminary formative periods that may take years. The self, and mentally its representation within the ego, is reaching a fairly formed and crystallized stage. One of its characteristics, which will be more and more regularly applied, is where it believes it belongs and fits in the pecking order of life. The nature of object relations begins to be seen and to be predictable. I recently attended the fiftieth class reunion of my medical school. I was struck by how everyone was the same, much more than how different.

It is surprising, clinically and in life, how many roads lead back to the specific age of seventeen without commensurate focal attention having been paid to it. Clinical reconstructions and direct observations have pointed to and reinforced with convincing regularity the crucial nature of this age period. As in all things psychological, I am not speaking of a sharp line and would not wish to be held to such an expectation of precision. I do not wish to have to stop at each observation to acknowledge and pay homage to all development that has gone before and that will follow.

The observational data from which my reflections are drawn come from both sides of adolescence and from outside as well as inside the psychoanalytic situation. They stem from a combination of clinical reconstructions, direct observations, and life experiences. All patients past adolescence have been seventeen and reproduce critical material from that period, too often overlooked. My patients report about their children who are adolescents, and now some are bringing in thoughts about their grandchildren as adolescents. I also hear about and read about grandchildren of former patients whom I knew about when they themselves were younger. From more personal experience, we have all been seventeen. My children have also been seventeen, and, among my grandchildren, one is fifteen, one sixteen, and one was seventeen until a few weeks ago.

At the end of late adolescence, the adult is "born." I would note the metaphoric nature of this insight. We will not stretch the metaphor to the literal but recognize the vast difference from actual conventional birth and these similar but still only analogous ones. There is only one "real" birth and only one death. In many ways, however, the new young adult is as raw for his new role and functions as the newborn was for the challenges of the new world into which he arrived. Presumably, his mental functions have grown or are growing to be "mature." At least the world is getting ready to look at him, and expect of him, and demand of him, as if they were. The id and derivative affects have been tamed; the superego has been tried, tested, and shaped and is supposedly reliable. The ego has had time to institute a workable and effective inventory of defenses and is experienced enough to differentiate impulses that can be directed toward appropriate action from those that need to be deflected or defended against. Mastery is sufficiently at hand over internal instinctual demands and pressures, and over external limiting stimuli, so that the ego executor and moral agent is at the brink of being able to be held responsible for the person's deeds. All is close to being in order.

Or so the script goes. But at this age, as at all ages, regressions and progressions are intermixed, and the achieved state is stable in name only. Every stage of development, from the earliest to the end of the life cycle, bears imprints of former phases and portents of stages still ahead. Rapaport (1953) points out that in the stages of development of psychoanalytic theory, as in ontogenetic development itself, each phase borrows from the past and looks to the future. Regressions and progressions are the norm, not exceptional or pathological. Freud (1937) states, "Portions of the earlier organization always persist alongside of the more recent one, and even in normal development the . . . residues of earlier libidinal fixations may still be retained in the final configuration" (p. 229).

For a report that can stand alongside clinical observations as to this simultaneous backward and forward look, I will quote a page, not from a psychoanalyst, but from Booth Tarkington's (1916) book called, appropriately, *Seventeen*. The subject is hapless Silly Willy Baxter, to whom love has come for the first time during the summer of his seventeenth year:

> In the elder teens adolescence may be completed, but not by experience, and these years know their own tragedies. It is the time of life when one finds it unendurable not to seem perfect in all outward matters: in worldly position, in the equipments of wealth, in family, and in the grace, elegance, and dignity of all appearances in public. And yet the youth is continually betrayed by the child still intermittently insistent within him, and by the child which undiplomatic people too often assume him to be. Thus with William's attire: he could ill have borne any suggestion that it was not of the mode, but taking care of it was a different matter. Also, when it came to his appetite, he could and would eat anything at any time, but something younger than his years led him—often in semisecrecy—to candy-stores and soda-water fountains and ice-cream parlors; he still relished green apples and knew cravings for other dangerous inedibles. But these survivals were far from painful to him; what injured his sensibilities was the disposition on the part of people—especially his parents, and frequently his aunts and uncles—to regard him as a little boy. Briefly, the deference

his soul demanded in its own right, not from strangers only, but from his family, was about that which is supposed to be shown a Grand Duke visiting his Estates. Therefore William suffered often. [p. 20]

Times have changed, but not human psychology or development. This description is dated, but also timeless. The affects and their contents can be the same. Even soda-water fountains and ice-cream parlors, among other things, have reappeared.

In spite of the new "birth" being metaphoric, a new form has emerged, new enough and stable enough, as in Winnicott's (1951) phrase regarding mothering. It is new because it can now begin to be looked at as semipermanent—permanent because for the first time it can be expected to endure, "semi-" because it is open to change and evolution and there will still be many surprises. It is a time of integration and consolidation, of decisions of directions. Unconscious choices have hardened into character attitudes in major crossroads of behavioral patterns, a position on the spectrum of activity-passivity, a characterologic attitude toward object-relations, a turn toward an exclusive or at least dominant sexual orientation and identity. Jacobs (1987) refers to this age as a "discreet developmental phase." Deep unconscious patterns take shape in the relations between ego and superego, attitudes toward success-failure, achiever-nonachiever, leader-follower, winner-loser. To Freud's (1905) statement that the heir of the Oedipus complex is the superego, Blos (1962) adds that the heir of adolescence is the self (p. 136).

While the idea of "birth" at this age was metaphoric but the emergence of a new form real, the same is true with the separation that ensues at this stage. In the movement from child to "adult," celebrated at the entry to adolescence at bar mitzvah or bas mitzvah or any confirmation, "now I am a man" is an "as-if" anticipation of things to come. The same meaning at eighteen, however, is no longer a symbolic passage but the real thing. The boy now becomes a man, and the girl a woman, not an older boy with a symbolic fountain pen. At this phase it can be a car. And the separation that follows, or at least the prospect for that, is now real, not metaphoric. If anyone thought that separation-individuation of the mother and child at age one and a half was traumatic for both, one has but to view the affective reactions at this new and more final separation. It is not atypical for the young person to leave for college and never return to live at home again. Reactions of anxiety, mourning, and a gamut of related emotions, on both sides, may be conscious or reveal themselves by indirect symptomatic or other sequelae. It is difficult and ambiguous to state which of the two participants in the act of separation has been the active and which the passive one; the child-adult and the parents have shared a combination of both.

The legal age recognizing maturity and responsibility is an indistinct one, perhaps unconsciously reflecting the psychological ambiguity: the license to drive may come in different states anywhere from fifteen to eighteen, the right to vote at eighteen, the right to drink alcohol at twenty-one, the obligation to register for the draft and be subjected to the military at age eighteen. Girls can be given the pill in their early and midteens but cannot have their tubes ligated legally until twenty-one. Sexual activity is also now for real. With sexual consummation taking place even years earlier, the facing of the possibility of parenthood is also becoming more open and expected. The accepting of adult responsibility is becoming more common in the young male, to whom it has always been biologically less obligatory than the female. Besides the fate of sexual impulses, the ego's status vis-à-vis the vicissitudes of the aggressive as well as the sexual drives is a determining factor in the intrapsychic and, reflectively, the interpersonal activities of the newly established and independent self.

A woman in her fifties has an obsessive preoccupation with anxiety over social interaction, to the point of suffering from a social phobia. Every actual or potential social exchange, whether with the most mild and innocuous or the most authoritative individuals, is regarded as a confrontation involving the possibility of attack, humiliation, and traumatic helplessness. The patient reacts with severe anxiety over aggression, fearing first that her own ever-present anger will come out and be visible and that the inevitable retaliation will reduce her to a state of crumbling and collapse.

The severe pregenital mother-child psychopathology on which this syndrome was built was held in abeyance during her childhood years by a psychological withdrawal, a shyness and reticence by which she withheld all but the most necessary contacts. She was saved, she felt, from exposure and punishment only by her loved and loving father, whose positive attitudes toward her sustained her in her daily life, even though he was mostly absent. The character stance of quiet, submissive withdrawal, covered by a social pseudocompliance, took a definitive and stable form during her late adolescent years, when she left home for a boarding school and assumed what was to be her lifelong interpersonal patterns. A pseudocompensation prevailed until college and then marriage, when the increased social contacts that could no longer be staved off undid her defenses of withdrawal and avoidance and subjected her since then to social anxiety toward any or all of her displaced objects.

An important formula in the status of self-esteem during this as in other periods of life is the relation between the ego and the ego-ideal. The distance between the latter and the self-representation within the ego, with regard to superego functioning and the status of object relations, is a crucial one for the state of mental well-being, as described by Jacobson (1953, 1964), Sandler (1960), and Sandler and Rosenblatt (1962). This has also been stressed, although differently, by Gedo (1979), Kohut (1971, 1977), and in most nonanalytic theoretical systems (e.g., Branden 1971), but without the role of the id and the interrelations of all the psychic structures to each other. Jacobson (1953) described self-esteem as the gulf between or concordance of the wishful concept of the self and the self-representations.

What can be striking to any observer is the almost universal discrepancy between such an inner self-representation and the achievements in "actuality," to use Erikson's (1962) term. The formative years, preoedipal and oedipal, coming to a consolidated position in late adolescence, produce an internal conceptual image of the self that ignores, distorts, or alters reality and lives an independent existence with almost no relation to the state of one's actual significance and status in the outer world. Ongoing achievements in adult years do not impinge and have little if any dynamic power in affecting or counteracting a negative self-image formed and hardened from childhood through adolescence. Case after case bears this out in a way that never ceases to impress and surprise me. Empirically, this occurs also where parental input has been satisfactory. The opposite also occurs, but less often—a grandiose image. Almost always this is the result of reaction formation. Arrogance is usually due to insecurity.

The goal of psychoanalysis is to undo the impermeability of the pathologically structured self-representation, to allow subsequent events to influence and correct it. I have the feeling with some patients that, at a deep formative ego level, they took care of "actual" reality first, built up a solid physical and material base, and unconsciously decided to take care of the self-image later. This they now come to analysis to do. It is not always an easy task. It may, however, be easier than the other way around, where the image comes first and the reality perhaps never.

It is impressive, when one sets his sights to be aware of it, how often a definitive event in neurosogenesis involves the period of passage through the seventeenth year. A patient in treatment for many years comes back repeatedly to the onset decades ago of his obsessive, ruminative panneurosis, which he always remembers as having started when he was seventeen years old, visiting his grandfather in another city and studying there for his college entrance exams. His grandfather, who, like his parents, always expected big things from him, was especially doting and loving. An A student until then, the patient remembers studying late at night, his grandfather sleeping in the next room, when the thought suddenly struck him that he would fail, that his whole life would be ruined, and he felt that he was going crazy.

This was the first of the panic attacks he was to suffer recurrently for many years. The charged and fertile background of his formative years, with the gradual buildup of increasingly less controllable sexual and aggressive impulses, have since become known in all their traumatic quality. And the vicissitudes of his severe neurosis, reaching most of the time to a borderline state, have been lived, experienced, and treated with variable and unstable success. But the time of onset has always had its own meaning along the lines I have been describing. In perspective to the total neurosis, it is akin to the day residue, which is the precipitating stimulus of a dream. But, since this is not an event but an age, it has three-dimensional meanings of its own, actually with all the components built in of his chronic anxiety and depressive state.

Another patient returns often, whenever she pauses to take an overview of her life development, to the time, at age seventeen, when she left her homeland and her family abroad to come to the United States to study. Although it was not planned that way, she never returned to live there again. Not only her career but also her further character development, with the anxiety and symptoms that it enveloped, stemmed from that decision and action as a major focal point of her life. As her own oldest son is now approaching that same age, the patient is even more acutely aware of that period of her life and the crucial determining directions to which it led.

References to this age come up clinically as one listens. Just as I am writing this, a patient reports two dreams, both featuring the number seventeen. In one dream, the patient arrives at his analytic hour seventeen minutes early. He walks in without waiting to be admitted and sees the analyst lying on the couch, with the covers over him. He has probably just received a massage. In the second dream, a pretty girl is making up to him. He is tempted but upset, feeling she is too young, probably seventeen. If she were eighteen, it would be okay, but seventeen is dangerous.

Both dreams relate to incestuous conflicts in his early life and repeated in the transference. The analyst dream points also to primal scene oedipal material, also displaced to the transference. The patient is now in his forties, having conflictful and frustrating times with women. These go back to oedipal wishes, conflicts, and fears. He is also chronically worried about certain possibly illegal financial behavior. If he were below the legal age, that is, seventeen, not eighteen, he could be excused. Up to seventeen, oedipal fantasies and other crimes can be entertained with some excuse. After that, or in his present life, their current derivatives into adulthood cannot be tolerated by his superego without severe anxiety and guilt. Seventeen is the last year of innocence and protection.

All roads seem to lead to seventeen, from an apparently wide unconscious knowledge of the nodal point that exists at that time. In Arthur Miller's *Death of a Salesman,* seventeen-year-old Biff comes on his errant father in the hotel room. Crushed and discovered, the father tells the story of his failed life to his son: "When I was 17, I layed down, and never did anything again." In a television program about being young again, a forty-year-old expresses the wish to be seventeen. In Nazi Germany, the storm-troopers looked for youths of seventeen, old enough to do the job but at an age when they could still be indoctrinated.

In the recent film *Back to the Future,* produced by Steven Spielberg, which touched a receptive nerve in a large audience, a boy of seventeen is depicted who reacts with dismay as he is caught in a crisis of identification with a weak, cowering, and ineffectual father. "I am no good at confrontations," the father laments as an excuse for his recurrent disgraces and humiliations. Through a series of magical interventions, the boy is catapulted back to the year in time when his father himself was seventeen. Through some zany incidents, the boy maneuvers to have his father take a different position and character trait on the scale of activity-passivity in relation to the town bully who mistreats and humiliates him. At the last moment, when the father, at the time of wooing the mother, was submitting as he had in reality in the past to the aggressive acts of his constant tormentor, the son, turning down an oedipal seduction by the mother on the way, peps up the father as though with an injection of adrenalin and instigates him to fight back. The scene shows the father, heretofore puny, cowardly, and silly, begin suddenly to tighten and expand his fist, much as in a Popeye maneuver and, suddenly gaining strength and stature, strike the bully down with one blow.

With this one turn from passivity to aggression, the father's total subsequent life is altered, as he wins his wife now not through an accident of just being there but through his heroic act. Time is then reversed, and the father, many years later, appears now as a confident, potent, and aggressive male with the erstwhile bully working for him, polishing his car in an obsequious role. The mother, rather than being alcoholic as she became in the original development, is now an attractive, active, successful, and proud woman. The boy now has two positive parents to identify with as he proceeds with his own new development. The course of life has been altered by the seventeen-year-old redirecting his father at seventeen. In a recent paper (Rangell 1986), I summarized the course of behavioral events and their outcomes as being brought about by a combination of psychic determinism, autonomous ego will, and chance. Spielberg altered the original brew and the ratio of these ingredients in determining the directions of the behavior of his characters and changed the course of their lives.

Seventeen is the king of the hill among the teenage crowd. All things being equal, he is the "big man on campus" of that particular cohesive age group. Of course, things are never equal, so that a rough fifteen- or sixteen-year-old can easily dominate a passive ("wimpy") seventeen-year-old in the pecking order. But, at fourteen, fifteen, or sixteen, the youth is pointing upward. At eighteen, the big man leaves his position behind and is at the bottom of the heap among the young grownups. There is a magazine called *Seventeen*. Its readership consists mostly of girls twelve and older. It is girls because they avowedly want the boys; boys do not openly admit the opposite at quite that young age. The magazine is a source of instruction for those who would study the status of impulses, defenses, and group organization at that age. Intimate questions are laid out and answered for all to see, privately: to or not to? inner concerns about body, thoughts, and affects; herpes, vaginal infections, smell, looks, how to walk, sit, talk; problems of body ego, of object relations, of comparisons on the social scale. An ad proclaims, "Playboy tampons." The first open flowering of internal dilemmas of the kind put more resignedly by the older adult population in later years for the advisers to the lovelorn to answer.

Times change, but they also do not. In the columns of *Seventeen,* girls are told that, as their mothers told them, you can still say "no." Alongside an article on how to deal with embarrassing parents, the best and most stylish dress one girl could find for a dance was a dress of her mother's in mothballs in a chest in the attic. She wore it proudly. Twelve- and thirteen-year-olds take the pill, and some become pregnant. The magazine debates the pros and cons of abortion. The choice is no longer automatically for it. Boys are taught and are beginning to accept the responsibility of parenthood.

Clothes change from skin-tight pants and the "sweater girl" look to father's loose and hanging shirts or coats—or to Guess, Benetton, or Salvation Army clothes and back to tight-fitting pyjama-looking outfits again. My grandson has worn a tuxedo—and a red tie—to a prom. My sons would never have conceived of being in that position (neither did I, at that age). He was invited by the girl. That was also something that never happened to me. And they went by "limo." But teenagers do not rush now to get a license to drive a car, which I cannot understand or identify with. It is cool now to wait and to be driven by others. In my time, one "borrowed" father's car for little rides two years before it was legal. The symbols have changed, but not the conflicts or inner goals or psychological mechanisms; I made the same observation recently about dreams (Rangell 1987).

While in the quest for a "real" separation these individuals seem to strive fiercely for independence, the tendency to cling to each other and remain in groups is still apparent. As much dependence is manifest now as at any earlier or later period in life. Although separation-individuation has taken place in the early years, object attachment remains forever, as Mahler (1972; Mahler and Furer 1968; Mahler, Pine, and Bergman 1975) pointed out during rapprochement and beyond, and Freud (1937) before her with respect to the "adhesiveness of the libido," which at times makes analysis interminable. Bowlby (1969, 1973, 1980) pointed to the same phenomenon of attachment behavior, as did

Kohut (1971, 1977) with his self/object and as I described in terms of figure-ground in the need to cling (Rangell 1954, 1955) or the derivative universal "need to belong" manifested in the psychology of groups, small and large (Rangell 1975, 1976, 1980). A prototype for these was the classic work of Hermann (1936) on clinging.

Fads, up to the most dangerous cults, have always drawn heavily on the vulnerable teenage group. Styles, fashions, and tastes change—uniformly and together. Hair becomes long, then short—in all, not one alone. There is protest outwardly against family closeness, but closeness with others is sought as much. Where the goal is to shock by being different, teenagers become conforming to each other. One lad told his mother that he is embarrassed that his parents are still together; all his friend's parents are divorced. His friends have two homes to go to; he has only one. Teenagers with mohawk haircuts walk around together. Musical styles change, in unison. The Beatles, now the Boss, fill the stadium. But, again, underlying mechanisms are more stable. The music changes from the Charleston to rock and roll, or jazz, or country music, but all play to the chords of the body and the id. Films (now videocassettes) that make the most money are those directed toward the teenage audience. Producers know that teenagers are the most cohesive and predictable group. The tough, the cool, the loose, the soft porn (sexual and aggressive), sells the most.

As an apt description of the social affinity of this age group, how they "stick together" against the common enemy or the outsider, I will quote another excerpt from Tarkington's *Seventeen*. (Note here the importance of body size, the tenuous control of the body in space, of one's movements, actions, and of their effects on others.) Willy has just been introduced by Johnny Watson to his "big fat lummox of a cousin," who comes on too strongly to the magic girl everyone wants:

This severe phrase of theirs, almost simultaneous in the two minds, was not wholly a failure as a thumb-nail sketch of Mr. George Crooper. And yet there was the impressiveness of size about him, especially about his legs and chin. At seventeen and eighteen growth is still going on, sometimes in a sporadic way, several parts seeming to have sprouted faster than others. Often the features have not quite settled down together in harmony, a mouth, for instance, appearing to have gained such a lead over the rest of a face, that even a mother may fear it can never be overtaken. Voices, too, often seem misplaced; one hears, outside the door, the bass rumble of a sinister giant, and a mild boy, thin as a cricket, walks in. The contrary was George Crooper's case; his voice was an unexpected piping tenor, half falsetto and frequently girlish—as surprising as the absurd voice of an elephant.

He had the general outwardness of a vast and lumpy child. His chin had so distanced his other features that his eyes, nose, and brow seemed almost baby-like in comparison, while his mountainous legs were the great part of the rest of him. He was one of those huge, bottle-shaped boys who are always in motion in spite of their cumbersomeness. His gestures were continuous, though difficult to interpret as bearing upon the subject of his equally continuous conversation; and under all circumstances he kept his conspicuous legs incessantly moving, whether he was going anywhere or remaining in comparatively one spot.

His expression was pathetically offensive, the result of his bland confidence in the audible opinions of a small town whereof his father was the richest inhabitant—and the one thing about him, even more obvious than his chin, his legs, and his spectacular taste in flannels, was his perfect trust that he was as welcome to every one as he was to his mother. This might some day lead him in the direction of great pain, but on the occasion of the "subscription party" for Miss Pratt it gave him an advantage.

"When do I get to meet that cutie?", he insisted, as Johnnie Watson moved backward from the cousinly arm, which threatened further flailing. [p. 130]

Self-centered and asocial actions exist side by side with the noble and altruistic. The intrapsychic balance is a conflictual tug between two poles. The id is on one side, pressing always to be heard. But the superego at the other end can be as strong. Idealism has always been the stamp of youth; idealists are the same young people who are prey to drugs or other paths to immediate expression and satisfaction. The ego, between the two psychic structures, can be effective as well as overwhelmed. One young man is a student arbitrator and on the ethics committee in his school, to judge and decide about others in trouble, because he is considered to be the most "fair." A patient tells of a crucial time in his inner thoughts and later his life that occurred when he entered junior high. After feeling anxious, depressed, and rejected for a number of years (probably during his whole latency), moving into the new school, he remembers almost consciously—or preconsciously and probably unconsciously too—deciding that people would be nice to him if he were nice to them. He began, at first self-consciously and deliberately, then automatically, "to be nice" to others. Not long afterward, he became president of the class in his young teens, a feat he repeated when he became student body president of a large college some years later. He has since gone on to a successful political career. It will be no surprise to add that, in analysis, he was dealing with "a jelly center," a core of unconscious anxiety that stood in his way in all his upward moves.

In a period that calls for such massive integration, the ego can be overwhelmed as easily as it can be sufficient to its task. As Blos (1962) states, "Late adolescence is a decisive turning point, and consequently is a time of crisis" (p. 130). Since Erikson (1950, 1956), this has been known as an "identity crisis." Just as with psychic trauma (Rangell 1967), the outcome now too depends on the ratio between the ego capacities and the stimuli that impinge, the demands on it from three sides, the instincts, the superego, and the external world. Fragility of the ego vis-à-vis the pressures on it makes breakdown and decompensation at this age a common experience. This has been accelerated, not decreased, with technological advance, in which the human dimension becomes lost rather than furthered. Waelder (1967), surveying the sweep of civilization through a psychoanalytic lens, has stated that history is an alternation of excesses and that progress has as many victims as beneficiaries.

Braatoy (1934) has emphasized the high psychic mortality of the postadolescent period. The suicide rate among fifteen- to twenty-four-year-olds increased over 50 percent from 1970 to 1980 and has become a serious public health concern. The dynamic backgrounds for this are complex, occurring as much at times of apparent success as in states of obvious material and psychological deprivation. Choices made may be not for the child (this term no longer seems appropriate chronologically, but psychologically it can still hold) but for the father or mother. Good grades in college, admission to a professional school, a promising start, a seemingly ideal situation, and then suicide from an undiscovered and undisclosed depression is a not uncommon sequence. The son has been living out the parents' ambitions, not his own. I have seen this happen with tragic suddenness in a seemingly successful medical student. A similar syndrome, but with a less drastic outcome, was seen in a young professional tennis champion, fulfilling his father's frustrated wishes, until analytic treatment succeeded in altering the course of his life to more ego-syntonic goals.

Once again, as at age two, intergenerational rifts and a clash of interests between parents and child assume major proportions. Interpersonal conflicts now as always are internalized into intrapsychic ones. The prospect of a more definitive external separation and its accompanying intrapsychic fantasies and anxieties are a dominant issue requiring urgent and current solutions. Separation now will no longer be symbolic or metaphoric but will connote an air of actuality and an intention of finality. These conflicts can lead to satisfactory resolutions by adaptive choices or successful compromises or, where conditions are unfavorable, to unresolvable impasses with pathological up to malignant results.

Problems of love, work, and ideology are in the balance, the most crucial decisions that will determine future life. The directions taken and paths unconsciously chosen are determined by current internal and external conditions, grafted on the character traits, formative intrapsychic modes, and interstructural relations established and operative since the earliest years. Old patterns shine through and old influences exert themselves, added to by inputs from the gamut of development thus far. Again, it is psychological and somatic together and early structural determinants in both the psychic and somatic sense. I saw a photograph of a young man recently whom I had not seen since he was a child and thought it was his father as I knew him years ago. Identical features of voice, posture, attitudes, and affect accompany similar, and sometimes identical, body frames, all coming together at successive maturational phases. Nurture and nature continue reciprocally active even in their late derivatives and effects.

Will there be integration and synthesis, Hartmann's (1939, 1950) and Nunberg's (1931) main criteria for normality and mental health, or will the ego's efforts result in pathological splitting and fragmentation? Besides separation and depression, the gamut of etiologic anxieties can be at work. Oedipal-castrative anxiety plays a central role in the onset of psychopathology at this as at any other period. In fact, it can be revived with great intensity. Even in choices of illness, however, at this age in life, the tendency to cling to and to identify with others reveals itself. Where hysteria was the contagious mental illness in finde-siècle Vienna, this has been replaced in today's culture by the prevalence of anorexia or anorexia-bulimia, particularly in young girls. The same contagiousness occurs in these illnesses, as Freud (1896) showed is responsible for hysteria by unconscious identification. Although dominantly oral on the surface, the etiologic background of the eating disorder syndrome today is determined by the entire spectrum of oedipal and pregenital fixations and regressions, as shown by Fischer (1985) and Ritvo (1983).

With respect to sexual choices and pathology, homoerotic activities and relationships in the early teens are not as significant for future psychosexual solutions as those that take definitive shape and recur with regularity in later adolescence. Sexual identity and patterns that become evident now acquire a more stabilized and enduring state. I am analyzing a patient now in whom a decisive direction of enduring homosexuality took place at seventeen. Another young man underwent a homosexual crisis and panic at the same age from which he seems to be moving now to a heterosexual choice. It is ironic that the somatic affliction of AIDS should be an accompaniment or sequel to this new current wave of sexual freedom, as an equally contagious somatic sexually related condition.

What I have said about relative finality of psychic constellations during this period of life does not, of course, mean that conditions and relationships will not be continually open to change. Development and maturation have a long way to go. Sexual as well as other conflicts or unfinished tasks have a lifetime ahead of them. Masturbation fantasies during adolescence, considered by the Laufers (Laufer 1976; Laufer and Laufer 1984) as centrally indicative of the status of both intrapsychic life and object relations, presumably have more opportunity beyond adolescence of being carried over from fantasy to reality. That this is never completely accomplished is well known to writers and is a common observation of psychoanalytic clinicians. A gulf between unconscious fantasy and reality is a given of psychic life. This might also be credited with playing a major role in human creativity, the urge toward it and the fact of its achievement. Or there can also ensue "the syndrome of prolonged adolescence" (Blos 1954).

Evolution, gestations, and even new later constellations continue throughout the life cycle, as described by Erikson (1950) and by others since. Changes, surprises, and unexpected outcomes occur at any time. A newly appointed college president describes how he was disturbed and involved with drugs during adolescence. A man under forty, who is already a legendary business and financial success, returns to a high school reunion where he was a "loser" and low in the ranks of achievement. There was a well-known song after World War II about the private who, after the war, became president of the New York Stock Exchange. Psychoanalysis is relevant and can be effective only because of the continuous if not permanent openness to change.

Early conditions and determinants will out. A patient has twin sons now in their thirties. From birth on, the first born, who was physically less robust than the second, was nevertheless the leader and more aggressive of the two. He was always the initiator of their common activities. The twin who was born second, although he could knock over the first and could do anything better that required physical strength, "tagged along" and was always the passive follower. The first became a successful rock-and-roll star. The second led an inadequate and drifting life and has recently been hospitalized as a schizophrenic. The mother suffered from frequent migraine headaches, was reserved and withdrawn, and for years was addicted to sedatives and pain-relieving medication. The rock star gradually slipped into a severe and chronic cocaine addiction and is in as serious trouble as the more decompensated younger of the twins. Both now have different forms but equal intensities of emotional disabilities.

Freud himself did not arrive at his monumental achievements until his thirties and forties. Earlier connections, however, were not absent. In what I consider a remarkable group of letters of Freud's (1969), the earliest to be preserved and the latest to be discovered, young Freud, then sixteen to eighteen years old, describes his feelings to his friend, Emil Fluss, on his return to Vienna after having visited his place of birth, Pribor in Moravia, which he had left when he was three years old. Looking back at the mind of this teenager from the present retrospective view, I will quote my observations on these letters made in the opening address to the International Congress held in Vienna in 1971 (Rangell 1972). This was the first Congress held in the birthplace of psychoanalysis and the first return of Anna Freud to Vienna since the Freuds left it in 1938. The purpose of this quote is to connect seventeen with forty:

A number of remarkable characteristics are already revealed in this searching young mind:

(1) He is already seen to subject his affective stirrings, his feelings and excitements, his "first love" [to Gisela, his friend's sister], to introspection and to describe them in words in terms of the secondary process. (2) He seeks to convey his thoughts in a communication which is private, special, unlike any other. The opening letter addressed to "Dear new friend" is marked 'confidential'. (The recipient changes some years later from Fluss to Fliess!) (3) This communication is characterized by a search for the truth: "I shall confess the unvarnished truth to you—but to you alone." (Already the basic element of psychoanalysis.) (4) But there also needs to be complete trust, the basic trust. "I trust that no one will be allowed to see what was not meant for him to see," or else—(5) there is another more usual type of communication: "All you would hear would be smoothed-tongued platitudes that won't tell you anything."

There are already some profound harbingers of things to come. (6) "I enjoy tracing the closely knit web of connecting threads which chance and fate have woven around us all." Or (7) "How admirable is the fine instinct with which nature has endowed us." Or (8) discounting the role of accidental circumstance when his friend and the latter's girl friend happen to meet, he is convinced "of the inscrutable workings of a divine power".

(9) Even more prophetic, and in keeping with a central theme of this paper: "I have a good deal of reading to do—among them Sophocles' *Oedipus Rex*"! (His paper on this was rated "good", the only one in the class.) (10) And, recognizing already the complicated results of such knowledge, "You deprive yourself of much that is edifying if you can't read all these, but on the other hand you retain that cheerfulness which is so comforting about your letters."

Even a sense of his own destiny does not escape him. (11) "—So now I would counsel you (about these letters) preserve them—bind them together—guard them well—you never know"! (12) And finally there is a more ominous reference to the future, which comes back to our subject: he refers to a recurrent toothache. "It was a last feeble eruption of an erstwhile mighty crater. The last quiver from a region of my body that has for a long time been in open rebellion against peace and order in my system. I am referring to my teeth. Where others live to eat, I live to ruin my teeth. And where others eat to live, I suffer from toothache to live. Thus my life is inextricably bound up with toothache which will consequently stay with me for as long as I live" (!)

It was precisely there, pinpointed with uncanny accuracy at that tender age, that Freud half a century later was to begin his long, silent struggle against pain and inner destruction which was to continue for the last sixteen years of his life. And it was here again, from looking into the processes of his own inner life struggles, that Freud came up with insights with which all men could identify and which applied to all mankind.

All this was already there. Today, a hundred years and 27 International Congresses later—the promise of that 16-year-old youth did not go unfulfilled.—The cohesive theory of human behaviour which proliferated from his enjoyment in "tracing the closely knit web of connecting threads" has become the common heritage of the intellectual world. [Pp. 3–4]

Thinking of Freud, one is reminded how much can happen long after one's teens and twenties. These excerpts, however, also demonstrate how seventeen continues into the rest of life.

NOTE

An earlier version of this chapter was presented as the plenary address to the annual meeting of the Chicago Society for Adolescent Psychiatry, Lake Geneva, Wisconsin, February 23, 1986.

REFERENCES

Blos, P. 1954. Prolonged adolescence: the formulation of a syndrome and its therapeutic implications. *American Journal of Orthopsychiatry* 24:733–742.

Blos, P. 1962. *On Adolescence: A Psychoanalytic Interpretation.* New York: Free Press.

Bowlby, J. 1969. *Attachment and Loss.* Vol. 1, *Attachment.* New York: Basic.

Bowlby, J. 1973. *Attachment and Loss*. Vol. 2, *Separation, Anxiety and Anger*. New York: Basic.

Bowlby, J. 1980. *Attachment and Loss*. Vol. 3, *Sadness and Depression*. New York: Basic.

Braatoy, T. 1934. *Manner zwischen 15 und 25 Jahren* (Men between 15 and 25 years of age). Oslo: Fabritius & Sonner.

Branden, N. 1971. *The Psychology of Self-Esteem*. New York: Bantam.

Breuer, J., and Freud, S. 1893–1895. Studies on hysteria. *Standard Edition* 2:1–319. London: Hogarth, 1955.

Erikson, E. H. 1950. *Childhood and Society*. New York: Norton.

Erikson, E. H. 1956. The problem of ego identity. *Journal of the American Psychoanalytic Association* 4:56–121.

Erikson, E. H. 1962. Reality and actuality. *Journal of the American Psychoanalytic Association* 29:179–219.

Ferenczi, S. 1930. The principle of relaxation and neocatharsis. In M. Balint, ed. *The Selected Papers of Sandor Ferenczi*, vol. 3, *Final Contributions to the Problems and Methods of Psychoanalysis*. New York: Basic, 1955.

Fischer, N. 1985. Anorexia nervosa and unresolved rapprochement conflicts—a case study. Paper presented at the International Symposium on Separation-Individuation, Paris, November 3.

Freud, S. 1896. The aetiology of hysteria. *Standard Edition* 3:189–221. London: Hogarth, 1962.

Freud, S. 1905. Three essays on the theory of sexuality. *Standard Edition* 7:125–245. London: Hogarth, 1953.

Freud, S. 1937. Analysis terminable and interminable. *Standard Edition* 23:211–253. London: Hogarth, 1964.

Freud, S. 1969. Some early unpublished letters of Freud. *International Journal of Psycho-Analysis* 50:419–427.

Galenson, E., and Roiphe, H. 1974. The emergence of genital awareness during the second year of life. In R. C. Friedman, R. M. Richart, and R. L. Van der Wiele, eds. *Sex Differences and Behavior*. New York: Wiley.

Gedo, J. E. 1979. *Beyond Interpretation: Toward a Revised Theory for Psychoanalysis*. New York: International Universities Press.

Hartmann, H. 1939. *Ego Psychology and the Problem of Adaptation*. New York: International Universities Press, 1958.

Hartmann, H. 1950. Comments on the psychoanalytic theory of the ego. In *Essays on Ego Psychology: Selected Problems in Psychoanalytic Theory.* New York: International Universities Press, 1964.

Hermann, I. 1936. Sich-anklammern, auf-suche-gehen. *International Zeitschrift für Psycho-Analysis* 22:349–370.

Jacobs, T. J. 1987. Chairman's address to panel "Psychoanalysis of the Young Adult: Theory and Technique" [in panel report by J. F. Chused]. *Journal of the American Psychoanalytic Association* 35:175–187.

Jacobson, E. 1953. Contribution to the metapsychology of cyclothymic depression. In P. Greenacre, ed. *Affective Disorders.* New York: International Universities Press.

Jacobson, E. 1964. *The Self and the Object World.* New York: International Universities Press.

Kohut, H. 1971. *The Analysis of the Self.* New York: International Universities Press.

Kohut, H. 1977. *The Restoration of the Self.* New York: International Universities Press.

Laufer, M. 1976. The central masturbation fantasy, the final sexual organization, and adolescence. *Psychoanalytic Study of the Child* 31:297–316.

Laufer, M., and Laufer, M. E. 1984. *Adolescence and Developmental Breakdown.* New Haven, Conn.: Yale University Press.

Lorenz, K. 1950. The comparative method in studying innate behavior patterns. In *Symposia of the Society for Experimental Biology,* vol. 4. Cambridge: Cambridge University Press.

Mahler, M. S. 1972. Rapprochement subphase of the separation-individuation process. *Psychoanalytic Quarterly* 41:487–506.

Mahler, M. S., and Furer, M. 1968. *On Human Symbiosis and the Vicissitudes of Individuation: Infantile Psychosis.* New York: International Universities Press.

Mahler, M. S.; Pine, F.; and Bergman, A. 1975. *The Psychological Birth of the Human Infant: Symbiosis and Individuation.* New York: Basic.

Nunberg, H. 1931. The synthetic function of the ego. In *Practice and Theory of Psychoanalysis.* New York: International Universities Press, 1961.

115

Rangell, L. 1954. The psychology of poise—with a special elaboration on the psychic significance of the snout or perioral region. *International Journal of Psycho-Analysis* 35:313–333.

Rangell, L. 1955. The quest for ground in human motivation. Paper presented to the first western divisional meeting of the American Psychiatric Association and the West Coast Psychoanalytic Societies, October 29.

Rangell, L. 1967. The metapsychology of psychic trauma. In S. S. Furst, ed. *Psychic Trauma*. New York: Basic.

Rangell, L. 1972. Aggression, Oedipus, and historical perspective. *International Journal of Psycho-Analysis* 53:3–11.

Rangell, L. 1975. Man in a group. Third Robert Waelder Memorial Lecture to the Philadelphia Association for Psychoanalysis, October 17.

Rangell, L. 1976. Lessons from Watergate: a derivative for psychoanalysis. *Psychoanalytic Quarterly* 45:37–61.

Rangell, L. 1980. *The Mind of Watergate: An Exploration of the Compromise of Integrity*. New York: Norton.

Rangell, L. 1986. The executive functions of the ego: an extension of the concept of ego autonomy. *Psychoanalytic Study of the Child* 41:1–37.

Rangell, L. 1987. Historical perspectives and current status. In A. Rothstein, ed. *The Significance of the Interpretation of Dreams in Clinical Work*. Workshop Series of the American Psychoanalytic Association, Monograph no. 3. New York: International Universities Press.

Rapaport, D. 1953. On the psychoanalytic theory of affects. *International Journal of Psycho-Analysis* 34:177–198.

Rapaport, D. 1959. *The Structure of Psychoanalytic Theory. Psychological Issues,* Monograph 6. New York: International Universities Press.

Ritvo, S. 1983. Eating disturbances in an adolescent girl. Paper presented to the panel on "The Child/Adolescent Psychoanalyst at Work, with a Focus on Female Sexuality: Adolescent Case" at the thirty-third International Psychoanalytic Congress, Madrid, July 26.

Roiphe, H. 1968. On an early genital phase: with an addendum on genesis. *Psychoanalytic Study of the Child* 23:348–365.

Roiphe, H., and Galenson, E. 1972. Early genital activity and the castration complex. *Psychoanalytic Quarterly* 41:334–347.

Sandler, J. 1960. On the concept of superego. *Psychoanalytic Study of the Child* 15:128–162.

Sandler, J., and Rosenblatt, B. 1962. The concept of the representational world. *Psychoanalytic Study of the Child* 17:128–145.

Stern, D. N. 1983. Affect attunement: mechanisms and clinical implications. Paper presented to the second World Congress of Infant Psychiatry, Cannes, March 29.

Tarkington, B. 1916. *Seventeen*. New York: Harper & Row.

Tinbergen, N. 1951. *The Study of Instincts*. London: Oxford University Press.

Waelder, R. 1967. *Progress and Revolution*. New York: International Universities Press.

Winnicott, D. W. 1951. Transitional objects and transitional phenomena. In *Collected Papers: Through Paediatrics to Psycho-Analysis*. New York: Basic, 1975.

Winnicott, D. W. 1957. *Mother and Child: A Primer of First Relationships*. New York: Basic.

PART II

DEVELOPMENTAL ISSUES: TRANSITION TO YOUNG ADULTHOOD

EDITOR'S INTRODUCTION

Psychiatrists increasingly are called on to address problems in the young adult population. It is becoming clear that the transition from the adolescent years into young adulthood is associated with increasing stress. Young people entering college seem to be taking it more seriously. Those who do not pursue a traditional educational track in young adulthood seem to be more aware of their isolation. It is also clear that there is an increasing population of chronically, emotionally ill young adults.

Psychiatrists who are skillful with adolescents are particularly well poised to deal with the population of young adult patients. Their development of clinical techniques to deal with the troublesome adolescent population puts adolescent psychiatrists in a good position to be helpful. In recognition of this fact, the American Society for Adolescent Psychiatry focused a recent annual meeting on the topic of young adulthood. The meeting addressed developmental psychology, commonly occurring psychopathological syndromes, and approaches to treatment. This meeting was the first one focused entirely on this particular age group.

Robert L. Arnstein begins the section on adolescent development with an overview of normal transition to young adulthood. Arnstein uses his extensive clinical experiences at the Yale University Health Services and his extensive knowledge of the literature to present an elegant perspective. He first describes the theoretical and clinical work of major contributors in the field in order to outline current concepts of the transitional process into young adulthood. He addresses the psychological, cognitive, social cultural, educational, and vocational aspects. He outlines current knowledge about differentiation of this developmental process among young men and young women. He describes data-based studies that follow young people through the young adult transitional phase and into adulthood. He concludes the chapter with a cogent synthesis of his own about the key issues in this phase of life.

Ruthellen Josselson focuses on identity formation in adolescents and the implications for young adulthood. She clarifies that it is a crucial normative task on which young people base their sense of themselves as well as the vision of the structure of their lives. She defines identity as a largely unconscious organizing structure that integrates aspects of the self and provides continuity across the life span and life experiences. She clarifies that, to form an identity, an individual must experience some crisis in previously held ideas derived from the ascribed identity of younger periods. She describes four groups that have been previously defined through direct assessment of young people: identity achievement; foreclosure; moratorium; and diffusion. Josselson uses case material to illustrate the differences among these states.

Sidney Weissman, Rebecca Cohen, Andrew Boxer, and Bertram Cohler deal with the complex self-psychological perspective of the adolescent's transition to young adulthood. Their extensive review of key self psychology concepts helps clarify its relevance to this period of life. The authors look at this complex issue from the perspective of parents and conclude that the stresses that can accumulate during this period can derail the individual from developing a cohesive self-system.

Edward M. Hallowell, Jules Bemporad, and John Ratey begin the section on psychopathology with their chapter on depression in the transition to adult life. The authors noticed an increasing number of young adults in their study who presented with significant depression. They confirmed their impressions with surveys of other clinicians who worked with this age group. They further documented the seriousness of depression in this age group through epidemiological studies. They addressed the question of why the transition from adolescence to adult life in contemporary society can lead to seriously depressed states. They believe the current cultural climate may not be the cause of the plight of the patients in this age group, but this climate certainly intensifies the anguish of transition from youth to maturity. Case material is used to document how this transitional period of life can be particularly vulnerable to affective disorders.

Leona L. Bachrach draws from her sociological experience to address one of the most troublesome problems in the young adult group—substance abuse. Her chapter on sociological factors associated with substance abuse among new chronic patients explores this subject extensively. She particularly addresses the service needs (and service deficits) of the group of young adult chronic mental patients who are victims of substance abuse. She describes the so-called new chronic patients who are widely recognized as being volatile, difficult to reach, difficult to serve, and extremely stressful to mental health service systems. She first reviews the seminal contributions to the definition of the young adult, chronically mentally ill. She clarifies that what distinguishes these new chronic patients from chronic mental patients from the past is not their diagnostic distribution per se but rather their aggregate demand for services and their unique effect on the psychiatric service system. She clarifies that they are approaching the service system "with a vengeance." The drug involvement of this population is of particular concern because it represents a problem for which the psychiatric services system has failed. Her chapter leads to logical conclusions of what can be done to help this group of troublesome and troubled patients.

Charles Krasnow's chapter on Joseph Conrad's *The Shadow Line* approaches the issue of deviation from normal young adult development from the perspective of literature. Joseph Conrad's short novelle was written in 1915. Krasnow illustrates why it is a masterful and artistic rendering of the transition from late adolescence to early adulthood. The author describes how Conrad's novel provides a rich "museum" of late adolescent developmental conflict.

Rosa Linda Espinoza and Annette Ehrlich study personality, family relationships, and moral development in Chicano and black adolescent gangs. The authors make direct comparisons between gang members and nonmembers as well as between blacks and Chicanos. Espinoza and Ehrlich found significant differences among gang members and nonmembers in areas of impulse control, sense of right, subjects clustered in the areas of parental education, number of parents, and numbers of family members. The authors conclude that poverty is a major contributing factor to gang membership but that it is by no means the only factor. Personality problems requiring psychotherapy emerge as a second factor.

Lloyd Wells addresses a problem of developmental delay in a very

123

special population—medical students. He writes that many medical students are psychologically developed only at a late adolescent level of development. He notes that some are encouraged by the nature of the medical school experience itself to remain immersed in adolescent issues. He uses case material from his own extensive clinical work to document this risk of delayed psychological development and describes techniques for helping medical students enhance the rate of psychological development consistent with that of their professional role development.

David Dean Brockman begins the section on treatment with a chapter on psychoanalytic assessment of young adults. Dr. Brockman carefully dissects the process of assessment of young adults to determine the need for and the type of psychotherapy. He describes the process of assessing adult sexual object choice, serious commitment to a career, and the degree of consolidation of the structures that will compose the young adult personality and uses clinical venues as a way of outlining psychoanalytic assessment of young adult men and women.

Eugene H. Kaplan also uses a psychoanalytic developmental frame of reference. He focuses particularly on the issue of career change in early adulthood. His review of other contributions to an understanding of young adult development is extensive. The author concludes that career change in this period of life may both reflect and facilitate the reworking of unconscious conflicts.

Hilary Ryglewicz and Bert Pepper describe compromised development, the complex plight of young adults with mental/emotional disorders. They look at the developmental process, both normal and atypical, of young adults identified as having serious mental or emotional disorders. Their developmental courses have been affected in multiple and complex ways during their growth and development because of having to grow up with a debilitating problem. Ryglewicz and Pepper discuss treatment and program planning for serious long-term disorders in the community. They conclude that the treatment plan must contain habilitation efforts that approach the adaptations dysfunctional copying efforts and missed developmental opportunities of this group.

The last chapter in the special section focuses on an emerging national trend in the treatment of the population described earlier by Bachrach. The chapter by M. Susan Ridgely, Howard Goldman, and John A. Talbott on treatment of chronic mentally ill young adults with substance abuse problems is a cogent statement of the current state and emerging direction that exists in America today. They point out that the state of the art in treating chronic mentally ill young adults is not well advanced. When one considers the additional problem of addressing substance abuse among this population, the authors believe that it would be more accurate to describe the development of treatment as in its infancy, characterized more by trial and error than by implementation of established treatment protocols. Yet there are encouraging new trends. These trends have been delineated by a collaborative effort of the federal Alcohol, Drug Abuse, and Mental Health Administration (ADMHA) and the University of Maryland Task Force on Chronically Mentally Ill Young Adults with Substance Abuse. Although this project is still in process, the authors' chapter represents an extensive interim report on the state of treatment programming and training.

JOHN G. LOONEY

9 OVERVIEW OF NORMAL TRANSITION TO YOUNG ADULTHOOD

ROBERT L. ARNSTEIN

In presenting an overview on the normal transition to young adulthood, the first problem is the definition of "normal," "transition," and "young adulthood." Although it always seems rather unimaginative, if not obsessive, to spend too much time worrying about definitions, with this particular subject definitions become crucial. I learned from reviewing the empirical and theoretical literature that, depending on one's discipline, one's research method, one's subject pool, and one's values, answers emerge that are very difficult to relate one with another. Thus, while it is both accurate and current to talk about a biopsychosocial approach, it is not so easy to include all three in an integrated conceptual framework. Therefore, perhaps the most useful thing that I can do is to describe briefly some of the theoretical and empirical work of major contributors in the field and, by so doing, set the stage for the chapters about specific aspects that will follow. Many of these chapters, judging by their titles, will expand on points that I can only allude to in passing.

With regard to the definition of normality, I will cite Offer and Sabshin's (1974) differing concepts: they discuss normality as average, normality as utopia, normality as health, and normality as transactional systems. These are important concepts to keep in mind because much of the confusion on the subject comes from a failure to be clear about the type of normality one is discussing.

The definition of transition implies a concept of human development that originally derives from the observation of certain biological events happening in standardized progression. This progression begins in utero and is followed by postuterine growth and change, with events occurring in a more or less orderly sequence. The span of time, however, over which particular events may occur in human life inevitably widens with age, and some events that are social in nature or only loosely tied to biology can occur in no predetermined order, for example, parenthood and peak physical growth or family formation and adult work role.

Human growth and development have been divided into roughly labeled age periods so that words such as "childhood," "adolescence," "young adulthood," "middle age," and "old age" convey some loosely agreed on meaning. Two caveats, however, must be mentioned. The first is that recent changes in the average life span have probably changed the ages assigned to the later periods. Second, there are those who feel that while some of the periods are biologically demarcated, such as puberty marking the end of childhood, some are culturally influenced, and adolescence specifically is one of the latter (Prelinger 1974). Although there may have always been a period between childhood and full adulthood, some would question its significance, and most would certainly feel that adolescence has been extended by increased educational demands and postponed financial independence. Young adulthood is usually considered to be the stage when the human organism has reached "maturity"—in itself a complex term.

Maturity can be measured along biological, intellectual, sociocultural, and psychological timelines, but these do not necessarily proceed at an identical pace. Each may also be influenced by individual life experience, by the culture to which the individual belongs that establishes social role expectations, by historical events that may impose specific external forces, and by the biological timetable of the individual. These influences are further affected by such matters as gender and social class, and, historically, they have varied considerably in different eras and have differentially affected certain social groups, such as minorities (Mays 1986), within the larger society.

Biological development is obviously important. Timiras (1978) points out that the human is composed of a series of abilities and biological systems that reach peaks at different times. Unless illness, malnutrition, or gross neglect supervenes, these abilities and systems will develop more or less regardless of emotional development, intellectual capacity, or sociocultural setting and reach their peaks by the individual's twenties, although, depending on the skill or ability being measured, some may reach peaks earlier. Female swimmers and gymnasts, for example, often seem to achieve maximum proficiency in their early teens.

Intellectual development also has an initial biological thrust but in its later stages will probably depend more on educational efforts and application. Piaget (1977), a major figure in studying intellectual development, has described various levels of intellectual functioning and declared that the highest level, formal operations, is possible by the age of fourteen and is usually completed by age sixteen. Thus, one can say that intellectual development is completed well before the end of adolescence. Various investigators have questioned the general applicability of his findings, but, whatever the validity of his conclusions, it seems fairly clear that knowledge almost inevitably increases with age up to a point and that capacities that are enhanced by experience, such as judgment, may take much longer to reach a peak.

The psychological or emotional development is the most complex and is the one that we are most concerned with in this special section. There have been two main forms of investigation. One is the psychoanalytic, in which information is derived from the psychoanalysis of children and adults; in other words, the data are gathered primarily from patient populations. Initially, on the basis of these data Freud proposed a theory of psychological development that applied to early childhood, and later psychoanalysts have extended developmental theory to include adolescence and the transition to adulthood. It must be emphasized, however, that this theoretical stream focuses on development in the unconscious and basically conceives of the process in terms of derived mental constructs, such as ego, superego, and self and theories of energy attached to mental representations of infantile objects. The other main source of information comes from nonpatient populations that are studied by more direct methods, such as questionnaires or structured interviews that focus on conscious feelings and experiences. Not surprisingly, it is often difficult, if not impossible, to reconcile the two sets of data. Although both research methods may be valid, they are tapping two different sources of information about two different levels of experience, one overt and one essentially inferred.

The sociocultural dimension varies most from society to society and may even differ from social group to social group within a society. Often, there are behavioral markers, or rites of passage, that signify entrance into a more advanced sociocultural status, eventually defined as adulthood. Many such behavioral markers are defined by simple chronological age. In the United States, age alone is used to determine when one is eligible to vote, drink, drive, serve in the military, work, and marry without parental consent, to name just a few privileges or obligations, each representing a different dimension of adulthood. Even here, however, there are variations because the designated age may differ in different states and, in some cases, vary with gender for certain actions, such as marriage. Other steps—for example, educational advancement—are determined not by age but by the completion of a defined number of school credits. Because, however, the sociocultural standard that defines adulthood often stresses readiness to fulfill certain social roles, such as a work or family role appropriate to the society, there is an implication that the educational task will be completed. Yet, in our contemporary world, where education may continue uninterruptedly until the individual's late twenties or beyond, it is difficult to claim that someone of this age is not an adult. Furthermore, the social role expectations of a society may differ for males and females and change over time. At the turn of the century, female college students were a distinct minority but are now, I believe, a slight majority. As recently as forty years ago, Parsons (1949), in a description of the adult role for urban women, wrote: "The woman's fundamental status is that of her husband's wife, the mother of his children" (p. 274). This description now seems incomplete, if not totally obsolete, and to some quite objectionable.

There are, of course, interactions between these measures so that one may have reached an adult standard of intellectual or biological maturity and not the same degree of adulthood as defined by emotional or sociocultural measures. Thus, one can be biologically able to bear or father a child but not emotionally ready to raise it. Conversely, one may not be filling a work role but nevertheless be engaged in fulfilling an appropriate marital and parental role.

In regard to young adulthood, there is general agreement about the age at which one should reach it—at some point between seventeen and twenty-two—but no real agreement about a succinct and coherent definition of the state in psychological terms. Most investigators and clinicians have focused attention on the tasks of adolescence that must be completed in order to achieve psychological adulthood. I have summarized these as follows: (1) separation from parents, (2) ego synthesis or identity formation, (3) development of a capacity for intimacy, (4) achievement of genital primacy, (5) change in object relations, (6) stabilization of character structure, (7) development of a time perspective, (8) development of a capacity for friendship, (9) commitment to a set of life goals encompassing vocation and work role, and (10) achievement of an effective moral code.

This list represents a considerable condensing and interpretation of a large body of observations by many individuals. Thus, depending on one's theoretical convictions and particular training, one may have different words for these concepts or disagree with aspects of their application. These seem, however, to be the tasks that are most frequently mentioned by the principal writers on the subject.

The transition to adulthood will inevitably be influenced by cultural attitudes toward family structure, social class stability, occupational choice, and individual psychological characteristics valued by the culture. In the United States, where a considerable degree of independence is highly valued, the most frequently cited psychological task that must be achieved is separation from parents. Offer and Offer (1975) state: "The establishment of a self separate from the parents is one of the major tasks of young adulthood. The adolescent must disengage himself from parental domination" (p. 167). Lidz (1968) says: "The transition from adolescent to adult behavior involves becoming a person in one's own right, not simply someone's son or daughter" (p. 344). In cultures in which independence and mobility, both geographic and social, are subordinated to the expectation that the next generation will remain in the same location and line of work, separation from parents may be a less important psychological step. Even in the United States the value is not omnipresent. The parent who attempts to thwart an adult child's independence is a not infrequent stage character, usually comic.

A major task, primarily elucidated by Erikson, involves identity formation (as related to adolescence), which includes how one sees oneself as well as how others see one. This task is embedded in Erikson's (1950) description of life crises, which are roughly correlated with life age periods. The crisis correlated with adolescence is described as "identity versus identity confusion." Inevitably, this developmental task interacts with the separation task because forming one's own identity, by definition, implies some degree of separation from parents. It does not, however, necessarily signify outright rebellion, and underlying values may be transmitted from one generation to the next.

131

When talking about this subject, there is always a temptation to recall one's own life—a temptation I shall not resist. Although I do not pretend to be normal by anyone's standard, I grew up before the identity crisis had been invented, which was unfortunate because, without an identity crisis to have, I was forced to consider several more serious diagnoses. In college, matters became so unsettled that I tried a brand of psychoanalysis that seemed to have helped my older siblings, and, when that failed, I took the more desperate step of getting myself admitted to law school. Fortunately for the legal profession and me, an unlikely deus ex machina came along in the form of the original peacetime draft lottery, which I won, and so I was drafted into the Army prior to Pearl Harbor. That gave me roughly five years to think it over, and, by the time I was discharged, my thinking, at least about my vocational identity, was considerably clearer.

Another task, the development of a capacity for intimacy, is related to the achievement of genital primacy and the establishment of a satisfactory gender identity and sexual orientation. This task, again, owes some of its elaboration to Erikson (1950), who designated intimacy versus isolation as the dominant conflict of the young adult life stage. Although many theorists feel that the ultimate basis for adult gender identity and sexual orientation has its roots in earliest childhood, the late adolescent–young adult period is one of considerable sexual experimentation, and it is difficult not to feel that this experimentation influences the individual's eventual adult sexual adjustment. Blos (1979), in particular, states that the attainment of a clear sexual identity is crucial to the transition to adulthood because, he feels, if sexual ambiguity prevails, maturation in all spheres will be hampered. The capacity for intimacy, of course, involves more than simply gratifying sexual activity. It involves, in addition, the ability to engage in a relationship of trust and a degree of emotional openness.

On a rather different level of psychic development, several authors (e.g., Blos 1979; Wolf 1980) stress the fact that the individual must disengage from the infantile object representations, usually of the parents, and shift cathexes to nonincestuous objects as part of the transition to a mature primary love relationship. In observable terms, this may involve initially a shift to an adult outside the family, sometimes a teacher, a coach, or the parent of a friend, who fills a quasi-parental role. This attachment is then followed by a shift to a peer in what may be a transient "crush" or infatuation, and, eventually, a deeper relationship may be established, often with a new partner. Adatto (1980) applies Winnicott's concept of the "transitional object" but states that in the adolescent situation that object tends to be a human being. This shift in love relationship is, of course, interrelated to all the tasks already described and may evoke parental opposition, often from the opposite-sex parent. I have already referred to stock stage characters, but I must mention a real one, the mother of a friend, who told me that, when she was introduced to her mother-in-law-to-be, an imposing grande dame, she was greeted with the statement, "My dear, I want you to understand that it's nothing personal, but I'm determined to hate anyone my son marries."

Several authors stress the tasks of the stabilization of character structure and the development of a time perspective. The former is described by Blotcky and Looney (1980) as a "stabilization of the psychic apparatus" (p. 191) with improved consistency in both drive regulation and harmony of ego defenses. The latter is described as a feeling for oneself in relation to past, present, and future, with its implications of societal and personal expectations.

Although less often mentioned specifically by developmental theorists, longitudinal studies document the importance of a capacity for friendship, so I feel that it should probably be included as a significant developmental task. Interestingly, it seems to correlate not only with general measures of mental health and successful transition to adulthood but also with the ability to establish a satisfactory primary, romantic relationship.

Finally, there is the general need to establish a set of life goals, which task encompasses vocation and anticipated work role, presumes the capacity for commitment and the achievement of an acceptable moral code, and requires sufficient confidence and self-esteem to permit the individual to pursue the goals chosen. Kimmel and Weiner (1985) quote Havighurst as dividing the task in two and describing it as "acquiring a set of values and an ethical system as a guide to behavior—developing an ideology" and "desiring and achieving socially responsible behavior" (p. 18).

This is perhaps a good moment to mention one major area of divided opinion—the difference in adolescent developmental process as it applies to males and females. As is so often the case, much of the earlier work on normal development evolved from observations on males. Recently, there has been increased focus on adolescent development in females, and several clinicians have questioned whether the separation process should be given the same prominence in females that it has in males. Chodorow (1978), Gilligan (1982), Klein (1986), and Miller (1976) all feel that there is a real difference in ideal female development and that, consequently, a different standard of adulthood should be used as a measure. Instead of the independence or autonomy that is often set as a goal in the separation process, they stress a self-in-relation theory with "self-development for women [occurring], not through a progressive series of separations, but through the experience of evolving empathic relationships" (Klein 1986, p. 27). Here again, however, one would need to ask whether this difference results from biology or from sociocultural expectations. In an era of sociocultural change, will the developmental process be affected?

Inasmuch as this is an overview, I feel it is appropriate to mention briefly the main proponents of the classic theories of the psychological transition to adulthood. They are not the only important investigators, but space precludes a more extensive review.

Erikson (1945, 1946), already cited in relation to identity, first introduced the concept as a result of his observations of two American Indian tribes, and he initially seemed to stress social identity—that is, how the Indian child learns the identity that he or she is to achieve as an adult member of the community. He gradually elaborated the concept to include both internal and external components. His definitions of identity changed some over time, but one (Erikson 1946) involved "the immediate perception of one's self-sameness and continuity in time; and the simultaneous perception of the fact that others recognize one's sameness and continuity" (p. 363). Simultaneously, he developed an epigenetic approach and constructed stages of a life cycle characterized by crises or turning points leading either to normal development or to pathology. A whole research industry has grown up around these stages, and there has been a considerable range in describing the nature of identity. Marcia (1966) reconstructed Erikson's concepts of moratorium and crisis into quadripartite states and developed scales to measure foreclosed identity, moratorium, achievement, and identity diffusion.

A second major contributor to adolescent development is Blos, who stressed what he called "the second individuation process of adolescence" (1967, p. 163), referring back to Mahler's concept of the separation-individuation process in childhood. Blos feels that this process in adolescence involves disengagement from internal objects, which can be achieved only by "ego and drive regression" in the service of development. He comments that this is the only time that regression occurs in the process of healthy development. He goes on (Blos 1979) to describe four conditions that are necessary to progress to adulthood. Sexual identity and individuation have already been mentioned; the other two are residual trauma and ego continuity. Although Blos initially derived his theory from observations on males, more recently he has modified his theory to describe female adolescent development, and he differentiates between the two by stating that, while the adolescent boy must resolve the positive and negative Oedipus complex, the girl's regressive pull is to the preoedipal mother (Blos 1980).

Anna Freud (1963), who was one of the pioneers in delineating adolescent development, proposed a theory of development that was based on discrete developmental lines. She describes several, including id and ego, and states that "notions of average normality . . . expect a fairly close correspondence between growth on the individual lines" (p. 262). This implies that progress can proceed differentially on the individual lines, but she also states that, if there is too much disharmony in the advance along each line, there is likely to be pathology. She is one of the principal proponents of the idea of "turmoil" as a normal, and probably essential, event in healthy adolescent development.

Kohut (1971), in describing his psychology of the self, feels that the primary narcissism of early childhood must be transformed into mature self-esteem and the archaic idealized parental images into mature values in the transitional process. Wolf (1980), in a commentary on Kohut's work, describes "the transformation from preadolescent idealized parental images to the post-adolescent idealized ethics and values" (p. 48), which, if accomplished, indicates that the individual has achieved a cohesive personality. Kohut also cites "wisdom" and "humor" as two qualities related to maturity and states that the central task of adolescence is the reorganization of the self.

Hartmann (1958) is another important theorist who, in his work on ego psychology, has contributed heavily. He discusses the task of adult development in terms of adaptation, which he defines as "primarily a reciprocal relationship between the organism and its environment" (p. 24). In his discussion of mental health, Hartmann proposes the concept of "preparedness for *average expectable* environmental situations and for *average expectable* internal conflicts" (p. 55). He stresses that adaptation is not simply a matter of compliance with external demands; rather it requires integration of internal, psychological forces with external, social pressures.

Neugarten (1969, 1971) has been a major writer on the subject from a sociocultural perspective. She feels that "a social clock must be superimposed over the biological clock in the study of lives" (1971, p. 85). She states that, although the norms vary for different groups, for any given group norms are closely related to actual occurrences and that, in fact, the norms act as a system of social controls (Neugarten 1969). She also points out that, in age periods when major changes, such as marriage and parenthood, may occur, age can be misleading because these events will in themselves have an effect on personality and on the process of maturation (Neugarten 1971).

Most of the foregoing theories are derived largely from clinical work. There is, however, another important body of data based on nonpatient populations studied by one or another research design. Some are longitudinal, some cross-sectional, and some retrospective. Research methods include interviews, questionnaires, projective tests, and demographic data and various combinations of these information-gathering techniques sometimes enhanced by derived indices, such as personality scales.

Offer and Offer (1975) studied a group of males from the beginning of high school through their fourth post–high school year. They described three groups that followed three different passages through adolescence—the continuous growth group, the surgent growth group, and the tumultuous growth group. While all groups were within the normal range, only the latter displayed the turmoil often described as characteristic of adolescence. Silber, Hamburg, Coelho, Murphey, Rosenberg, and Pearlin (1966) studied a small cohort of high school seniors into college and stressed the importance of coping strategies that facilitated the transition. Vaillant (1977) conducted a long-range followup study on men who had been part of a study started when they were normal Harvard students. He described his findings in terms of mechanisms of defense, feeling that the healthier individuals used mature defenses, which he lists as sublimation, altruism, suppression, anticipation, and humor. He feels that the profile of an individual's use of mature defenses correlates closely with health and maturity. Gould

(1972) developed cross-sectional groups for different age periods and found the group for the young adulthood period to be characterized by a feeling of being established, autonomous, and separate from the family. He felt that they were engaged in the work of being adults.

Various other studies have produced interesting observations, such as Heath's (1979) follow-up study of Princeton undergraduates. This stresses the general ability to establish friendships as important to psychological health as well as correlating strongly with the capacity to maintain an intimate relationship in marriage. Levinson, Darrow, Klein, Levinson, and McKee (1978) reconstructed life histories of middle-aged males and found remarkable correlation in the maturing experience. Kohlberg and Kramer (1969) studied moral development and constructed a hierarchy of stages. The Oakland Growth Study (Block 1971), the Berkeley Guidance Study (MacFarlane 1964), and the Fels Institute Study (Kagan and Moss 1962) were conducted with cohorts followed from birth to adulthood, with varying and sometimes conflicting conclusions. A Fels Study finding was that culturally supported gender characteristics, such as aggressiveness for males and dependency for females, were quite stable over time.

At this point, I think I should attempt to summarize and add a few thoughts of my own. First, setting and context are important factors. In our society, young adulthood may be thought to start at seventeen to nineteen, when individuals have completed compulsory schooling. Two paths then form: one for those who go on to college and one for those who do not. The latter will find jobs, enter the military, or assume more household responsibility and will, thereby, be undertaking adult social roles and tend to be regarded as adults. Those who enter college will not be assuming full adult social roles, but they will have greater independence and, in many ways, will be expected to behave as adults.

In addition to the social role, there is unquestionably a process of psychological maturation during which the individual, one hopes, will achieve a reasonably coherent and separate personality. Psychoanalysts believe that this process is primarily unconscious. Schafer (1973) states: "Genuine emancipation seems to be built on revision, modulation, and selective acceptance as well as rejection, flexible mastery, and complex substitutions and other changes of aims, representations, and patterns of behavior" (p. 45). In describing another aspect of the process, the need to transform the so-called inner world, particularly the "archaic infantile world," he is quite forthright in saying that it will be slow and that he does not know exactly how it happens.

On a more overt level, one observes that late adolescence and young adulthood are periods when the individual must and does make many conscious choices. Some of these are in the service of experimentation, but experimentation will, presumably in turn, lead to more final choices about occupation, marriage, friends, religion, and style of life. Wittenberg (1968) and Hartmann (1960) speak of a philosophy of life or weltanschauung. This suggests that an essential accomplishment is the development of a personally acceptable code of behavior that is satisfying to the individual and sufficiently consonant with the surrounding society to avoid major disruptions. The capacity for commitment—that is, the ability to make choices and to close off other possibilities—is almost always a necessary ingredient, and for many the closing off is the most difficult aspect of the transition. It is also important to be able to cope with setbacks and/or stresses and not become demoralized. Experimentation almost by definition implies that one will make mistakes, and the ability to maintain perspective on the experience and to rebound is essential.

One can reasonably ask whether, assuming that there are both conscious and unconscious events that must occur, they go on simultaneously or whether one must or may precede the other and, if so, which comes first. Thus, does a move away from home, for example, begin the process of disengagement from infantile object ties and, thus, lead to experimentation with new relationships, or do new relationships cause loosening of internal ties? E. Prelinger (December 1986, personal communication) suggests that there are always both conscious and unconscious components to each step in the separation process. Furthermore, it is important to note that, although I have been writing as though these events get settled once and for all, this is not really accurate. They frequently recur in at least partial form throughout adult life and require reworking.

It is tempting to close with a summary list of those qualities that must be achieved in order to be seen as having reached normal young adulthood. Having reviewed the literature, however, I am wary because I began to be suspicious that each list tended to include those qualities that authors ascribed to themselves in actuality or fantasy. Thus, my list would probably say more about me than about normality. Instead, I will quote one of Heath's (1979) subjects, who spoke of the need to stop pretending that you are something that you are not and "to face yourself in the mirror." This, to me, implies an acceptance of oneself, both one's accomplishments and one's deficiencies, an attitude of some self-respect, and, by extrapolation, a willingness to deal with others straightforwardly and without pretense.

NOTE

This chapter is based in large measure on "Young Adulthood: Stages of Maturity," in *Normality and the Life Cycle*, ed. D. Offer and M. Sabshin (New York: Basic, 1984).

REFERENCES

Adatto, C. P. 1980. Late adolescence to early adulthood. In S. I. Greenspan and G. H. Pollock, eds. *The Course of Life: Psychoanalytic Contributions toward Understanding Personality Development,* vol. 2, *Latency, Adolescence, and Youth.* Washington, D.C.: National Institute of Mental Health.

Block, J. 1971. *Lives through Time.* Berkeley, Calif.: Bancroft.

Blos, P. 1967. The second individuation process of adolescence. *Psychoanalytic Study of the Child* 22:162–186.

Blos, P. 1979. *The Adolescent Passage.* New York: International Universities Press.

Blos, P. 1980. Modifications in the traditional psychoanalytic theory of female adolescent development. *Adolescent Psychiatry* 8:8–24.

Blotcky, M., and Looney, J. C. 1980. Normal female and male adolescent psychological development: an overview of theory and research. *Adolescent Psychiatry* 8:184–199.

Chodorow, N. 1978. *The Reproduction of Mothering.* Berkeley, Calif.: University of California Press.

Erikson, E. H. 1945. Childhood and tradition in two American Indian tribes. *Psychoanalytic Study of the Child* 1:319–350.

Erikson, E. H. 1946. Ego development and historical change. *Psychoanalytic Study of the Child* 2:359–396.

Erikson, E. H. 1950. *Childhood and Society.* New York: Norton.

Freud, A. 1963. The concept of developmental lines. *Psychoanalytic Study of the Child* 18:245–265.

Gilligan, C. 1982. *In a Different Voice*. Cambridge, Mass.: Harvard University Press.

Gould, R. L. 1972. The phases of adult life: a study in developmental psychology. *American Journal of Psychiatry* 129:521–532.

Hartmann, H. 1958. *Ego Psychology and the Problem of Adaptation*. New York: International Universities Press.

Hartmann, H. 1960. *Psychoanalysis and Moral Values*. New York: International Universities Press.

Heath, R. 1979. *Princeton Retrospectives*. Princeton, N.J.: Princeton University, Class of 1954.

Kagan, J., and Moss, H. A. 1962. *Birth to Maturity*. New York: Wiley.

Kimmel, D. C., and Weiner, I. B. 1985. *Adolescence, a Developmental Transition*. Hillsdale, N.J.: Erlbaum.

Klein, R. 1986. Commentary on values and college women's development. *Journal of College Student Psychotherapy* 1:25–29.

Kohlberg, L., and Kramer, R. 1969. Continuities and discontinuities in childhood and adult moral development. *Human Development* 12:93–120.

Kohut, H. 1971. *The Analysis of the Self*. New York: International Universities Press.

Levinson, D. J.; Darrow, C. N.; Klein, E. B.; Levinson, M. A.; and McKee, B. 1978. *The Seasons of a Man's Life*. New York: Knopf.

Lidz, T. 1968. *The Person*. New York: Basic.

MacFarlane, J. W. 1964. Perspectives on personality consistency and change from the Guidance Study. *Vita Humana* 7:115–126.

Marcia, J. E. 1966. Development and validation of ego identity status. *Journal of Personality and Social Psychology* 3:551–558.

Mays, V. M. 1986. Identity development of black Americans: the role of history and the importance of ethnicity. *American Journal of Psychotherapy* 40:582–594.

Miller, J. B. 1976. *Toward a New Psychology of Women*. Boston: Beacon.

Neugarten, B. L. 1969. Continuities and discontinuities of psychological issues in adult life. *Human Development* 12:121–130.

Neugarten, B. L. 1971. Introduction to the symposium: models and methods for the study of the life cycle. *Human Development* 14:81–86.

Offer, D., and Offer, J. B. 1975. *From Teenage to Young Manhood: A Psychological Study*. New York: Basic.

Offer, D., and Sabshin, M. 1974. *Normality.* New York: Basic.

Offer, D., and Sabshin, M., eds. 1984. *Normality and the Life Cycle.* New York: Basic.

Parsons, T. 1949. Age and sex in the social structure of the United States. In C. Kluckhohn and H. A. Murray, eds. *Personality in Nature, Society, and Culture.* New York: Knopf.

Piaget, J. 1977. The stages of intellectual development in childhood and adolescence. In H. E. Gruber and J. J. Voneche, eds. *The Essential Piaget.* New York: Basic.

Prelinger, E. 1974. Crises of identity. In M. D. Keys, ed. *The Identity Crisis.* New York: National Project Center for Film and the Humanities.

Schafer, R. 1973. Concepts of self and identity and the experience of separation-individuation in adolescence. *Psychoanalytic Quarterly* 42:42–60.

Silber, E.; Hamburg, D. A.; Coelho, G. V.; Murphey, E. B.; Rosenberg, M.; and Pearlin, L. D. 1966. Adaptive behavior in competent adolescents: coping with anticipation of college. *Archives of General Psychiatry* 5:354–365.

Timiras, P. S. 1978. Biological perspectives on aging. *American Scientist* 66:605–614.

Vaillant, G. E. 1977. *Adaptation to Life.* Boston: Little, Brown.

Wittenberg, R. 1968. *Postadolescence.* New York: Grune & Stratton.

Wolf, E. S. 1980. Tomorrow's self: Heinz Kohut's contribution to adolescent psychiatry. *Adolescent Psychiatry* 8:41–50.

10 IDENTITY FORMATION IN ADOLESCENCE: IMPLICATIONS FOR YOUNG ADULTHOOD

RUTHELLEN JOSSELSON

Identity formation is a crucial normative task of adolescence, for it is in this realm that young people base their sense of themselves as well as their vision of the structure of their lives. Identity is a largely unconscious organizing structure that integrates aspects of the self and provides continuity across the lifespan and across life experiences. Identity is what we want to be recognized as in addition to what we learn about how we are recognized. It is our trust in our meaning for and place in our world, our confidence in our continued relationship to that world.

To be an adolescent is not yet to have such a place: one must meet the requirements of others while dreaming of what one may become. To be an adult is to stake out a place, to take a role in life, no longer subservient, now choosing and responsible. Identity, in that it involves renunciation of what is not chosen, becomes then a template for the making of adult decisions. As the life cycle progresses, identity becomes amplified and differentiated, often fundamentally modified, but it can never be undone. Choices made become part of the individual's history. Previous identity must always be integrated with the new. The identity formation period, then, is a critical time. It is the hatching period of the adult.

Erikson (1956, 1968) has provided us with a rich and evocative theory of identity formation and related these processes to other aspects of ego development. Marcia (1966) devised an empirical interview-based approach to study identity formation among nonclinical populations of adolescents. This research paradigm, known as identity status research, focuses on the dual axes of crisis and commitment outlined by Erikson. To forge an identity, the individual must experience some crisis in previously held ideas derived from the ascribed identity of childhood. The young person must consider options of occupational and ideological choice. Then, having weighed possibilities, perhaps experimented with different choices, the young person, at the close of adolescence, must make commitments that become the core of this newly wrought identity.

Using the dimensions of crisis and commitment as the central axes, Marcia defined four groups on the basis of the presence or absence of crisis and commitment.

1. *Identity achievement.* These are the young people who have explored options and then decided, committing themselves to ways of being.

2. *Foreclosure.* These young people are ones who have made commitments in the absence of a searching or crisis phase. They have carried forward either parentally derived expectations or childhood plans and beliefs without subjecting them to question or scrutiny. Their identity formation is premature, rooted in earlier (preadolescent) phases of development.

3. *Moratorium.* These are people actively in a crisis or testing phase. They are struggling to make commitments but have not yet found what feels right as "my way."

4. *Diffusion.* Following Erikson, these young people are experiencing neither crisis nor commitment. They have abandoned childhood resolutions but are not struggling for new ones. They are drifting, avoiding the identity formation task.

Two decades of research with these groups has shown them to be distinct and internally coherent (for a review of the research, see Marcia [1980]). Identity achievements have been shown to be the healthy, mature young people, highest on such variables as self-esteem, self-direction, resistance to conformity pressure, and so on. Those diffuse in identity consistently bring up the rear of the developmental continuum. They are high in anxiety, low in ego development, and most undifferentiated in sex-role orientation. The foreclosures and moratoriums are more difficult to make general statements about because, in these two groups, the sexes differ. Male moratoriums, those actively in crisis, behave on objective measures much the same way male achievements do. Thus, for males, achievement and moratorium are the two "high" statuses. Among females, however, the foreclosures behave much like achievements, with moratoriums resembling diffusions on personality measures. I mention this only briefly because it is important to keep in mind that there are important differences in the way in which men and women experience the identity formation stage.

We have just begun to understand the relation between late adolescent identity formation and the experience of adulthood. Until now, we have assumed that healthy adolescent development presages positive adult development, all the while remaining optimistic that those who do not do their developmental work during adolescence may yet find a second opportunity in early adulthood. Without longitudinal data, we have been at a loss to know how the modes of passage through adolescence shape later growth. The material I will be discussing is drawn from a twelve-year follow-up study of thirty-four randomly selected college senior women. These subjects were classified into the four identity status groups and intensively interviewed. The purpose of the study was to understand the psychodynamic antecedents of identity formation in a nonclinical sample of young people and to learn about how different styles of identity development shape adulthood. I will begin a summary of my longitudinal findings by presenting a case, one of the moratoriums, to illustrate an identity crisis in process and to serve as a marker for the differences among the groups.

Millie in College

Millie was a perky, cherubic-looking young woman who came to the interview dressed in the "hippie" garb that came to symbolize the era of the late 1960s. Millie was raised in a New York suburb, the middle of three children. Neither of her parents had attended college, but they wanted her to have as much education as possible. She ventured away from home to a large, private university in Philadelphia.

Millie had expected that she would become a nurse like her mother but found that she did not "have the temperament." Since then, she had switched her major three times. After giving up on nursing, she applied for a physical therapy program but could not get accepted into the program because of her grades, so she opted for a psychology major. This, she found, was making her "get too much into myself," and she was afraid that more psychology would "screw me up," so she changed again to biology. This made sense to her because she had begun to think in terms of doing cancer research as a result of two summers she had spent working in a nursing home. Having developed a close relationship with one particular dying woman, she became quite upset about the ravages of cancer and thought that she might like to take part in searching for a cure. After a few semesters of biology courses, however, Millie was becoming very upset at the idea of killing frogs in her physiology class and had come to realize that she would not have the stomach to do cancer research. She wished she had just gone into teaching, but it was too late. Of her future occupation, she said, "I think I'd like to be a bum. I've felt really tied down by school, and I'd like to start doing some traveling. I don't want to settle down in a job right now since I've been settled down in school for so long. I feel like I've missed a lot, and I'd like to just get a job like a waitress and just travel around and meet people and be exposed to things. I'd like to learn a little about life before I settle down into a routine."

Millie was not sure about the prospect of marriage, but she said that she would probably marry eventually. "I don't like to think of myself as forty years old and unmarried, but right now I can't imagine it. I can imagine loving someone or living with someone, but as soon as there is a legal bond—that this is the way it's going to be—I get scared." As for children, she said, "I don't want my life to be my children. I want my own life. I've seen too many parents—like mine—who have put their whole lives into their children and then when the children grow up, they're lost. You've got to realize from the start that eventually they're going to leave."

Raised in the strictest Catholic tradition, she had become increasingly aware of the church's "hypocrisy." When she noticed that many people were going to church only to see what other people were wearing, she stopped going to church. "I know my parents would like me to go to church, and I'd like to do it for them, but I couldn't because I'd be a hypocrite and I'd be deceiving them into thinking I'm a good Catholic girl again when I'm not." But she was not sure what to believe instead. "I do want to believe," she said, "because just to believe in reality is not so nice because there are a lot of things in reality that are not so nice." She tried to develop a personal ethical system but became stymied when she thought about how she might raise children. "I went to Catholic schools, and those things are ingrained in me. I can cut down the Catholic church, but when I hear someone else do it, I get really defensive."

Millie had had intense political struggles in regard to involvement in antiwar protests. "I was believing what people were saying—that you can give up your grades for people who are over in Viet Nam dying. You can make a sacrifice for them. And I felt, 'Yeah, that's what I'm going to do.' But there's no correlation between me not going to class [during the student strike] and them dying over there. It's not doing them any good. And I really got screwed. And nothing came of it. The summer came and everyone went home and that was it. And I had three incompletes. I'm apathetic now. I really did get involved, and all I could see was I was getting screwed and nothing was coming of it. I don't know what I'd do now. Things aren't the way I'd like them to be in my ideal society."

On the question of premarital sex, Millie had very definite views. In her opinion, "Someone who is twenty-two and a virgin is perverted." In formulating her own standards, she felt that "you shouldn't make love just to satisfy your animal desires." The first time she had intercourse, it was with a man she loved and hoped to marry. "He changed my ideas because I used to be so inhibited. He changed my whole way of life because I used to be very superstraight and closed-minded." She defined her new sexual values as based on what she "feels for a person" but worried that "there are a lot of guys who can't handle a sexual relationship and will just think that the girl's a slut." She had gotten over the idea "that if you have sex before you're married, you go straight to Hell," but she confided that her parents would "freak out" if they knew about her sexual behavior.

Approaching college graduation, Millie remained in a highly conflicted moratorium state. Uncertain about occupation, religion, politics, or sexual standards, Millie exemplified a "pure" moratorium (in terms of the groups of this study). She had made no commitments in any identity-related aspect of her life but was struggling for them through exploration, trial and error, and thought.

Asked to describe herself, Millie began talking about her persistent conflict over being a child or an adult. "I don't think I act my age. I think I act like a kid. Maybe it's that I don't act the way I thought I

would act at this age. I used to think that when I was age twenty—
I don't know—that I'd walk around discussing Plato or something."
This feeling that things in the present—especially the way she was—
were not what she had hoped for or expected was a continual theme
that occupied her reflections on herself. One of her early memories
manifested the same feeling of wish for and fear of the privileges of
the next stage: "The day before I went to kindergarten, which I was
really looking forward to—very apprehensive but very excited about
being a 'big girl.' And my mother said I had to get up at 7 A.M. and I
began to think twice about it." Even as a child, she remembered wanting the advantages of growing up but fearing the obligations.

Part of this conflict stemmed from Millie's quest to be right about
things. She had little to say about her childhood except that she was
always a very good girl. She remembered her early life as a harmonious,
secure environment in which she was just like her parents (who were
like everyone else's parents, and all the other kids were just like her).
Success was easy. Her movement into the more complex world of
college startled her because there was no longer the ready, ubiquitous
social agreement that she was always right. In her words, "It starts
when you're little. You think your parents are gods. Then you find out
they're only human, but you still believe what they say because they
are your parents. . . . The more I learn, the more middle of the road
I become, and it's hard that way because I like to have the answers.
But it seems like that's the way it's going—that you just can't say that
this is right and this is wrong."

Millie described her parents as having been affectionate and generous. She felt that her mother often gave her more than she deserved
and felt very guilty about this. Her father, whom she saw as strong,
silent, and stable, was the authority at home, and she was frightened
of him. He set definite limits for her, and she never felt able to disobey
him. The atmosphere at home seemed to have been one of living up
to fairly stringent internal and external demands. "I always want to
run away, but I never do. My mother once told me that if you shirk
responsibility once, you'll just do it all the time, so I never do." But
responsibility, especially responsibility for things she had not yet claimed
as her own, weighed heavily on Millie.

As a result of these internal and external pressures, Millie always
hungered for structure, for something she could bounce against to test
if she were right or wrong. In high school, she would become very

dependent on the boys she dated, trying to live up to what they wanted her to be. Then she would get very depressed when they would break up with her.

When she first entered college, she had felt adrift at the loss of structure and fell in love with a boy who was to be the focus of her life for the next three years. He was, like her father, a strong, authoritarian figure who set out to mold her and teach her. However, he was sadistic about this, poking fun at her middle-class attitudes, beating her occasionally, leaving her frequently. He entertained himself by shocking her with his foul language, his use of drugs, and his increasingly "far out" friends. Millie described him as a "freak," and her parents, after one look at him, despised him. Consequently, Millie became caught in a complex struggle between her parents and her boyfriend, unable to give up her dependency on either of them. "I was torn between my parents and him and I couldn't condemn them for their motives because they only wanted the best for me and everything I did was wrong and everyone was always mad at me and there I was in the middle." While she was grateful to her boyfriend for having opened her to new ideas and making her less dependent on her parents, she simply shifted her conflicted dependency needs onto him. She idealized him as she had once idealized her parents and tried in every way to gain his approval. Not long before the interview, he had left her once more, this time definitively, and Millie found herself longing for him or, at least, "to be completely in love with someone and to be near people who mean a lot to me." But she had come too far from home simply to return. What she was yearning for was someone to take the choices away from her and provide the answers. Again, she felt a sense of failure because she was never able to fulfill her boyfriend's expectations of her.

As the end of college approached, Millie was dealing with the impending separation from her friends who were going off in different directions. She was not sure what to do. As she thought about her future, she had to confront the distance in outlook she had attained from her past. She said, "I have a different attitude about life. It's strange because the more I think about it, the more confused I get as to what I want to do with myself, where I think I'm going. It's scary in that sense, but it's good in the sense that I'm not just living a life that's already been made for me—like I'm not just falling into a rut that I just didn't even question—that I'd just go to college, get married, live in suburbia, and be a housewife, and naturally I would be a virgin until I got married." Asked how she saw her life five years hence, Millie replied, "I hope I'll have the answers to a lot of questions I'm asking myself now like, 'What is life?' and 'What are people?'"

There was cause to worry about Millie at the end of college. Her struggle for individuation seemed to be failing. Instead of being able to dispense with authority and make reality-based decisions, she was engaged in a search for authorities to comply with or rebel against. While she had managed to disengage from the content of the internalized demands of her childhood, she nevertheless was seeking new goals phrased in the same tone of absoluteness. In trying to grow away from her parents, she unconsciously chose someone who would impose opposite demands with equivalent force to those that her father once imposed on her. Notice, for example, the very totalistic statement she made to justify her sexual behavior—anyone different from her is "perverted."

Millie also felt unable to live up to her own expectations, unable to be "as big a girl" as she wished. Uncertain of herself and not valuing any of her own capacities or accomplishments, Millie seemed unable to conceive of herself as existing as an individual. Her life seemed centered on how people were reacting to her as she vacillated between pleasing them and shocking them. Her self-esteem derived from the approval of others; there was no sense that anything in herself was competent in its own right. Because she did not trust herself, and because she feared her own impulses, Millie felt the need for someone to keep her on leash and make her into someone. But, at the same time, her wish to be her own person prevented her from striking the bargain and becoming what someone else wanted her to be.

Millie at Thirty-four

When I saw Millie at age thirty-four, she was pregnant, relaxed, and talkative. In contrast to her earlier interview, there was much less intense conflict and less internal struggle. At present, she is mainly focused on her family, her three-year-old daughter and her husband. But she got to this life circumstance by a circuitous route.

Millie tried a number of things, but everything failed. She spent her early adulthood in several different occupations, from driving a cab to computer work. She had many disappointing relationships until she finally, hesitantly, married. Having already had several abortions, she decided to carry through a pregnancy, quit work, and make a career of mothering. Too many times, Millie felt that she had had the "wind knocked out of my sails" by disappointments in her jobs, in her friends, in humanity. As a result, Millie grew closer again to her family and became grateful to them. With them she could count on the love and protection she assumed she would find but failed to find in the larger world. Most important, she has moved closer to them internally, feeling that the values they gave her, the way they raised her, was the right way after all. She thinks lovingly of her parents as her heritage, the sense of where she came from, and they are among the most important people in her life.

What she has become by age thirty-four, she has become largely by default. Not knowing what else to do or to believe, she has taken what is available and tried to adapt to it. She is clearly disappointed in herself for not working but is bravely trying to rationalize a career out of motherhood. She will teach her children the Catholicism she tried to escape because she was unable to find another belief system that works for her. She has increasingly come to feel that the world may not be a nice place and that she may have no meaningful place in it. Now her hopes are that she can somehow create a nice world for her children.

At age thirty-four, Millie is still very much in search of self-esteem, now hoping to find it in motherhood. She has never adequately internalized a sense of self-worth, partly because her dreams have been so far from what she was capable of accomplishing. This conflict over self-esteem is epitomized in the earliest memory she reported in this later interview: "Being in kindergarten, we were cutting out shamrocks. The teacher asked me to cut out the shamrock and I was so impressed that she asked me to cut it out. This was going to be the best shamrock the world had ever seen. I was being so careful that I was going too slow, and she ended up coming over and taking it out of my hands and saying, 'OK, we'll let someone else do this.' I was crushed."

This very poignant memory encapsulates the psychological struggle Millie has experienced throughout her life. The theme of the "best the world has ever seen" has pervaded Millie's psychological life since childhood, and she has never quite figured out how to put her actions and aspirations together. She dreams of greatness and is continually disappointed to find herself only real.

In a very major sense, Millie appears to be trying to go home again. While it is difficult to say percisely where she ought to be ranked in identity status, she seems to be trying to return to a foreclosure position. Maybe all those old values were right after all, thinks Millie, as she tries to make a life for herself much like her mother's—taking care of children and home, getting involved in the church, and doing crafts. Her failure at making a clear life-style of her own leaves her at least grateful that she has internalized something else to fall back on, and this is what she, like several other moratorium women, has done.

Discussion

There are deep and important differences in the psychodynamic constellations of the four groups as they enter the adolescent task of identity formation. For foreclosures, preoccupations with security, founded in an early and intense attachment to one or the other parent, shape a reluctance to "leave home" emotionally and to rework familiar and safe patterns. These young people sidestep rather than undertake the adolescent challenge. Firmly tied to parentally based superegos, they are inhibited in impulse expression and rigid in their defenses. What becomes of the foreclosures as they enter adulthood? By age thirty-four, they remain pretty much the same psychologically as they were at age twenty-one. Among women, foreclosures become purveyors of the heritage, carrying on family and religious traditions, remaining in the occupations they chose as late adolescents but decided on as children. They recreate the lives they had known as children and rest secure.

Identity diffusions have a more complex journey, but the follow-up data show that most do not seriously resolve their diffuseness into early adulthood. Lacking in necessary aspects of ego functioning, these young people have too few solid internalizations out of which to shape an identity. Leaves blown by the wind, they await fortune to structure their lives and provide them a way to be. With the identity diffusions, we are more in the realm of psychopathology than normality. Stuck with unresolved earlier problems, these women do not bring to their adolescence enough inner psychological resources to address identity decisions seriously (for a fuller discussion of this group, see Josselson [1987]).

The identity achievements have, as predicted, the most auspicious outcome. Young people who went through a generally mild but definite period of exploration during college, they were able to consider alternatives and make commitments by the time of graduation. Adulthood for them has, in general, brought further refinements of identity but within the confines of the self-chosen identity of late adolescence. Less rigid than the foreclosures, identity achievements are more able to tolerate uncertainty, anxiety, and guilt. But few of them have highly dramatic exploratory periods such as we saw in Millie. Their growth takes place incrementally and quietly as they struggle to integrate new aspects of themselves that may fundamentally modify the old.

The moratorium status at the end of college is an unstable one. Such women take the greatest risks in terms of making of themselves something quite different from what they had been. This creates enormous problems of guilt and uncertainty. Because they have ventured so far from shore, they are the most vulnerable, and some, frightened by the currents, merely swim home again. Others, given fortunate circumstances and useful social supports, go on to achieve identities formulated on their own terms.

The longitudinal data of this study show that the separation-individuation phase of adolescence is critical to identity formation in adulthood. Although women individuate less than men, they vary in how much they seek to become individuated selves. A continuum of separation-individuation underlies the four identity status categories; in fact, these categories themselves may be no more than an artificial way of dividing that continuum. At one end lie the foreclosures, those who have not separated or individuated very much. If one remains a foreclosure by the end of college, one's future life is quite predictable unless untoward events block the chosen path and force reconsideration. At the other end are the diffusions, who have separated and individuated too much, too early. They did not internalize enough identity-forming structure from their parents to be able to crystallize a workable identity.

The moratorium women were the most insightful and open to change of the four groups. They seemed to have the acuity of vision, the responsiveness to social problems, and the psychological closeness to great philosophical questions that have so often been sentimentalized by observers of youths. They were, above all, aware of choice and often paralyzed by their awareness. Emotionally attuned to options, these women knew that they could design their own lives but frequently wanted to choose both sides of a contradiction. Moratoriums, who would be placed nearer the diffusions on the separation-individuation continuum, have a strongly internalized sense of who they are supposed to be, but they try to break away from this self too drastically, too painfully. Some are able to bear the pain and move on to achieved identities. Others become overwhelmed and return to essentially foreclosed positions.

The identity achievements, in between the foreclosures and moratoriums, tend to separate from their childhood selves gradually and incrementally, preserving relatedness at each step. Their growth is best described as a process of ongoing rapprochement: moving forward, touching base, and moving forward in a rhythm that continues into adulthood.

What, then, determines the path through the identity formation phase that the adolescent will take? Foreclosures as young girls had harmonious, gratifying relationships with their families. They were "good girls," doing what was right, dominated by the superego. For them, the adolescent task jeopardizes a too harmonious inner balance, and so they seek to avoid the psychological tasks of adolescence by recreating an environment in which the old balance can continue to be effective. They experience no push to individuate and may be harshly critical of others who seek greater self-definition.

The identity achievements start with a similar ego-superego configuration, but the superego never had as much of a monopoly on self-esteem. Although no more talented than the foreclosures, they tend to value competence more for its own sake than for its role in pleasing others. They also have more capacity to tolerate anxiety and guilt, which occur when they do not please others or meet their own inner standards. They experience more stress and pain than the foreclosures but gain in flexibility.

The moratoriums attempt to battle their superego head on, denying at times that it exists at all. But they cannot quite bring themselves to give up the experience of being good. As a result, they tend, during late adolescence, to swing back and forth, trying to hold on to the loving functions of the superego with one hand and to abolish it with the other. The extremes of identity confusion among the moratoriums during college are the outward sign of the intensity of the internal separation-individuation struggle, despite their conscious denials and externalizations of it.

The diffusions are confronting a struggle of a different kind. Lacking the building blocks that the other statuses are trying to rearrange, they are questing for parts of the self that they failed to develop at earlier times of their lives.

Conclusions

Identity development reaches a critical peak during adolescence. The pathway chosen through this phase, in part determined by earlier psychological development, has profound implications for adulthood. Those college students who are achieved, foreclosed, or diffuse in identity in their final year of college are likely to remain so, at least through age thirty-four. Once the psychosocial period for exploration and first commitments has passed, young people are somewhat frozen into the style they had followed unless external circumstances force massive reorganization. Development not undertaken or not successfully traversed during adolescence is not easily reworked in later life.

The phenomenon of "going home again," of undoing tentative steps toward independence, can be viewed most clearly in longitudinal data. What appears to be a hopeful period of exploration and crisis in adolescence can founder if the young person reaches too far or if adequate social supports are not available. The separation and individuation necessary for identity development must occur at an optimal pace and with significant others available to validate the emerging identity elements.

NOTE

This chapter is based on a speech delivered at the meeting of the American Society for Adolescent Psychiatry, April 1987. Full results of this study have been published in Ruthellen Josselson, *Finding Herself: Pathways to Identity Development in Women* (San Francisco: Jossey-Bass, 1987).

REFERENCES

Erikson, E. H. 1956. The problem of ego identity. *Journal of the American Psychoanalytic Association* 4:56–121.

Erikson, E. H. 1968. *Identity, Youth and Crisis*. New York: Norton.

Josselson, R. 1987. Identity diffusion: a long-term follow-up. *Adolescent Psychiatry* 14:230–258.

Marcia, J. E. 1966. Development and validation of ego identity status. *Journal of Personality and Social Psychology* 3:551–558.

Marcia, J. E. 1980. Identity in adolescence. In J. Adelson, ed. *Handbook of Adolescent Psychology*. New York: Wiley.

11   PARENTHOOD EXPERIENCE AND THE ADOLESCENT'S TRANSITION TO YOUNG ADULTHOOD: SELF PSYCHOLOGICAL PERSPECTIVES

SIDNEY H. WEISSMAN, REBECCA S. COHEN, ANDREW M. BOXER,
AND BERTRAM J. COHLER

To set the stage for addressing the parents' experience of their children entering young adulthood, we will review, from the perspective of self psychology, the child's experience of adolescence, which is ushered in by major biological and psychological changes. Piaget (1967) and others (see Brown 1988) have also established that, in addition to experiencing these changes, the adolescent begins to use the developing capacity for symbolic and abstract thought in identity formation.

From the perspective of psychology of the self, adolescents endure major shifts in self-experience. These include changes in the body and the experience of sexual desires. Moreover, the capacity to make new kinds of judgments and decisions is constantly expanding in different cognitive domains and to varying degrees. This new cognitive capacity, when present, enables the adolescent to assess parents, peers, ideas, and ideals in a conceptual manner. Further accretions of self structure, during which the self has taken over parental functions (transmuting internalizations) coupled with cognitive growth, produce changes in the nature of adolescent selfobject experience.

The concept of the selfobject is critical to understanding self psychology. The selfobject construct was initially developed by Kohut (1971) to describe a specific transference relationship that he observed in the psychoanalysis of certain patients. As his observations continued, the selfobject construct was extended to normal development.

The intrapsychic operation in which one individual (object) attains psychological intactness and self-esteem regulation by use of an aspect or attribute of another individual (object) in a specific situation or relationship is referred to in psychology of the self as a selfobject relationship. The individual may or may not be aware of the importance of the other in maintaining psychological equilibrium. Evolving selfobject needs are seen as critical throughout life from the perspective of self psychology. Wolf (1980) describes a developmental line of selfobject relationships.

In adolescence, new selfobjects will be based less on the concrete attributes of the selfobject, as was true in latency, and more on the symbolic and more subtle attributes of the selfobject. These new selfobjects represent idealizations, goals, and desires integrated into an evolving harmony with the adolescent's expanded abilities and ambitions and are known as idealized selfobjects. Because of the continuous physical and cognitive growth of adolescents, we can anticipate that they will seek these new selfobjects outside the family.

The idealized selfobjects, by providing models for current and future activities, serve as a guide for growth and for exploration of the world. New selfobjects will render the adolescent less reliant on the earlier mirroring-type selfobjects to sustain essential self-cohesion in stressful situations. The Offers' work (Offer and Offer 1975; see also Boxer, Solomon, Offer, Petersen, and Halprin 1984) has indicated that the models usually chosen by adolescents are surprisingly similar to those of their parents. For most adolescents, the new idealized selfobjects are transferred versions of the mirroring selfobjects, but they appear now in more abstract, idealized forms. In some cases, however, the dynamics of the family and an adolescent's unique needs will lead to selfobject choices that are at variance with earlier ones. In such instances, adolescents' "new" ideals will put them into conflict with their parents.

If the new selfobjects are required for the purpose of mirroring, the adolescent will be locked into relationships that do not promote effective and sustained growth. For example, this is evident when a teenager becomes involved in a drug-using peer group. Here, these are peers to stabilize the adolescent's and their own shaky selves by the use of substance and the mutual mirroring that occurs in the process. Although these friends or groups may be presented as "idealized figures," closer examination reveals that they are growth inhibiting. They are usually

156

mirroring selfobject relationships in which the experience sustains the involved adolescents' vulnerable self systems by surrounding them with individuals like themselves.

We do not intend to imply that selfobject experiences fit hierarchically into certain periods of development and not others. On the contrary, throughout the life cycle, one is involved in various combinations of selfobject experiences. However, we suspect that at critical phases the primary or past selfobject experiences will shift and that new or updated ones will be acquired. Selfobject experiences, which had been essential to maintain psychological equilibrium at a previous stage, now become internalized aspects of the self. This process is known as transmuting internalization. Successful adolescents enter young adulthood with increased internalized structures that enable them to acquire and eventually sustain future goals. From the perspective of self psychology, this means a cohesive self, one with ideals and ambitions in harmony with abilities. Of course, there is no clearly established time for this to occur, and certainly not all young adults will have achieved this integration. Therefore, family and society often provide sustaining selfobject functions to stabilize less cohesive self systems. The very nature of extended preparations for careers may require continued need for parental participation. This, however, is distinct from the psychological process of expansion of self. There can be an extended need for parental mirroring experiences simultaneously operating as a young adult uses school or workplace to acquire internally transmuting selfobject functions gradually.

Adolescent Psychopathology

Within this brief outline of self psychology, let us consider adolescent psychopathology, where an enfeebled self existed prior to adolescence. Such adolescents present various long-standing symptomatic behaviors and a history of fragmentation. They will attempt to establish mirroring selfobject experiences with any objects available to maintain cohesion in order to remain stable and functioning. They will appear to the outside world as immature and unable to explore in an effective fashion. Because of a fragile self and a constant need for assurance, they will tend to develop idealizing selfobject experiences with other, similar adolescents. They will tell their parents that these friends are "special." Seemingly, they can appear to have entered into idealizing selfobject relationships and pursue adolescent tasks. Clearer observation will indicate that they and their friends have mirroring-type relationships that serve to prevent effective new explorations of the world. This, we would submit, is also true when the selfobjects are various rock groups or television personalities that dominate rather pervasively the adolescents' lives. The adolescents seek either outside affirmation of the self or a merger with a group to maintain cohesion and, thus, cannot address other developmental tasks. For the more typical adolescent, such groups serve as transitory selfobjects and are not idealized to the exclusion of other idealizing experiences. The disorders that we see in adolescents with inadequate self systems can be described as disorders of self-regulation or cohesion. Such pathology is a manifestation of an attempt to stabilize a faulty self system. Selfobjects, which these adolescents seek, may stabilize their life situations but will not always lead to effective growth.

Another disorder is present in those children who enter adolescence with self systems that are cohesive but that become disorganized for some period of time under the stresses of adolescence. These adolescents may appear to be similar to the first group. Here, a diagnostician must carefully obtain an adequate history and assessment of current functioning to determine more certainly that the adolescent had functioned previously at a more integrated level. This evaluation should include a review of selfobject experiences. In these adolescents, we postulate that we will find more subtle and complex selfobject experiences, serving both mirroring and idealizing functions. Often, an idealized selfobject other than the primary ones can serve to isolate a teenager from expanded repertoires of selfobject relationships, which will make possible a self-integration that includes appropriate sexual organization. For example, the premature, intense sexual coupling seen in early adolescence can interfere with an effective entry into the world outside the family. One can sustain cohesion by replacing the early selfobjects, thereby cutting off further development.

An unfortunate issue of adolescent pathology, which we recently have been asked to address, is the growing number of adolescent suicides. Historical trends would seem to have argued that, with the declining number of adolescents in the general population, there would be less strain on the resources available to teenagers (Holinger, Offer, and Ostrov 1987). Thus, we would have concluded that there would be a sustained reduction in the suicide rate. This was the case until the mid-1980s. Since then, however, the rate has increased. Earlier, we noted that some adolescents entered this phase without a cohesive self system. They continued to utilize mirroring selfobjects to maintain cohesion and self-regulation. It seems that, in the current era of satellite television, the widespread coverage of tragic suicide pacts on one coast can be experienced by teenagers on the other coast with the same immediacy as if the events occurred a mile from their homes. Seemingly, every disturbed teenager is a neighbor to every other such teenager in today's America. Thus, vulnerable teenagers can respond to the adolescent who suicides as a reflection of themselves.

The suicide victim's activity provides psychological cohesion for the vulnerable teenager by providing the needed mirroring or merging experiences. Thereby, the sense of aloneness is mitigated. Such youths do not always meet DSM-III-R criteria for major affective disorders but are adolescents with varied types of character pathology. To be effective as clinicians, we must understand the nature of the pathological selfobject relationship that the disorganized, fragmented teenager forms with the suicide victim. Thus, we can develop a treatment and prevention strategy for intervention—for example, we must prevent the vulnerable teenager from establishing a selfobject relationship with suicide victims. We should assume that, with modern telecommunications, a multiple suicide will attract national attention. We should identify the unique components apparent in a suicide victim and determine the ways in which they can be experienced as potential idealizing functions or selfobjects by vulnerable adolescents. Additionally, we can provide help to schools, educators, and parents to be mindful both of the pain experienced by the specific child who died and of its possible effects. The aim of consultation should be to diminish idealizations of the suicide victim so as to sustain children in distinguishing their selves from that of the victim. Should a teenager be unable to sustain such differentiation, we must emphasize to all involved that the need for psychotherapy may be indicated.

In anticipating the tasks of young adulthood, an assessment of the stresses on high school students is indicated. The stresses can accumulate to derail a fragile adolescent from developing a cohesive self system. The capacity for decision making is involved in the process of selecting a suitable college and the kinds of activities to engage in and in dealing with an upsurge of sexual impulses. Frequently, the decision-making process about sexual activity and career planning may modify the stress as structure is strengthened by appropriate self-selfobject relationships. Such aspects of this process may be confronted before an effective self has been established. Although there are today smaller cohorts of teenagers, it is clear that we have increased the pressures on them, and the result can be observed in the breakdown of the self systems of many adolescents. This breakdown has led to increased psychiatric hospitalizations among our youths and a heightened risk of suicide in both adolescence and young adulthood.

In considering the adolescent process, the diagnostician becomes immediately involved in the assessment of adolescents' links to their family or, more specifically, their relationship with their parents. Their newly developed intellectual capacity enables adolescents to see more clearly the complex relationship between their parents and to view the distinction between the parents' marital relationship and their parental relationship with their children. Elsewhere, Cohen and Weissman (1984; Weissman and Cohen 1985) have written about the relationship between coparents and child. This relationship, the parental alliance, encompasses the unique relationship that maintains the focus of all three members on the developmental needs or experiences of the child. This parental alliance as a process develops prior to birth of a child. With the arrival of the child, it becomes a triadic system in which all members focus around the developmental needs of the child. This alliance and its stability become essential for adolescents. It contains the complex selfobject relationships that link them to their parents. In that aspect of the alliance, which contains the interactions of the parental couple, adolescents can observe and experience directly the continuous negotiations between parents on their behalf. They can observe that idealizations are neither unilateral nor static as two parents can idealize each other, agree with and rely on each other, and, yet at other times, strongly and deeply disagree but still value each other. In adolescents' observation and experiencing of this parental alliance, they both observe and experience affectively the vicissitudes of the human relationship, which provides much of the foundation of their later life relationships.

The parental alliance during adolescence (or childhood) has special significance in divorce. Adolescents can observe that in the marital relationship their parents may be in conflict but that some parents can separate parental concerns from marital ones and still use each other as idealized selfobjects in dealing with their children. The most profound breakdown in a parental alliance that young adolescents may face is in a custody battle. The involvement in such a dispute interferes with the essential selfobject experiences a child needs with each parent. The requirement to select one parent inevitably disrupts the idealization of the other parent.

Notably, the adolescent's enhanced cognitive capacities give additional meaning to the psychological concept of idealization. In the absence of the capacity for symbolic and abstract thinking, the idealizations of the child tend to be concrete expressions of positive characteristics of the idealized object. Negative views are kept psychologically separate. In adolescence, the child now has some new increased capacities to have a variety of idealized views of the parent and at the same time to maintain other views. A major task of adolescence is to integrate these diverse views of the parents into a new cohesive picture. The parental alliance provides a matrix out of which the adolescent can develop this new view of each parent. At the conclusion of adolescence, the individual can transform the earlier idealizations into an empathic appreciation of the psychological totality of the parents.

The Parents' Perspective

We have discussed adolescence from the perspective of the child. We will now address the issue of the adolescent from the vantage point of the parent. Elson (1984) has proposed that the appropriate way to view the relationship of the parent to the child, and the ensuing changes that occur in the parent as the child changes, is as a double helix. Just as the actions of the parents lead to changes in the self of the child, child rearing creates changes in the selves of the parents. In other words, the parents partially define a component of their selves by the relationship with the child. Earlier, we have proposed that the framework in which to examine the experiences of parenting is in the parental alliance. As already indicated, an effective parental alliance contends with the developmental needs of the child and sustains each parent to function effectively within this framework. The parental alliance is distinct from the marital alliance but is obviously, at times, influenced positively or negatively by the marital alliance. For example, a custody fight indicates disruption in both alliances. The parental alliance creates the matrix in which parenthood occurs. The individual parent addresses

161

an adolescent child's specific needs depending on the sex of the child and that parent's unique expectations for the child. The parent's past is played out in relationship with the specific talents and needs of the child, in concert with the parallel issues that the coparent brings to the adolescent period parenting experience. Others have written on how the parents of adolescents are asked to address the developing sexuality of a child at a time when they are dealing with changes in their own reproductive capacities (Cohen and Balikov 1974; Boxer et al. 1984). Furthermore, a child becomes a mature adult, with increased cognitive and physical capacities and an unknown, potentially promising future, when the parents must address the unique limitations in their own life situations—for example, their respective careers or their marriages.

These counterexperiences, or narrowing of opportunities in the face of widening opportunities for offspring, create ample tension and difficulty for the parent. The parents may seize on the child's future as a reparative experience and expect the child to attain all that they were unable to do. The parents, thereby, confuse their needs and ambitions with the child's and may push or lead the child toward a specific direction, in the belief that they only want the best for the child.

In early adolescence, parents have the opportunity to observe the child taking on the first attributes of adulthood. The child oscillates between not needing the parents and great dependency on them. The parents experience a similar oscillation, not knowing if they are dealing with a twenty-five-year-old or a five-year-old. The self of the parent must be flexible to experience these diverse shifts. Furthermore, the parent will be obliged to confront the child's deidealization as the one person who could control, interpret, and manage the child's entire world. The parent is expected to know empathically that this deidealization process is essential for the child to develop an effective, realistic, and coherent view of the parent and the world. To test their newfound cognitive abilities and to distinguish themselves from their parents, adolescents often challenge the parents' conceptualization of the world. Parents who fail in experiencing this as a transformational process tend to need the mutual earlier idealizations. Consequently, children can become vulnerable and dependent when it is essential that they become assertive in their own behalf.

Another risk for parents is to compare their own adolescent accomplishments as far above or below those of their children. Envy or disappointment may result. Additionally, with the child's physical growth, attainment of secondary sexual characteristics, and interest in the opposite sex, the parent has the pleasurable experience of the child's entry into a new developmental period. Because this particular period heralds new autonomy, engagement with the world largely outside of the family, the parent will now confront an uncharted course. The custodial parenting of carpooling is simpler than waiting up for children to come home from a first date. Thus, a new set of developments is required in the self of the parent. The parents must accede to a loss of control. Uncertainties await parents' experiences of themselves as parents. Moreover, the contemporary middle-class adolescent has liberal amounts of money to spend, and sexual activity occurs earlier than it did in the parents' adolescence. This may lead parents to challenge the views of the child as well as direct parents to review their own adolescence.

Although society has focused generally on the needs of the adolescent who goes through a transitional, tumultuous period, a closer examination reveals that the parent goes through a similar experience. The task of parenthood during this period is for the parents to continue to provide stabilization for the child and concurrently stabilize themselves. Here again, the parental alliance provides the sustaining support and psychological nurturance to withstand the deidealization and assaults from the once-loving child. Although this had been significant for parental stabilization in earlier developmental periods, it becomes more essential in adolescence. With the sustaining matrix of the parental alliance, the parent can more readily begin to experience the child as an independent source of initiative and, thereby, is able to provide the essential support to further sustain the child's growth.

During the intermediate phase of adolescence, the teenager begins to struggle more visibly with the shape of life in the future. In middle high school, the special talents of the child become more manifest. Academic performance is evaluated, career interests emerge, and the type of university to attend (or other future plans) is considered. Here, it is natural for adults to wish to be affirmed, or mirrored, by having the adolescent pursue their (the adults') careers. If these have been ungratifying ones, the parent may attempt to discourage the child from following a similar course. Thus, we observe the continuing demands made on the self of the parents. They must be able to acknowledge, appropriately affirm, and idealize the talents and abilities of a particular child and to disentangle their unfulfilled capacities and achievements

163

from the true attributes, wishes, and needs of the child. Most often, genetic endowments and the sharing of experiences and values, which had produced idealizations of the parent, will lead the child to pursue a course not markedly dissimilar to those of the parents. The parents, however, must resist the urge to direct. Designing and shaping are the tasks of the adolescent. In the parent of the middle adolescent, we can observe a shift in the self as a parent sustains an empathic stance with the evolving needs of the child. Earlier, parents could more clearly trace the success or failure of their "attunement" and connection to their children—because the demands were simpler, the clues were easier to see. Now, however, parents are being asked to empathize with the apparent needs of an almost adult, of one who strives to act and function as an adult but who as yet does not have the ability fully to proceed on that course.

We know now that effective empathy, or the process of providing an effective selfobject experience for another, requires some feedback or acknowledgment. Many years ago, clinicians assumed that the mothers of autistic children were detached because, when they were observed with their children, they appeared to be cold and aloof. Today, we know that the mothers' aloofness was a result of the child's inability to respond to the mother's attempt to sustain interaction. The aloofness is a withdrawal by the mother from the child's inability to acknowledge her presence. This process, regarding the child's influence on the parent, is part of what has been termed reciprocal socialization (Cook and Cohler 1986). The parent of the middle adolescent experiences a similar process. The child must solidify a self that can be sustained cohesively without perpetual reliance on the parent. Consequently, children may no longer respond affably to their parents' ongoing involvement with them. The parents of the autistic child must not withdraw their response to the child's apparent lack of interest or to not knowing what or how the child feels. It is the parental alliance that sustains the parent in this experience.

The Transition to Young Adulthood

At the last stage of adolescence, parents and child arrive at a watershed. Both generations experience doubt as to the child's readiness for launching—rather like the countdown for a spaceship, when all are poised in wait for action or delay. Unlike a rocket launch, however, we have no blueprint or checklist to determine a child's psychological equipment. There will be a significant degree of tension in the parent-child relationship, even in those situations in which all seems well. Now the parent must be prepared to address the child as an adult capable of making independent decisions, often with an awareness of a child's incomplete state of self. Furthermore, the child still remains dependent on the parent, and some are financially dependent for many years to come. The parent may be placed in the difficult situation of having to sustain a child who may pursue activities in which the parent does not agree.

The tasks of young adulthood for middle- and upper-class offspring are largely linked to two issues: (1) the pursuit of education and career training and (2) the establishment of an enduring sexual relationship. When these have been established, one can expect that the child is ready for peer-like interaction with his parents. This marks the beginning of a child's capacity to recognize the unique attributes of the parents with their assets and frailties. This indicates that the capacity for empathy has been established. Additionally, the child is now ready to provide stabilizing selfobject experiences for parents when a family crisis occurs.

Although a mutually empathic interrelatedness is not possible until young adulthood, parents must receive gratifying responses from children in order for them to sustain child rearing that is empathic with the developmental needs of the child. Here, again, Elson's (1984) concept of the double helix demonstrates that parents continuously change and grow in tandem with interactions with their children.

The child's capacity to empathize with the parents brings about an alteration in the parental alliance. In earlier years, the coparents served as empathic stabilizers for each other as the child's development unfolded. The young adult, as noted, is capable of providing a selfobject experience should a parent need one. This is apparent in the face of a serious illness or death of a parent. The young adult provides a variety of sustaining selfobject supports for the other parent for stabilization of the latter and the family. Indeed, this major change becomes the basis of the newly evolving relationship between child and parent when the child reaches adulthood. As numerous new life events unfold, the role of the parental alliance for child and coparents may be blurred. Any one of the three may provide an essential selfobject function for the other at a given moment. Children do not act as parents to their

165

parents. Rather, the children's new capacities allow them to become self-selfobjects to a parent because of their empathic attributes. When such empathic shifts have occurred, intergenerational bonds have been transformed so that family attachments are sustained. These new bonds persist within a peer-like status between parents and adult children. Linkages between them are sustained despite differences in developmental levels, geographic distances, and socioeconomic variations and even despite the multifarious effects of recent cultural and social changes.

From the clinical situation, the larger picture, which the research of the past two decades has drawn into focus, is often obscured. Parent–young adult solidarity emerges in the foreground as an important interpersonal bond in American culture (Cohler and Geyer 1982; Greene and Boxer 1986). The previous psychoanalytic paradigm indicating that separation and distancing from the family are the requirements and/or hallmarks of maturity is not congruent with the research findings. While during this period a child's assertion of self-initiative may result in unique career choices and selections of sexual and marital partners very different from those of the parents, the self-experiences of both generations continue in the process of transformation. Furthermore, choices that differ from parental "maps to maturity" need not be acts of rebellion. As new young adults move in an energetic fashion to achieve their goals and expand values and ideals, parents are not necessarily catapulted into a depleted state or into an unrelenting struggle to prevent this autonomy from occurring; nor are they extruded from the young adults' real and psychological lives.

First, this process, as stated, takes place over time, during which the parental selves, sustained and expanded by the parental alliance, have become enriched, more flexible, and able to look ahead to a pleasing and gratifying future, less restricted by active child rearing. This is critical in view of the increased life span that has become part of the current parent generation's internal map of the life course. Second, some new options for women have captured the fancy of middle-aged women, who look ahead to acquiring new skills and personal fulfillment. Moreover, a third factor, that of the mounting cost of higher education, has made middle-aged men and women both confront the realistic need for two parent incomes. A resilient parental alliance can provide the vitality and hope for a woman entering, or reentering, the labor market. This is not an aspect of the popularly debated issue, Can women have it all? but one of a new dimension of achieving family goals and values within a flourishing parental alliance.

Repeated research findings indicate that most mothers do not anticipate and experience the empty nest but look ahead to this phase with anticipation and hope (Campbell, Converse, and Rodgers 1976; Glenn 1975; Greene and Boxer 1986; Neugarten and Datan 1974). A new psychological interdependency occurs within the parental alliance, and a new maintenance of parental bonds and independent functioning can result for both generations. The double helix is ever operating within the framework of the triadic parental alliance. What must occur, essentially, is that both generations become responsive to their new mutual capacities for expanded initiatives as a peer-like parent-child bond evolves. Inherent in this process is the reciprocal task for both generations in transforming their former mutual idealizations into new forms of admiration. Physical departure from the home is not the underlying issue; rather it is the reworking of idealizations within both generations by which each is sustained as the anticipated shifts or stresses occur.

For the young adult, simultaneous role changes pile up, for example, new self-responsibilities in school, work, career, or vocational choice, more intimate love relationships, marriage, and parenthood. The parent generation, however, is not repudiated but is often relied on for support. The shifts experienced by the young adult self, as it seeks new objects, often create needs for aspects of parental approval, for example, touching home base occasionally.

In the clinical situation, we are often confronted by an intergenerational picture in which all members experience self-deficits and, therefore, the process is aborted or interrupted. The parent whose stability (need for mirroring) is invested in a child is bound to experience the latter's forays of self-initiative as disruptive and/or depleting. Similarly, the young adult whose advancing capacities cannot be sustained without parental partnering, both mirroring and idealizing, may lose vigor, feel depleted and hopeless, and experience inhibition in various sectors of life, for example, the proverbial areas of love and work.

We will, now, briefly review the effect of some psychosocial trends. Serious study of the effect of parental divorce on young adult offspring has just begun. In a recent study (Cooney, Smyer, Hagestad, and Klock 1986), it was reported that all freshmen in the year studied whose

167

parents were involved in recent divorces experienced a range of re-actions—from mild stress and a drop in academic functioning to more serious depression and eventual return to the home for either school or work. Indications were clear that the daughters reacted more than sons to mothers' needs and experienced more stress. Another phe-nomenon, known as the returning young adult syndrome (Schnaiberg and Goldenberg 1986), is being reported whereby career shifts, eco-nomic changes, self-deficits, divorce, and serious mental illness require return to the parental home. Many parents report distress because these returns had not been expected either financially or emotionally.

Special mention should be made of the effects of the reactions of mothers and young adult daughters in anticipating the effects of the new career options for women. Many mothers, who espouse ideals for upward mobility and achievement for daughters, react with depletion-type experiences as the daughters embark on life-styles that cannot mirror their own. Many daughters experience depression and inhibition as they are unable to receive idealization from their mothers. Fur-thermore, many such daughters fail to grant their mothers the self-initiative or determination they seek for themselves and continue to need parental mirroring. It is as though their mothers must continue a type of "idealizing" of their lives—which essentially amounts to mirroring-type approval—in order for them to succeed. Another ob-served clinical reaction in young adult women is guilt over abandoning or cheating their mothers should their variant life-styles create deple-tion states in them. Such mothers are unable to experience pleasures in their daughter's adult status because "difference" is experienced as "deviance."

Clinical Case 1

A twenty-eight-year-old doctoral student had gone into therapy at age twenty-three because of loss of vitality and enthusiasm for com-pleting doctoral work in a biological science. She completed that ther-apy, married a young man not as accomplished as she, but remained unable to complete her work. She came from a typical suburban en-vironment, and the academic career she chose displeased her parents, particularly her mother. Her father was more distressed that her hus-band, also an academic, could not ensure a high financial status. The patient presented with depression and anger that neither a previous therapist nor her husband had been useful in sustaining her self-esteem. She had postponed completing her own work by attaching herself to an admired female professor and became involved in the latter's work to the neglect of her own. She enjoyed the closeness with this woman, who was very cultured as well as important in her field. In spite of the disapproval of her academic advisers, she could not interrupt her work with the professor. The therapy focused less on oedipal issues and competition problems with father than on the patient's narcissistic vulnerabilities created by mother's inability to feel pleasure in the daughter's pursuits and to idealize her unique choice of life. This young woman had a lifelong history of self-vulnerability manifested in excessive need for approval and admiration. She remained stable as long as the mutual parent-child idealizations were intact. As the need arose for transformation of her mirroring needs into unique idealizable values and goals, she failed because she could not sustain cohesion without a mirroring selfobject. As the patient's self became firmer, it became necessary that she relinquish her arrogant grandiose fantasy that mother should become changed and model her (mother's) life, recreational pursuits, and personal tastes to match (mirror) the patient's. Many such untransformed grandiosities appeared in both generations. As the therapy proceeded, the patient modified her needs for a mirroring relationship and committed herself to a realistic career choice. Amusingly, she chose a higher-earning job in industry than could ever be achieved in academe and was quite cognizant of her "own bourgeois values." Also, the marital relationship improved as the patient's cohesion was solidified. She and the mother were able to establish a relationship in which each accepted generational value differences, largely because the patient became empathically tuned into the parents, who were planning their retirement.

Clinical Case 2

The following case example will highlight how leaving home to attend college precipitated a depression in both mother and daughter. The primary patient, an eighteen-year-old woman, was the fourth child in a sibship of five. Her parents are both professionals. The patient left home to attend a small college a short drive from her parent's home. Immediately on beginning college she had difficulty. During the first months, she had difficulty focusing on her studies. Eventually, she stopped attending classes, remained in her room, and spent most of her time in the dormitory. Although the first semester was not going well, she returned to school after the Christmas vacation. Two weeks after her return to school, she took an overdose of a tranquilizer and was hospitalized.

The past history revealed that as a high school student she was quite involved in managing the family home. It was the patient who frequently did all or most of the grocery shopping. She, in fact, functioned as mother and housekeeper for her siblings and for her mother. The prospect of leaving for college made her anxious. She was concerned about how her mother would handle the home in her absence. Increasingly, she became preoccupied with these concerns about her mother. She did not know with whom to talk, and the agitation increased. On returning home at Christmas, she observed that her mother was not doing well and concluded that it was her fault. In her absence, her mother had indeed become depressed and lost over twenty pounds. She returned to school, frightened and guilty, isolated herself further from peers, and finally overdosed.

The overdose was clearly a call for help. The initial thrust of the therapy was to address the patient's relationship with her mother and how the patient had functioned as an essential selfobject for her mother. By sustaining her mother, she confirmed her own fragile sense of self-esteem. In her absence, mother became depressed because of the lack of the essential selfobject functioning that the patient had provided. The patient became depressed because she did not experience the affirmation that caring for her mother supplied.

Needless to say, the father was essentially absent and had abdicated the supporting role to his daughter. In this family, in which both parental and marital alliances were absent, the father supported the daughter's maintenance of the mother's stability. More than merely sustaining the wife, the daughter was expected to preserve the father's functioning by protecting his need to remain outside the psychological functioning of the family. In essence, she performed sustaining selfobject functions for both parents.

The therapy focused on strengthening the patient's fragile self-esteem and exploring the enmeshment with her mother. It became clear that it was essential for the mother to obtain her own therapy, which she did. The salient issue in this case demonstrates how parents can utilize the competencies of a child to sustain their own functioning. Furthermore, as the adolescent caretaker leaves, the vulnerable parent inevitably becomes depleted and depressed. The child's self, which is affirmed by maintaining the parent, becomes clinically depressed.

In this family, the parents did not have an effective parental alliance in supporting the child; also, a deficient marital alliance directed that mother looked to the only daughter for various supports. The treatment focused on involving the father in a developmentally appropriate way with the daughter and engaging him more effectively to take responsibility for his wife's needs. After two years of therapy and three months of hospitalization, the patient completed her education at a different university. Presently, she is planning to attend graduate school.

Discussion

In the clinical situation, we often observe the absence of the parental alliance. It has been well documented that a continuous parental alliance when parents divorce is critical for the favorable development of children and adolescents. Although a critical developmental problem is not at stake, a young adult often reexperiences the pain of an absent parental alliance in the process of making graduation, wedding plans, and so on. If the earlier years were filled with the traumas of an absent parental alliance, such as in many divorces, a young adult awaiting a critical life event (such as a graduation or marriage) can experience a depleted affective state, though it may be transitional.

The widely accepted changes in the pathways to adult status for women, no longer a simple transferring of dependence from parents to husband, are requiring revised perceptions of how the new young adult generation will work, marry, and eventually parent. Although there will be class variations that give shape and contour to content and timing, most sectors of the parent generation will be affected. Once again, the parental alliance is effective in sustaining parental self-esteem systems as continuous shifts occur. As the high divorce rate continues, new permutations will inevitably occur because both generations may experience disrupted marital and parental alliances. We suspect that we will see more of this in the clinical situation. Wallerstein (1986) reports that her ten-year follow-up study of divorce indicates that, if the marital disruption occurs when women are forty or over, they tend to be disadvantaged in rebuilding their lives, psychologically and socially.

171

Undoubtedly, this will have an effect on adolescents and young adults, particularly females.

In the clinical situation, we see the distortions in self-efficacy that appear as young adults must act toward self-initiative. They must be able, moreover, to integrate the consequences of this for themselves as well as for their parents. Very often, as the nuclear self becomes firmer, changes in young adults help parents recognize that they must relinquish their directing roles and find new ways to reconnect with offspring. Thus, the children's firmness can become useful to the parents. The double helix continues to operate. Such, of course, will not prevail when the parent generation is seriously depleted and/or grandiose.

Conclusions

We have outlined the continuous process of self-transformation that occurs so that parents, adolescents, and young adult offspring can not only sustain but reshape their interdependence, their selfobject needs for each other, and the achievement of various alliances with individual parents and/or parental partners. We have suggested that many parents find enrichment and pleasure as their children move ahead to achieve self-directed lives. We have presented a review of the newly beginning research to support our argument. Additionally, we have presented clinical problems that manifest when the transformations are interrupted because the selfobject status of children and parents cannot conform to the developing tasks of young adulthood.

REFERENCES

Boxer, A.; Solomon, B.; Offer, D.; Petersen, A.; and Halprin, F. 1984. Parents' perceptions of young adolescents. In R. S. Cohen, B. J. Cohler, and S. H. Weissman, eds. *Parenthood: A Psychodynamic Perspective*. New York: Guilford.

Brown, T. A. 1988. Ships in the night: Piaget and American cognitive science. *Human Development* 31:60–64.

Campbell, A.; Converse, P. E.; and Rodgers, W. L. 1976. *The Quality of American Life*. New York: Russell Sage.

Cohen, R. S., and Balikov, H. 1974. On the impact of adolescence upon parents. *Adolescent Psychiatry* 3:217–236.

Cohen, R. S., and Weissman, S. H. 1984. The parenting alliance. In R. S. Cohen, B. J. Cohler, and S. H. Weissman, eds. *Parenthood: A Psychodynamic Perspective*. New York: Guilford.

Cohler, B. J., and Geyer, E. S. 1982. Psychological autonomy and interdependence within the family. In F. Walsh, ed. *Normal Family Process*. New York: Guilford.

Cook, J. A., and Cohler, B. J. 1986. Reciprocal socialization and the care of offspring with cancer and with schizophrenia. In N. Datan, A. L. Greene, and H. W. Reese, eds. *Life-Span Developmental Psychology: Intergenerational Relations*. Hillsdale, N.J.: Erlbaum.

Cooney, T. M.; Smyer, M. A.; Hagestad, G. O.; and Klock, R. 1986. Parental divorce in young adulthood: some preliminary findings. *American Journal of Orthopsychiatry* 56:470–477.

Elson, M. 1984. Parenthood and the transformation of narcissism. In R. Cohen, B. Cohler, and S. H. Weissman, eds. *Parenthood: A Psychodynamic Perspective*. New York: Guilford.

Glenn, N. D. 1975. Psychological well-being in the postparental stage: some evidence from national surveys. *Journal of Marriage and the Family* 37:105–110.

Greene, A. L., and Boxer, A. M. 1986. Daughters and sons as young adults: restructuring the ties that bind. In N. Datan, A. L. Greene, and H. W. Reese, eds. *Life-Span Developmental Psychology: Intergenerational Relations*. Hillsdale, N.J.: Erlbaum.

Holinger, P.; Offer, D.; and Ostrov, E. 1987. Suicide and homicide in the United States: an epidemiological study of violent death, population changes, and the potential for prediction. *American Journal of Psychiatry* 144:215–219.

Kohut, H. 1971. *The Analysis of the Self*. New York: International Universities Press.

Neugarten, B. L., and Datan, N. 1974. The middle years. In S. Arieti, ed. *American Handbook of Psychiatry,* vol. 1. New York: Basic.

Offer, D., and Offer, J. 1975. *From Teenage to Young Manhood: A Psychological Study*. New York: Basic.

Piaget, J. 1967. *Six Psychological Studies*. New York: Random House.

Schnaiberg, A., and Goldenberg, S. 1986. From empty nest to crowded nest: some contradictions in the returning-young-adult syndrome. Paper presented at the annual meeting of the American Sociological Association, New York, August 31.

Wallerstein, J. 1986. Women after divorce. *American Journal of Orthopsychiatry* 56:65–77.

Weissman, S. H., and Cohen, R. S. 1985. The parenting alliance and adolescence. *Adolescent Psychiatry* 12:24–45.

Wolf, E. 1980. On the developmental line of selfobject relations. In A. Goldberg, ed. *Advances in Self-Psychology.* New York: International Universities Press.

12 DEPRESSION IN THE TRANSITION
TO ADULT LIFE

EDWARD M. HALLOWELL, JULES BEMPORAD,
AND JOHN J. RATEY

Over the past decade, we have seen an increasing number of young
adults who present with depression in our clinical practice. These individuals were mostly successful, bright, and attractive, characteristics
that made their despair all the more irrational, yet poignant. While
quite aware of the higher prevalence of depressive disorders in socioeconomically deprived portions of the population, we were, and
continue to be, surprised at the magnitude of the dysphoria in such an
apparently enviable group of individuals as these young adults.

A further puzzling aspect of these individuals is a sense of emptiness
in their dissatisfaction and mental anguish. In contrast to the "classical" form of severe depression as described in older textbooks or as
still seen in more senior patients, in which the individual is tormented
by a sense of guilt or a conviction of personal malevolence, these young
adults do not particularly blame themselves for their plight. Rather,
while they convey a sense of shame over being depressed, which they
perceive as a manifestation of failure, they seem to complain of total
lack of meaning in their existence. They do not portray themselves as
great sinners or even as lacking one particular quality that would make
them feel justifiably adequate. What permeates their plight is a lack of
expectations from themselves and from their environment. There is a
hopelessness that is truly chilling in people so young and for whom the
future should still hold much promise. Some feel cheated by life or by
bad advice received in the past; others cannot understand their discontent; and still others do not even identify their being depressed,

being only aware of going through their daily life in a mechanical and detached manner.

In comparing notes with other practitioners, we were struck by the frequency that this type of patient was being seen by other colleagues as well. The frequency of this form of depression was further brought home to us in the works of Kohut (1977), who describes a modern form of "empty" depression. Others in the past have also elaborated on this form of dysphoria, but Kohut made this predicament a centerpiece of his theory.

We were finally convinced of the seriousness of this form of depression by results of epidemiological research studies on psychiatric illnesses, which were recently reported in the literature. This research involved a large number of centers across the country and studied the prevalence of various disorders in the general population. Major depressive disorders were found to be most frequent in young adults. This finding went against clinical lore that taught that severe depression was an illness of advanced age when hopelessness toward the future, regret for opportunities lost, lack of physical vigor, and accumulated losses of loved ones made this illness more justifiable and understandable. This finding of a greater prevalence of depression in young people also went against pure probability since older individuals, just by living longer, should have a greater chance of becoming depressed even if there were no developmental stage-specific predilection. Nevertheless, young adults showed the highest rate of depression—and severe depression at that (Robins, Helzer, Weissman, Orvashell, Grunenberg, Burke, and Regler 1984).

These findings matched our own observations and have caused us to look more closely at the transition from adolescence to adult life in contemporary society. Historically, adolescence has been seen as a time for troubled and troublesome individuals. Ever since Hall (1904) put adolescence on the map, this developmental stage has been characterized by stress, acting-out behavior, and high rates of psychopathology. Hall's seminal hypotheses were echoed by others who generalized to the whole population of teenagers on the basis of a relatively few disturbed youngsters who were being seen in psychotherapy. Further confirmation came from theoretical and research studies that suggested that during adolescence the emergence of genital sexuality upset the complacent equilibrium of the younger child and that true abstract thought made its appearance during this time, causing the individual to have to deal with unpleasant generalities of which, before, he could safely remain unaware.

In contrast, not much really new occurred during young adult life in terms of biology or cognition. This was the time to stop sowing one's wild oats and to settle down to sober, conforming, and productive adult life. Yet, as more studies were done on normal, and not disturbed, populations, adolescence began to look healthier and happier while young adult life appeared sicker and more miserable. Offer and Offer's (1975) studies on a sample of Chicago school teenagers revealed that the great majority progress through the adolescent years without much turmoil. On the other hand, retrospective studies of normal middle-aged adults often singled out young adult life as the most disturbed period of development. It would thus appear that this later stage may be the true Achilles heel of Western society.

It was to current society that we began to look for answers. One immediate possibility was that adolescence and all its former problems were being postponed for a decade or so as a result of prolonged schooling, later entry into the labor force, planned parenthood pushing child bearing and rearing into more mature years, and a greater afflu-ence allowing for a longer period of financial irresponsibility. If ado-lescence, as a developmental social stage, was created in the wake of the Industrial Revolution, was young adult life, as we know it, a result of a postindustrial, bureaucracy-predominated economy? Indeed, the gradual increase in age at which one finally gets down to the business of making a living has definitely created a class of "postadolescent adolescents." However, these were not the people we were seeing in our consulting rooms. Most had found their niche and make their mark. It was just this being settled, of feeling one had no alternatives, that so permeated their sadness. They displayed none of the sophomoric idealism of the younger folk and none of the optimism or fear that goes with it. Rather, there was a sense of cynical despair.

This pervasive malaise of having lost an essential part of one's moral, intellectual, or psychological self has been movingly portrayed in the film *The Big Chill*. The success, both critical and financial, of this movie attests to its ability to speak to young adults who closely identified with its protagonists. The film centers around a group of young adults who knew each other in college and are again united by the suicide of one of their group. Through a series of revealing psychological con-frontations, each character shows that he or she has left something

177

behind in college—that each has given up a vital part of himself or herself. Each has become aware of the cold indifference of the real world and of the cold indifference in oneself that has developed in response to that world. This is the big chill of the title, and its realization brings with it deep scars and deeper resentments. With the passage to adult life, each has lost the comfort and the spark of their former idealism. Our patients also complained of a troubled passage from adolescence to adult status, of a lost Eden of innocence suppressed beneath the harsh realities of the serious world.

We wondered if we were not witnessing a necessary coming to terms with life—a passage from the idealized to the real, from a life of principle to a life of compromise—that had always existed in the complexities of civilization. Indeed, there is evidence of the disenchantment that accompanied one's coming of age in the great literature of our forebears. However, one also senses that somehow it was easier then. Even in discussing this phenomenon with elderly or senior members of society, there is a recollection that, certainly, compromises were made and readjustments were necessary but that shared values or purposes smoothed the transition. The current cultural climate may not be the cause of our patients' plight, but this climate certainly intensifies the anguish of transition from youth to maturity.

From simply listening and attempting an understanding of what it means to be a young adult in today's world, we have compiled a list of factors that, according to these individuals, have played a role in shaping their inner lives. The list includes a multitude of "social facts" that were not really delineated as such but taken as a regular part of one's world. To an older "outsider," these factors do stand out; to our younger patients, they simply blend into the landscape of the eighties. We have found among contributory factors a lack of extended family; repeated moves in childhood; ambivalence in the mother's acceptance of her role; the influence of television on development in being the major representative of society; the cynicism of post-Vietnam and post-Watergate government; the decline of religion; the marked decrease of a sense of security in one's job or close personal relationships and, conversely, a corresponding decrease in a sense of loyalty to institutions or loved ones; an explosion of information that creates a constant anxiety over one's capabilities; a lack of respect for supervisors or senior citizens, who are perceived as dinosaurs rather than sages, and, with this disrespect, a fear of old age as representing obsolescence and uselessness; an absence of mentors or tradition; an ambiguity of sexual roles; and an ambiguity of the problem of evil with a relationistic condoning of immorality. It would appear that in the absence of, or at least in an age of decline of, traditional values, the self has assumed center stage.

As a way of developing our thesis—that we are seeing an overreliance on the self as a way of finding meaning in life and of creating and maintaining self-esteem—it is important to refrain from moralizing in elaborating the point. Once the phenomenon has been observed, it is inviting to veer off into a sermon on the selfishness of Yuppies, a sort of "O tempora, o mores!" expostulation. While that may even be edifying, it is not as interesting as the question of cause. Why, if Lasch (1979) is correct, has the "culture of narcissism" come to be? How has it grown out of what came before, and what are the implications for the understanding and treatment of depression in young adults? In order to develop possible answers to these questions and to illustrate our thesis anecdotally, we present some related clinical material.

Our first example derives from a meeting one of us had with the faculty of a private, coeducational elementary school in New England. The reason for the meeting was to discuss teaching as a career and for each member of the faculty to present parts of his or her own experience, both positive and negative. The school has a long history, so that two generations of teachers were represented, one group twenty-two to forty, the other forty to seventy-five. In addition, both sexes teach at the school.

The older teachers presented their stories first. The typical account was on the whole positive, affirming the traditional values associated with teaching, finding the work often exasperating and tiring but in the main rewarding and lively. "It has kept me young," many said. "I wanted a life of security and of teaching. That is what I have received."

The stories from the younger faculty differed considerably. Most expressed pleasure in actual teaching. However, most complained that teaching was only a small fraction of their job. There was a cynical sense of having been deceived into being glorified baby-sitters and a commonly expressed regret at not having chosen some fast-track, high-paying career. "We live in a time where it's the bucks that count," one said.

After selected faculty had presented their stories, there was group discussion. Strikingly, the younger group dominated. They did not want to hear from the older teachers. When one of the older group would speak, the younger group would visibly tune out so that soon the older ones would lapse into a wistful silence. As the discussion evolved, it became a kind of support group for helping the younger teachers cope with their general dissatisfaction with their careers.

In talking with these people individually, the older teachers expressed sorrow that teaching was not as gratifying to the younger ones as it had been to them. The younger teachers expressed anger and disappointment over their situation. "We're not a bunch of spoiled brats," one of them said. "It's just that the world is a very different place now than it was twenty-five years ago."

Now consider an individual case in psychotherapy. Mr. G is a twenty-six-year-old man who sought consultation because of problems in his romantic life. "The bottom line is that I'm unable to love anyone," he said in his first session.

The externals of his life sounded almost ideal. He was in perfect health and looked younger than his stated age. He was still an active basketball player, playing "just to show I'll never get old." He had built a highly successful business from the ground up. Five years of work had left him a very rich man in charge of a business he had created. He had an active social life, enjoyed sailing and tennis, and took regular vacations with his wife. His wife was attractive and capable. The only marital problem was Mr. G's growing unhappiness, the source of which he was unable to explain to his wife. So what was the problem? Why was he unhappy?

In looking more closely at his life, we found that he took pleasure in almost none of it. He told me about his work in approximately fifteen seconds, as if it were an everyday occurrence for a man to take himself from poverty to many millions by age twenty-six. When pressed he said, "Well, it's no big deal. It's basically dog work. What's it connected to? What does it mean? Nothing."

Basketball he used to like, but even that was becoming grueling because he pushed himself so hard. The tennis and sailing were "all for show," and the social acquaintances were "just that, acquaintances, people you have to have to make a business grow."

As for his wife, he said, "I feel sorry for her. I really do. I feel nothing toward her, and she deserves better than that. I have other women, and she pretends not to know, and I try not to show."

Growing up, he did not get much from his parents, both of whom had to work hard to make ends meet. "My father was basically a bastard. Still is. He told me I would never amount to anything, and as far as I'm concerned I still don't." Having relayed all this in a tense staccato-like voice, he asked, "Is there a cure for what I've got?"

As the therapy progressed, there emerged a pattern of repeated attempts to please the unpleasable, internalized father figure, with no soothing from the mother figure whom the patient rejected and devalued. He saw himself mainly in terms of an ego ideal that he could never live up to. Great achievements only left him hungry for more and too ashamed to reach out to others. Thus, he was chronically depressed, although highly successful. Rather than turning toward traditional sources of support—spouse, friends, community, church, clubs—he turned away from them, finding what they had to offer insipid and unreal. Repeatedly unable to acknowledge his dissatisfaction to anyone but himself, he grew ever more isolated, his genuine self severely mocking the social false self he adopted.

His depression and isolation begat desperation, which led to ever greater industry and activity, until he could bear it no longer and sought help. His appreciation of the irony of his situation—having it all but enjoying none of it—deepened as the therapy progressed, leading him to bitter condemnations of himself and thoughts of suicide. Inquiries as to whether he would act on his suicidal ideas led to curt, angry rebuffs of the therapist. "What do you care? Can you be sued if I kill myself? Will it hurt your reputation?" At the same time, the patient decided that he wanted to meet more frequently and that he wanted to solve his problems right away.

As we met more often, the patient began vigorously to devalue psychotherapy and the therapist. "Nice work if you can get it," became his mocking refrain for the job of being a psychotherapist. At the same time, he began to feel better. The thoughts of suicide abated as his anger found expression. One day, he made the following interpretation. "You know, coming in here and getting pissed at you feels a lot like what I do to myself every day. It makes me feel good, getting it off me and onto you. It's like you're a hooker and I can piss on you." He then associated to his wife and to his mother and began to feel sad over having rejected them, pissed on them. I reminded him that the refrain, "Nice work if you can get it," was a line from a love song.

Mr. G agreed that he had pissed on love, that whenever he felt it he scorned it. "Well, that is interesting," I said. "You used to say you never felt it at all."

Whereas Mr. G had presented as driven, self-absorbed, and feeling unable to love and empty, he now became quite filled—with anger and sadness. First he turned his anger on his father, then on the world. More and more, a genuine person was emerging from the shell.

As he began to connect more with his wife, she said she wanted a child, and he agreed. At this point, however, he became preoccupied with the dangers of current life, from pollution to AIDS, nuclear war, and the national debt. Over time this led to his becoming involved in a local chapter of an international disarmament organization. He said that his work there was better than therapy, and he began to find genuine meaning and support from that organization. It became a turning point in his psychotherapy and in his life.

He agreed to have a child. He cut way back on work and began to focus on his marriage and the disarmament group. He played less tennis but enjoyed it more. He developed—or regained, as he put it—a sense of humor, kidding and joking spontaneously. Although retaining an underlying pessimism about the world, he began to see reasons for hope. Soon he will terminate in therapy.

Turning to other examples, consider this material from the world of business. In our work consulting to various companies on the psychological issues of management, we are hearing of the pain involved in making layoffs and cutbacks, the agony of the process that is so euphemistically called "downsizing." At the same time, we are hearing of young people coming in, particularly to fields such as finance, corporate law, or high technology, who expect to make a great deal of money soon. These fast-trackers will give long hours and all the brain power they can muster, but they will not necessarily give, nor do they expect, loyalty, trust, or affection. They smirk at the idea of warmth in the workplace and trivialize it with demeaning terms like "touchy feely." When they come in for psychotherapy, their usual chief complaint is that of being on a treadmill or finding work cold, impersonal, and without meaning.

In making the transition from adolescence to young adulthood, the transition from college to career is the life-task equivalent. In fast-track business careers, we are seeing the transition managed cynically or, one might say, with psychological naïveté, in that these young people are not taking into account the psychic toll their pace will exact—and not only the toll their pace will exact but, more important, the lack of sustaining group identifications that go with it.

Their plan puts money above all else. To an ever-increasing number of adolescents, in our observation, success in adulthood means making a lot of money. The assumption is that whatever it takes to make the money, within the general bounds of law, will be worth it. When the money is made and the emotional depression hits, it is hard for these people to understand what went wrong.

Now, we are not implying that there is anything psychologically toxic about money. To the contrary, common sense alone reminds us that having money is better than not having money. However, what we are suggesting is that, owing to the general enervation and vitiation of heretofore fundamentally sustaining social institutions, young people are overloading personal success, particularly defined in terms of wealth, as a measure of self-esteem and happiness. There is much that is potentially self-deceptive in the whole process, much that is perilously subject to what Samuel Johnson (1749) called "The secret ambush of a specious prayer."

The depression in young adulthood then takes on the appearance of a grand masked ball. Everyone is dressed up and beautiful. No one recognizes anyone else. Everyone is in disguise, looking stylish and pleased. But behind the masks there is, at this masked ball, depression, ennui, and disappointment. All outward appearances contradict the inner sense of loss.

What loss could matter when so much has been gained? It is the loss of the dream, the loss of the sustaining ideal, the loss of the connectedness to something larger than self that affects these young adults so deeply. Fitzgerald (1920) evoked some of this mood at the end of *The Great Gatsby:* "And as I sat there brooding on the old, unknown world, I thought of Gatsby's wonder when he first picked out the green light at the end of Daisy's dock. He had come a long way to this blue lawn, and his dream must have seemed so close that he could hardly fail to grasp it. He did not know that it was already behind him, somewhere back in that vast obscurity beyond the city, where the dark fields of the republic rolled on under the night." It is out of the desperate attempt to regain that connectedness that has seen the epidemic growth of fad religions, fatuous causes, charismatic leaders, and a general cult of personality and attention to self such as this country has never seen before.

Although we are focusing on the transition to young adulthood, a stage recently popularized in the term "Yuppie" and portrayed in such movies as *The Big Chill,* the beginnings of this trend can be seen well before adolescence. Among many middle-class and affluent families, there is a preoccupation with children's achievements such that one wonders if kids can even play any more. There are admissions interviews for exclusive kindergartens. Parents angle and scheme to get their children into the right soccer camp or the best ballet school. Whereas families used to eat dinner together, now each member of the family is on his or her own schedule, dutifully trying to succeed. Just as the family is losing its ability to provide warmth and support, it is increasing pressure on children to succeed and achieve. The life of a child, particularly an affluent child, has become so fast paced, goal directed, and organized that there is little room for the relaxed meanderings of imaginative play or the high adventure of a day of playing hookey. It may be that the popular movie *Ferris Bueller's Day Off* was such a great hit because so many kids are itching to do it.

It is not surprising, then, to see many adolescents "tracked for success," to see money become a prime value, and to see depression commonplace when the transition is made to an age of full autonomy. It is not that anyone is to blame, that parents have become too selfish or children too ambitious, but rather that the same forces that are unpinning the rootedness of children, adolescents, and young adults are also having the same effect on their parents, forces mentioned earlier mainly having to do with the disintegration of meaningful group identifications. Parents still want the best for their children, and young people still bring the gusto and enthusiasm of childhood to whatever they do. It is rather that the changing social structures we have seen over the past three decades, while greatly enlarging economic opportunity, may not make for the greatest psychological health.

Having illustrated the situation with anecdotal material from the older end of the transitional period, let us briefly present the case of an adolescent heading into young adulthood. Susan P, a sixteen-year-old tenth grader, was seen in emergency condition following a suicide attempt. Susan was a very thin, strikingly attractive young woman who was a boarding student at a highly competitive preparatory school. Although she was very guarded at first, using indifference and nonchalance as a screen, over time she told an elaborate, intricately symbolic history of a series of feigned identities or conjured selves.

She had not wanted to go to boarding school. Once she got there, in the ninth grade, she felt tremendous pressure both from the general tone of the school as well as from herself to be someone special. Specifically, there was an English teacher at the school whom Susan fell in love with from afar, not having him in class, speaking to him only casually on the paths and in hallways. She found out everything she could about him from other students, other teachers, maintenance people, anyone. Over time she developed an ongoing melodrama around the teacher and his wife, whom she imagined to be a monster.

The situation went beyond a typical adolescent crush, if there is such a thing, as Susan began being different people on different weeks, one week a radical feminist, the next a reclusive Emily Dickinson, the next an aspiring Olympic equestrian. In fact, she was very good at playing these roles, and the school, teachers, and peers alike, rather than seeing her behavior as a sign of mental anguish, in fact looked forward to her weekly performances. She became the celebrity she had set out to be.

However, as the English teacher was not responding, she began to feel that she was not good enough for him, and she became enraged with the wife. This made her feel guilty, and she began to hurt herself, beginning with cigarette burns on the soles of her feet so that no one would notice, moving to smaller razor cuts on her wrists, finally culminating in the overdose.

In psychotherapy, what emerged, as one might expect, was that the drama at school was a displacement of feelings toward her parents. Even the roles she played had symbolic meaning. Her father loved Emily Dickinson; her mother scoffed at poetry, for example. But aside from the interesting particulars of the case, what was poignant, and for this chapter worth generalizing from, was her description of the desperate situation she saw herself heading into as she grew up.

Her mother, a housewife, had cautioned her from age three or four never to be a housewife. Father had told her from early on that she was special and would do great things, although she was not sure what. As the family moved often because of the father's business, Susan was sent off to boarding school as soon as possible, even though she felt a deep desire to remain at home, particularly with her father.

"The older I got the more I felt I was a misfit," she said. "I had no idea where I could fit in the world. I knew I was supposed to be great, whatever that means, and then when I hit this school with all its tradition and smart people, I could feel my mind almost snap. I just wanted to be warm and safe, and I thought Mr. Barklay [the English teacher] could do that for me. I felt ashamed of the part of me that liked horses and animals because that wasn't special or great. I felt ashamed of the part of me that was a woman. I felt so guilty and confused; I knew I was never going to fit in.''

Although her solutions were peculiar, her dilemma is not unusual. The role confusion, many women feel, is an issue still being worked out and having as much to do with social forces as intrapsychic ones. But the larger, more overriding problem Susan represents is the dilemma facing young men as well as young women. It is the dilemma of finding where one fits, the major developmental step from adolescence to young adulthood, without the social supports and directives that were present a generation or two ago.

Without social conventions and consistent directives, the main directive becomes simply success. Without religion, without extended and active family, without a sustaining group in general, the adolescent finds both the excitement of freedom of choice—we are living in a time of unrivaled opportunity to be whoever we want to be—as well as the burden of the self to live up to a host of expectations, both internally and externally imposed, often conflicted if not diametrically opposed.

Within many adolescents whose situation is not as desperate as Susan's and who, therefore, do not get help, there is a spring waiting to uncoil, a tension, a pressure to achieve beyond what is within their nature or disposition. In young adulthood, we see the depression that is the logical outcome of reaching a goal that was never meant to be. "Is that all there is?" It may be that this is nothing new. The pressure to find one's place and consolidate one's identity has caused stress and depression for as long as adolescence has been written about, and the prolongation of typically adolescent issues well into young adulthood is no recent phenomenon.

However, taking the end of the Viet Nam war as a point of reference, there has been significant rearrangement of formal and informal structures of interpersonal life. Many who began to come of age during that war found that when it ended they changed their values and goals quite dramatically, away from group identifications and affiliations toward individual achievement and a reliance on the self. The years of that war understandably engendered a mistrust in government, a questioning of the value of self-sacrifice, and a pleasure ethic that led to such labels as "the Me Generation."

Now, having pursued those self-oriented goals, and having achieved much material success, they are seeing more of the dark side of that approach, a depression among affluent young people who feel that their lives lack higher meaning while at the same time finding the conventional sources of such meaning worn out or obsolete.

We think of the young school teachers we presented earlier, earnest and idealistic on the one hand but angry and cynical on the other, wanting to go on teaching but feeling exploited and lacking the general supports the older teachers all but took for granted in their way of life. Or we think of our patient Mr. G, who as soon as he began to allow his real self to emerge became preoccupied with the dangers of the current world for himself and his child. Whether it be a mammoth national debt waiting to destroy us economically, or stockpiled nuclear weapons waiting to blow us up, or AIDS waiting to wipe us out in a plague, he saw so much danger as to wonder if life were not better lived in a cloud of driven selfhood.

Conclusions

All this is not so much the depression of the narcissistic personality, intrapsychically caused, leading to an inability to love as it is the depression of a society in flux, "wandering between two worlds," to use Matthew Arnold's (1852) phrase, "one dead, / The other powerless to be born." Our social structures have not caught up with the changes in individual freedom and opportunity. Many young people are finding, in their determination to have it all, that they have lost a great deal. One thinks of the words of T. S. Eliot (1935), "The last temptation is the greatest treason: / To do the right deed for the wrong reason."

REFERENCES

Arnold, M. 1852. The buried life. In M. H. Abrams, gen. ed. *The Norton Anthology of English Literature*. 2d ed. New York: Norton, 1968.
Eliot, T. S. 1935. *Murder in the Cathedral*. San Diego, Calif.: Harcourt, Brace, Jovanovich, 1964.

Fitzgerald, F. S. 1920. *The Great Gatsby.* New York: Scribner.

Hall, G. S. 1904. *Adolescence.* New York: Appleton.

Johnson, S. 1749. The vanity of human wishes. In M. H. Abrams, gen. ed. *The Norton Anthology of English Literature.* 2d ed. New York: Norton, 1968.

Kohut, H. 1977. *The Restoration of the Self.* New York: International Universities Press.

Lasch, C. 1979. *The Culture of Narcissism.* New York: Norton.

Offer, D., and Offer, J. 1975. Three developmental routes in normal male adolescence. *Adolescent Psychiatry* 4:121–141.

Robins, L. N.; Helzer, J.; Weissman, M.; Orvashell, H.; Grunenberg, E.; Burke, J.; and Regler, D. Lifetime prevalence of specific disorders in three sites. *Archives of General Psychiatry* 41:949–958.

13 SOCIOLOGICAL FACTORS ASSOCIATED WITH SUBSTANCE ABUSE AMONG NEW CHRONIC PATIENTS

LEONA L. BACHRACH

This chapter discusses the service deficits and service needs of a subgroup of chronic mental patients who have been the subject of considerable attention in the United States in recent years—the so-called new chronic patients who are variously described in the literature as being volatile, difficult to reach, difficult to serve, and extremely stressful to mental health service systems. Since I am a sociologist by training, not a clinician, my approach to the subject of these new chronic patients will be a contextual one, not a clinical one. Accordingly, my primary concern will be with the climate within which psychiatric and support services for these patients are planned and delivered, not with treatments per se.

In this country, new chronic patients are often called "young adult chronic patients" (Pepper, Kirshner, and Ryglewicz 1981). In England, the same individuals are more likely to be called "new long-term patients"—that is, patients who have long-term needs for psychiatric and support services but who, unlike earlier generations of chronic mental patients, will probably spend very little time, perhaps no time at all, as residents of state mental hospitals (Shepherd 1984; Wing and Morris 1981).

The topic of young adult chronic patients entered the psychiatric literature largely as the result of the substantial efforts of Pepper and his colleagues. These authors had articulated some very basic concerns that were beginning to trouble psychiatric service providers all over the country. In effect, Pepper and his colleagues told those service providers that they were not alone, that other people were just as bemused by the emergence of this patient population as they were.

Today, many clinicians and service planners continue to find Pepper's work seminal and valuable. Numerous articles and collections of papers on the subject of young adult chronic patients (e.g., Pepper and Ryglewicz 1982, 1984a; *The Young Adult Chronic Patient,* n.d.) have appeared in the literature. However, the concept is not without controversy (Bachrach 1984a; Wintersteen and Rapp 1986), and some individuals are adopting other terminology to describe these patients. Thus, even though I have myself published several articles with the term "young adult chronic patient" in their titles (Bachrach 1982a, 1982b, 1984a, 1984b), I have in recent years referred to these individuals simply as "new chronic patients" or "new long-term patients" (Bachrach 1986), largely because Pepper's original cohort and others like it have begun to age. Some of those patients are now in their forties, are growing older, and continue to experience the kinds of problems I shall be describing in this chapter, even though they are no longer young. That should be a warning to us.

A Deinstitutionalized Generation

Who exactly are these new chronic patients? Practically every reference to them in the literature comments generally on the fact that they have a wide variety of serious problems and more specifically mentions substance abuse as a major problem. Beyond this, these patients appear to have the same range of illnesses that other chronic mental patients do. They are most often diagnosed with schizophrenia, although many are manic depressive; and, in some communities, substantial numbers are diagnosed with personality disorders.

Thus, what distinguishes these new chronic patients from chronic mental patients of the past is not their diagnostic distribution per se but rather their aggregate demand for services and their unique effect on the psychiatric service system. These patients are approaching the service system in a whole new way—one might even say with a vengeance. It is not at all surprising that a program administrator in the state of North Carolina has referred to them as a "mutant strain" of psychiatric patient (E. Thomas, personal communication, 1981)—mutant not in any biological or genetic sense but simply in terms of their effect on the psychiatric service system.

190

Yet, the arrival of these patients should not have taken us by surprise. We should have been able to see them and their very special problems approaching, for, to a certain extent, they were quite predictable. However, we had our blinders on, and we simply did not anticipate either their arrival or their full effect.

Why should we be interested in these new chronic patients as a separate entity? What is so special about them? The fact is that these patients represent a truly deinstitutionalized population. They are what deinstitutionalization is all about: they are the first generation of chronic mental patients who generally, since the onset of their illnesses, have lived exclusively in an era of deinstitutionalization. In other words, they are the generation that, in the optimism of the 1960s, was going to be the beneficiary of noninstitutional—and what we thought of then as nonrestrictive—care (Bachrach 1982b). Thus, the new chronic patient typifies the deinstitutionalized patient of today and also of tomorrow, and his or her problems in receiving adequate services reflect all the major problems that have come home to roost with the deinstitutionalization movement.

When these new chronic patients are enrolled in psychiatric services, they tend to be pervasive users of the service system. They use the full range of psychiatric facilities, so that we find them in state mental hospitals, in general hospitals, in community mental health centers, in private psychiatric hospitals, and in all types of outpatient psychiatric facilities.

At any given time, however, a substantial portion of the population of these new chronic patients is not enrolled in any psychiatric facility at all and so is essentially unserved by the psychiatric service system. Growing numbers of these individuals are vagrant street people (Prevost 1982), although, of course, not all street people are mentally ill.

Those new chronic patients who do utilize the psychiatric service system tend to do so in a "revolving door" manner, and they frequently move around among facilities. They often utilize the criminal justice system in addition to, or else in place of, the mental health service system and often end up in jails and other correctional facilities.

In many communities, these new chronic patients become general hospital emergency room regulars (Chafetz and Goldfinger 1984). However, their referral out of the emergency room to other facilities tends to be very problematic because these patients are often difficult to engage in treatment and because they appear to have no established

191

niche within the psychiatric service system. This is probably at least in part a function of certain characteristics that many of these new chronic patients share. They are described throughout the literature as having a high risk for suicide, very fragile ego development, and extreme vulnerability to stress and personal rejection. They are, in short, prototypical "difficult" patients whose needs often exceed the tolerances of service delivery agencies (Bachrach, Talbott, and Meyerson 1987).

Indeed, not all chronic mental patients of the 1980s fit this very general description. Some of today's chronic mental patients seem to respond quite favorably to services as they are being developed and offered in our deinstitutionalized service systems. This only makes the more difficult to serve new chronic patients—those who are characterized by volatility and noncompliance, those who insist on receiving, but who regularly reject, a wide variety of service interventions—stand out in bold relief.

Ely (1985) has written a characterization that fits at least a portion of this patient population whom she calls "schizopaths"—that is, "young adults who have been diagnosed as chronic schizophrenics but who, in remission, often present as character-disordered or sociopathic individuals. They regularly abuse drugs and alcohol and generally appear to be wending their way through life via manipulation, deceit, and bravado. However, this unsavory facade is quite fragile. These individuals do not have the emotional backup to sustain such characterological maneuvers. They are empty, sad, vulnerable people who desperately use every shred of ego strength available to them to survive" (p. 6).

Service Delivery Problems

As discussed, a common theme in the literature on these new chronic patients is the difficulties that they typically pose for clinicians and for service systems. Service providers throughout the United States seem to experience a great deal of trouble and frustration when they attempt to plan services for, and deliver services to, these individuals. Thus Harris and Bergman (1979) have written, "After several rounds of bouncing between hospital and community, no one expects these patients to change. They are treated perfunctorily by a staff that is too discouraged to do more than go through the motions" (p. 6). Similarly, an article by Robbins, Stern, Robbins, and Margolin (1978) describes these patients in New York City as being surly individuals whom staff perceive as "negativistic, difficult, and frightening" (p. 44).

These two descriptions from inner-city service settings, however, tell only part of the story, for new chronic patients are not an exclusively urban phenomenon. They are also found in suburban communities (Steyn 1981) and in rural places. Robert DeForge (personal communication, 1981), a county mental health official in Washington County, Vermont, reports that these patients regularly migrate into his very rural community from a variety of points along the Eastern seacoast. Once they arrive in Vermont, they impose severe stresses on the service system.

There seem to be two major reasons for the increasing prominence of these new chronic patients in the population in the 1980s. In part, they represent the group of individuals who probably would have been institutionalized twenty-five or thirty years ago. Today, very much as the result of deinstitutionalization policies and practices, these patients have assumed increasing visibility in the psychiatric service system (Bachrach 1982b). They are no longer confined to state mental hospitals for long periods of time. In fact, in many communities, a sizable portion of new chronic patients never enter state hospitals at all, as the result of what are sometimes euphemistically called "admission diversion policies." These policies, which deflect admissions away from state mental hospitals, are directly attributable to deinstitutionalization philosophy (Bachrach 1978). Yet, very often, the facilities to which new chronic patients might be diverted exist only in fantasy.

It is exceedingly important, however, to note that these new chronic patients are not entirely an artifact of deinstitutionalization. There is a second reason for their emergence, one that has to do with the changing demography of the United States. These patients are drawn largely from the postwar, baby-boom generation. Their numbers have been accumulating as successive cohorts of baby-boom babies have been reaching the primary ages for onset of the major psychiatric illnesses. In other words, these patients are having a marked effect on our psychiatric service systems in the United States today simply because there are a great many of them around and they are no longer hidden in state mental hospitals (Bachrach 1982b).

The Sociology of Patient Care

Obviously, these observations should be matters of profound concern to people charged with organizing and delivering care to chronic mental patients today. It would seem essential that an understanding of these matters precede service planning. But often, unfortunately, that kind of understanding is lacking, largely because planning authorities have generally paid little attention to the sociology of service delivery, to the broad context in which services are delivered to chronically mentally ill individuals.

More specifically, service planners have too often ignored the fact that, as the result of deinstitutionalization philosophy, the context of patient care has changed dramatically—and not always for the better. For better or worse, the state mental hospital in the "old days" provided clearly outlined rules of behavior for both patients and staff. Patients knew precisely who they were and what was expected of them, and their roles were well defined. They knew the "rules of the game."

By contrast, in today's systems of care, we give patients few clues about how they should behave. In fact, we have largely replaced such clues with mixed messages. We may, for example, instruct the patient to behave like a patient because he or she is a sick individual—but then fail to provide the structure or the milieu in which acting like a patient has any real meaning. Or we may ask the patient to accept the role of patient voluntarily for the benefits that that role will confer on him or her. But the patient role is one that is full of ambiguity, stigma, and diminished opportunity. We must not be surprised when the patient refuses to accept it.

Indeed, it seems as if, in the absence of a clearly defined patient role, today's new chronic patients look to one another for reinforcement. Not being primarily institutionalized, these patients now have peers outside the hospital with whom they share a common culture—a culture that tends to differ materially from the cultural exposures of most mental health professionals. Today's new chronic patients often live together in the community. Sometimes they travel together and serve to reinforce one anothers' pathologies. Now we are beginning to discover, often to our dismay, that their fertility experience is quite marked in some places and that they are beginning to have babies of their own (Pepper and Ryglewicz 1984b; Test, Knoedler, Allness, and Burke 1985).

Another mixed message that we give to chronic patients in our evolving psychiatric service systems has to do with some rather serious ambiguities about where they fit into society. One of the early goals for deinstitutionalization was to "normalize" patients, and, in fact, normalization continues to be a buzzword in some quarters today. Many professionals as well as civil libertarians like the sound of that word and what it implies: civil liberty and equal opportunity for people who, through no fault of their own, are chronically ill and disabled.

But what does it really mean to normalize people who have chronic and disabling mental illnesses? Are we, in fact, necessarily doing them a favor when we attempt to normalize them? Certainly, in some instances, the answer to this question must be a negative one. By promoting normalization for some members of the chronic patient population, we are merely delivering very confusing messages to them. These messages may even be, at least at times, potentially harmful ones.

It seems to come down to this in many cases: we have instructed our new chronic patients to do what everyone else does. And, for people who are chronically mentally ill and often young, doing what everyone else does may have some very special, and not always very happy, implications.

For example, doing what everyone else does might mean moving around a great deal, being geographically mobile. According to the Census Bureau, the age groups with the highest rates of geographic mobility in the United States consist of young adults. When we tell chronic patients to behave like other people their own ages, we are probably thus promoting gross migration patterns among individuals who are chronically mentally ill, who are desperately in need of continuity in their care, and who would almost certainly be better off staying in one place where they can establish a therapeutic relationship (Bachrach 1987). Doing what everyone else does might also mean, particularly among younger adults, using alcohol and street drugs recreationally. In addition to their primary mental illnesses, we find that these new chronic patients have a distressingly high prevalence of substance abuse.

Thus, although moving around from place to place and using alcohol and street drugs might be very normalizing, they are not good medicines for schizophrenia. It appears that the philosophy of normalization, whatever benefits it might confer on people who have chronic mental illnesses, has also created something of a monster in our mental health service systems.

Substance Abuse in the New Chronic Patient Population

The dilemma that these circumstances pose has been discussed by Bergman and Harris (1985), who describe the elements of comprehensive care for new chronic patients (see O'Connor 1987). These investigators show that 60 percent of their patients, all people who are severely and persistently mentally ill, have histories of substance abuse. What is especially interesting in the Bergman and Harris data is the finding that their patients deliberately and knowingly conform to the social norms that prevail in the neighborhoods where they live—norms that, in the words of these investigators, "condone substance use and, to some extent, substance abuse." When these patients use drugs, they thus consider themselves to be "a part of the neighborhood mainstream" (p. 53)—a very normalizing outcome!

Drug involvement is not merely something that is part of the mainstream culture; it has also become very much a part of the patients' own peer culture—hardly a surprising development. Bergman and Harris (1985) write that, although some of their patients may use drugs in an effort at self-medication, by far the major reason for their doing so is "to be part of a peer group." These patients clearly regard drugs as simply "an integral part of their social life" (p. 52), and they feel themselves to be under considerable pressure to participate in the culture of their peers.

Bergman and Harris have also found that their patients generally lack insight into the effects that drugs may have on the course of their illnesses. By and large, they are not aware that drug use can complicate already debilitating psychiatric conditions. Bergman and Harris (1985) explain the dilemma that is inherent in this situation: "Young adult chronic patients are also young adults. They find themselves struggling with the common social problems encountered in the late 20s and early 30s. Though they have typical reasons to use drugs (to be sociable or to relieve anxiety), they unfortunately have atypical responses to such use" (p. 53).

Often the psychiatric service system fails deplorably in its attempts to reach these new chronic patients. Indeed, it frequently creates insuperable barriers to care. One such barrier that merits particular attention is the categorical nature of many programs that serve—or *should* serve—new chronic patients. Being who they are and what they are, these patients easily fall through the proverbial service system "cracks." They do not belong in substance abuse programs because they are chronically mentally ill, and they do not fit in with other chronic mental patients because of what their exposure to alcohol and other substances does to them and to their behavior (Bachrach 1986).

New chronic patients, in short, are multiply disabled individuals whose many disabilities interact dramatically to limit their access to care. Some of their disabilities result from their primary psychiatric illnesses, but others are the tertiary disabilities described by Shepherd (1984) and Wing and Morris (1981)—culturally and societally induced disabilities that are external to the patients themselves and serve as major barriers to care.

The New Chronic Patient as a "Difficult" Patient

The problems associated with serving new chronic patients in today's psychiatric service systems are clearly related to their status as "difficult" patients—that is, patients who are noted for their treatment resistance and intractability. A recent review of the literature (Bachrach et al. 1987) suggests that there are actually three different sources of difficult patienthood, all of which are amply illustrated in the case of new chronic patients.

First, patients may be viewed as difficult because they have special attributes—special characteristics or behaviors—that differentiate them from other (i.e., nondifficult) patients. Thus, the literature generally portrays difficult patients as being more demanding, more puzzling, less likely to evoke empathy, more dangerous to themselves and others, more attention seeking and manipulative, more likely to polarize staff, more technically difficult as psychiatric cases, and more likely to misuse medication than nondifficult patients (Neill 1979).

Second, patients may be viewed as difficult because clinicians see them that way—because of a perceptual bias on the part of service providers (Link and Milcarek 1980; Smith and Steindler 1983; Stern and Minkoff 1979). Indeed, there is a reciprocity between the first and second sources of difficult patienthood so that, in practice, it is generally very difficult to separate specific patient attributes from the clinical context in which they occur. Indeed, patient attributes are difficult only contextually; they are troublesome only when they are understood to be troublesome. Specific attributes may thus be necessary, but they are most certainly not sufficient conditions for the definition of difficult patienthood.

Accordingly, a major portion of difficult patienthood resides in clinicians' expectations—in clinicians' idealized images of what patients ought to be. Jeffery (1979), a British sociologist, reports that hospital personnel generally classify patients as difficult when those patients break certain unwritten "rules" that dictate the course of their illnesses. Among these rules are that medical staff will be fully capable of treating the patient's illness, that the patient will regard his or her illness as an undesirable state that must be eliminated, and that the patient will cooperate fully with hospital personnel.

Finally, patients may be viewed as difficult because they are "system misfits"—that is, because they are individuals whose needs somehow exceed the capacities of the service system (Beeson 1983; Johansen 1983). This is particularly true with new chronic patients who are reaching maturity at a time when the psychiatric service system is undergoing radical change. Efforts to implement deinstitutionalization policy are still being tested, and the system is seeking an equilibrium that is proving more difficult to attain than the architects of the movement anticipated it would be. In this time of trial and error, the system of care often has little to offer new chronic patients. It even lacks a cohesive set of "rules" that might allow these patients to seek and establish their identity as patients. The inevitable mixed messages often encourage new chronic patients in behaviors like substance abuse that are nontherapeutic at best and destructive at worst. It is hardly surprising, given these circumstances, that these patients are often perceived as intolerable system stressors (Wilder and Karasu 1977).

Conclusions

New chronic patients are clearly individuals whose difficulties must be confronted in a variety of ways. They require therapeutic interventions that will modify the specific attributes that render them difficult,

198

but such therapeutic interventions represent only part of their needs. They also require clinicians who are able to tolerate them and who will attempt to work around and through their intractability. They certainly require service systems that can somehow neutralize, or at least minimize, the external barriers to their care (Bachrach 1982a).

It is thus critical, in seeking to meet the needs of these new chronic patients, to remember that many of the problems they face are related to the context in which care is provided. We cannot overlook these contextual sociological concerns if we mean to serve new chronic patients sensitively and effectively.

NOTE

Presented at the annual meeting of the American Society for Adolescent Psychiatry, Chicago, May 9, 1987.

REFERENCES

Bachrach, L. L. 1978. A conceptual approach to deinstitutionalization. *Hospital and Community Psychiatry* 29:573–578.

Bachrach, L. L. 1982a. Program planning for young adult chronic patients. In B. Pepper and H. Ryglewicz, eds. *The Young Adult Chronic Patient*. New Directions for Mental Health Services, no. 14. San Francisco: Jossey-Bass.

Bachrach, L. L. 1982b. Young adult chronic patients: an analytical review of the literature. *Hospital and Community Psychiatry* 33:189–197.

Bachrach, L. L. 1984a. The concept of young adult chronic psychiatric patients: questions from a research perspective. *Hospital and Community Psychiatry* 35:573–580.

Bachrach, L. L. 1984b. The young adult chronic patient in an era of deinstitutionalization. *American Journal of Public Health* 72:382–384.

Bachrach, L. L. 1986. The context of care for the chronic mental patient with substance abuse problems. *Psychiatric Quarterly* 58:3–14.

Bachrach, L. L. 1987. Geographic mobility and the homeless mentally ill. *Hospital and Community Psychiatry* 38:27–28.

Bachrach, L. L.; Talbott, J. A.; and Meyerson, A. T. 1987. The chronic psychiatric patient as a "difficult" patient: a conceptual analysis. In

A. T. Meyerson, ed. *Barriers to Treating the Chronic Mentally Ill.* New Directions for Mental Health Services, no. 33. San Francisco: Jossey-Bass.

Beeson, P. G. 1983. The bureaucratic context of mental health care. In W. B. Littrell, G. Sjoberg, and L. A. Zurcher, eds. *Bureaucracy as a Social Problem.* Greenwich, Conn.: JAI.

Bergman, H., and Harris, M. 1985. Substance abuse among young adult chronic patients. *Psychosocial Rehabilitation Journal* 9:49–54.

Chafetz, L., and Goldfinger, S. 1984. Residential instability in a psychiatric emergency setting. *Psychiatric Quarterly* 56:20–34.

Ely, A. R. 1985. Long-term group treatment for young male "schizopaths." *Social Work* 30:5–10.

Harris, M., and Bergman, H. 1979. *Coordination of Inpatient Hospitalization and Community Support Programs: An Integrated Systems Approach.* Washington, D.C.: St. Elizabeth's Hospital.

Jeffery, R. 1979. Normal rubbish: deviant patients in casualty departments. *Sociology of Health and Illness* 1:90–107.

Johansen, K. H. 1983. The impact of patients with chronic character pathology on a hospital inpatient unit. *Hospital and Community Psychiatry* 34:842–846.

Link, B., and Milcarek, B. 1980. Selection factors in the dispensation of therapy: the Matthew effect in the allocation of mental health resources. *Journal of Health and Social Behavior* 21:279–290.

Neill, J. R. 1979. The difficult patient: identification and response. *Journal of Clinical Psychiatry* 40:209–212.

O'Connor, J. 1987. Program connects community, chronically mentally ill. *Psychiatric News* (May 1), pp. 7, 34.

Pepper, B.; Kirshner, M. D.; and Ryglewicz, H. 1981. The young adult chronic patient: overview of a service population. *Hospital and Community Psychiatry* 32:463–469.

Pepper, B., and Ryglewicz, H., eds. 1982. *The Young Adult Chronic Patient.* New Directions for Mental Health Services, no. 14. San Francisco: Jossey-Bass.

Pepper, B., and Ryglewicz, H., eds. 1984a. *Advances in Treating the Young Adult Chronic Patient.* New Directions for Mental Health Services, no. 21. San Francisco: Jossey-Bass.

Pepper, B., and Ryglewicz, H. 1984b. Treating the young adult chronic patient: an update. In B. Pepper and H. Ryglewicz, eds. *Advances in Treating the Young Adult Chronic Patient*. New Directions for Mental Health Services, no. 21. San Francisco: Jossey-Bass.

Prevost, J. A. 1982. Youthful chronicity: paradox of the 80s. *Hospital and Community Psychiatry* 33:173.

Robbins, E.; Stern, M.; Robbins, L.; and Margolin, L. 1978. Unwelcome patients: where can they find asylum? *Hospital and Community Psychiatry* 29:44–46.

Shepherd, G. 1984. *Institutional Care and Rehabilitation*. London: Longman.

Smith, R. J., and Steindler, E. M. 1983. The impact of difficult patients upon treatment. *Bulletin of the Menninger Clinic* 47:107–116.

Stern, R., and Minkoff, K. 1979. Paradoxes in programming for chronic patients in a community clinic. *Hospital and Community Psychiatry* 30:613–617.

Steyn, R. 1981. Tomorrow's patients: our changing patient population. *Advance* (Virginia Department of Mental Health and Mental Retardation) (Summer–Fall), pp. 15–17.

Test, M. A.; Knoedler, W.; Allness, D. J.; and Burke, S. S. 1985. Characteristics of young adults with schizophrenic disorders treated in the community. *Hospital and Community Psychiatry* 36:853–858.

Wilder, J. F., and Karasu, T. B. 1977. Games institutions play: an exclusionary plot. *Hospital and Community Psychiatry* 28:459–460.

Wing, J. K., and Morris, B. 1981. Clinical basis of rehabilitation. In J. K. Wing and B. Morris, eds. *Handbook of Psychiatric Rehabilitation Practice*. Oxford: Oxford University Press.

Wintersteen, R. T., and Rapp, C. A. 1986. The young adult chronic patient: a dissenting view of an emerging concept. *Psychosocial Rehabilitation Journal* 4:3–13.

The Young Adult Chronic Patient: Collected Articles from "Hospital and Community Psychiatry." N.d. Washington, D.C.: American Psychiatric Association Hospital and Community Psychiatry Service.

14 JOSEPH CONRAD'S *THE SHADOW LINE:* FROM LATE ADOLESCENCE TO EARLY ADULTHOOD

Joseph Conrad's short novelle *The Shadow Line,* written in 1915, is a masterful, artistic rendering of the transition from late adolescence to early adulthood. For the adolescent clinician, *The Shadow Line* provides a rich "museum" of late adolescent developmental conflict and provokes a number of questions regarding this phase of human development.

On the surface, *The Shadow Line* is a simple tale. It tells the story of a young sailor with a secure position as a chief mate on a ship in the East Indies. He becomes overwhelmed with the ennui of his position and, in adolescent fashion, impulsively resigns. Though he can fault nothing on his previous ship—the owners, the crew, the ship itself—he feels driven to leave. He intends to give up the sea life and return to shore and "drift," without a clear goal. By chance, he is offered his "first command" (Conrad's alternate title for the work) and is forced, in assuming command, to experience a series of traumas and developmental struggles that bring him to a greater maturity.

His maiden voyage is marred by an outbreak of malaria, which leaves his crew weak and delirious. His supply of quinine, his only hope, has been tampered with and is useless. Moreover, the winds do not favor the young captain; he is plagued by utter calm for over two weeks, as his ship lies stranded at sea and disease overcomes his crew. He fights a parallel battle, too, with his crew's animistic belief in the supernatural. His chief mate, Mr. Burns, is of the belief that the ship has been cursed by its former captain. The old captain went mad and eventually died

© 1989 by The University of Chicago. All rights reserved.
0-226-24062-2/89/0016-0007$01.00

during the ship's last voyage, cursing the ship and its crew to drift endlessly. Since the old man was buried at sea, directly on the ship's present course, the chief mate attributes the dead winds and malaria to the ill intent of the "old devil." Thus, the hopeful young captain's "first command" becomes a death voyage; he steers a motionless boat with a slowly dying crew, lying stranded in the Gulf of Siam. The young captain must rely on his own strength, intuition, and "adolescent" experience as a seaman to bring his doomed ship to port.

Conrad's "The Shadow Line" and Late Adolescence

Technically, *The Shadow Line* is a novella, a form with some similarities to a short novel but without the novel's complexity and development. A novella is rather like a symphony composed in one movement; all its parts cohere, but its themes are less developed. *The Shadow Line* is structured into six chapters and is a brief work of only 133 pages. Several important aspects of the work are left ambiguous: the time of the work's setting, the time of its telling, and even the captain-narrator's name and age.

Now, *The Shadow Line* is certainly a tale of the sea. However, Conrad makes clear from the beginning that his story is no mere "sea-yarn" but rather a profound allegory of late adolescent development. In the introduction to *The Shadow Line,* Conrad (1927) writes: "Primarily the aim of this piece of writing was the presentation of certain facts which certainly were associated with the change from youth, care-free and fervent, to the more self conscious and more poignant period of maturer life" (p. viii).[1]

Furthermore, Conrad wrote *The Shadow Line* at a time in his own life when he was intensely preoccupied with issues of youth and maturity. In September 1915, Conrad's eldest son Borys, age seventeen, enlisted as a lieutenant in the British service. Conrad wrote that he actually had the plot of *The Shadow Line* in mind for a number of years, yet could finish it only in the several months after his son's enlistment. Indeed, Conrad wrote that this subject, the transition from youth to maturity, was "the only one I found it possible to attempt at the time" (p. ix). One can imagine that Conrad the father must have been intensely conflicted regarding his son's decision to enlist and in facing the threat of losing him in the war. In fact, he dedicated the work "TO BORYS AND ALL OTHERS—Who Like Himself Have Crossed in Early Youth the Shadow Line of Their Generation—WITH LOVE.'' It is almost painful to read this dedication, recalling Conrad's situation in the final months of 1915. And, if we return to *The Shadow Line* itself, the young captain's developmental conflicts spawned by command and the perception of human malice, disease, and plain bad luck all now take on a sober, biographical depth.

The work of writing *The Shadow Line*—the only work ''possible'' for Conrad at the time—must have allowed him to attempt to master his painful sense of separation from Borys and his fear of the loss of his son. Through his own reevoked experience as a young captain, Conrad could become ''like Borys,'' minimizing the distance through identification. In taking on the literary guise of a fatherly mentor in the persona of Captain Giles, Conrad could perhaps attempt to overcome the terrible passivity of being unable somehow to help his son. Perhaps, then, Conrad's consciousness of his son's crucial ''command,'' and of the larger issues of war and fate, allowed the writer to create a profound developmental allegory from the ''mere'' experiential events of his own life at sea.

Conrad's final revision of title for the work also implied his focus on development. His initial title, *First Command,* reflected a more biographical and relatively superficial aim. In fact, many of the events and characters within the work seem to derive from Conrad's own first appointment as a captain on the ship *Otago* in 1887. Later, however, he wrote that during the last months of 1915, while writing *The Shadow Line,* he experienced a ''change of mental attitude'' toward his material, resulting in the final title (Hawthorn 1985). The final title of the work gives a sense of refocus and delicacy to Conrad's material; the ''shadow line'' is the subtle crossroads of development, from youth to early maturity.

Conrad's developmental focus is also made plain in the novella itself. The work begins with motifs of youth and drift and ends with maturity and a sense of purpose. The narrator, the young captain, begins the work with some musings about his own youthful optimism: ''Only the young have such moments. . . . It is the privilege of early youth to live . . . in all the beautiful continuity of hope which knows no pauses and no introspection'' (p. 3). This foreshadows his later expansion of consciousness, a cardinal feature of late adolescence. However, early on he also anticipates his own painful development by alluding to the ''shadow line'' that he must cross, signifying the transition from adolescence to adulthood: "One goes on. And the time, too, goes on—'til one perceives ahead a shadow line warning one that the region of early youth, too, must be left behind" (p. 3).

In contrast, at the novella's end, after finally bringing his ship to port, the narrator tells Captain Giles that he feels not "tired"—but "old." He is no longer content to drift but tells Giles that, as soon as he can get a fresh crew, he will go back out to sea to finish his voyage. The matured "young" captain now has an aim and an evolved identity.

Based on Conrad's conscious intentions and on the work itself, the subject of *The Shadow Line* is the transition from late adolescence to early adulthood, the "shadow line" of the work's title. This chapter will discuss the rich variety of late adolescent conflicts that the young captain experiences on his "developmental voyage," with particular emphasis on the development of the self. I will then explore several developmental and literary concepts that the work provokes us to consider and, finally, extend an invitation for the adolescent clinician to study other literary works in the genre of bildungsroman, or "work of development."

Self-Development: Consciousness, Identity, Narcissism

As we examine the narrator's self-development and the functions of various characters in facilitating this development, it may be helpful to keep in one's mind's eye a normal late adolescent. Adatto (1980) and Ritvo (1971) have reviewed the phase-specific developmental tasks and conflicts of late adolescence. I will focus on several aspects of the line of self-development typical of late adolescence: the enlarging consciousness of the self and others, a consolidation of identity linked to life goals, and the transformations of narcissism, of grandiose strivings in fantasy into an ego ideal that may be implemented in reality. On the basis of *The Shadow Line,* I will also question the possible role of certain types of objects in facilitating the development of the self in late adolescence, objects that seem either to reflect or to contrast with aspects of the self. I will explore how, at least within the novella, both seem to promote self-development and raise questions requiring clinical validation. Finally, I will discuss the role of objects in late adolescence that seem "critical" to multiple lines of development.

The enlarging consciousness of the object world, the natural world, and the self is a hallmark of late adolescence. In the beginning of *The*

Shadow Line, the young captain's consciousness is limited and naive. He has little use for introspection or for divining the motivations of others. He quits his job impetuously, entirely on the basis of his affective state: his job was a "dreary and prosaic waste of days" (p. 7). Conrad makes clear that he considers this unthinking "caprice" a feature of "early youth" and a subject of conflict in late adolescence. The narrator gets his first brush with enhanced self-consciousness as he leaves his ship; his former crewmates question his leaving. The ship's woman-hating assistant engineer figures he is leaving "for some silly girl" (p. 6). The dyspeptic chief engineer assumes the problem could only be gastrointestinal and offers several bottles of medicine. Hence, externals—in the person of the narrator's crewmates—point the adolescent narrator toward his first limited introspection. Despite a good berth and pay, excellent ship, crew, captain, and owner, he now wonders, Why did I leave?

This expansion of consciousness continues on shore in Singapore, as the narrator runs into the sage Captain Giles. Giles, through persistent prodding and insinuating comments, leads the captain-to-be to face his ambivalence around leaving the sea life, an ambivalence he had repressed in order to return home. Moreover, Giles advises the narrator that he, Giles, is used to thinking things through. Because he is so conscious, "few things escaped his attention" (p. 22). The narrator then becomes conscious of the small plot going on around him to intercept his command. Giles' words provide a strong jolt to the narrator's naïveté, and the happenings around him at the hotel suddenly take on meaning. He becomes conscious for the first time of human greed and deception.

This is the first of many revelations around human nature and his own internal motivations. The young captain is subsequently able to perceive envy in the sour manner of the steamer captain who conveys him to his ship. Later, he recognizes a more hidden envy in his first mate, Mr. Burns. Ultimately, he becomes conscious of larger issues: he grasps the impartiality of disease and the impersonal bad fortune of dead winds. He recognizes the enormity of human malice when he learns that the former captain has tampered with the quinine, leaving him helpless to deal with his suffering crew. As he listens to the raving delirium of Burns, he becomes conscious of the capacity of human beings to regress to primitive superstition and animism.

In addition, though, the young captain gradually becomes more acutely conscious of himself: his affects of fear, helplessness, and remorse and his attempts at mastery. He feels his own regressive pull to explain his bad luck superstitiously. He recognizes his fear that he will die in the storm. And he becomes acutely, painfully aware of his guilt at not having checked the quinine supply before leaving port. Hence, the captain's earlier "beautiful continuity of hope," which knew "no pauses and no introspection," transforms gradually into a postadolescent consciousness of himself, others, and of natural events.

"Reflectors," "Foils," and the Narrative Self

Conrad the writer implies that the growth of the self occurs in two key ways: first, through life experience, the "brute force" of realities that require conscious introspection. Second, and perhaps most fertile for the adolescent clinician, Conrad implies that his hero's self-development depends crucially on objects that reflect, nurture, or contrast with aspects of the self. For instance, Captain Giles functions preeminently to facilitate the young captain's growing sense of himself as a seaman, ultimately as a captain. Giles functions, too, as an important object proper, leading to identifications within the narrator; he begins to "think things through," like Captain Giles.

However, *The Shadow Line* is also full of other characters—often in contrast with the young captain—who serve to promote his self-development. Burns, the raving, superstitious chief mate, the simpering steward, the self-important harbormaster—all contrast in some way with an aspect of the narrator's self and yet facilitate his self-development.

A number of Conrad's aesthetic devices may perhaps have analogues in normal adolescent development. The discussion that follows derives, in part, from the work of Kohut (1984), Wolf, Gedo, and Terman (1972), and other contributors to the theory of self psychology. Some definitions may first be in order to clarify the distinction between literary devices and developmental concepts and their interconnections and parallels. A "reflector" is a literary character who serves to reflect or resonate with aspects of the hero's self, thereby promoting self-development. A "foil" is a literary character who contrasts with an aspect of the hero's self or a wished-for aspect. The foil works by contrast, enhancing certain aspects of the self or diminishing certain negatively perceived aspects. A "critical persona" is a literary character who not only functions critically as "reflector" but ends up promoting multiple lines of the hero's development. Within *The Shadow Line,* for instance, Captain Giles is a critical persona, facilitating not only the narrator's self-development but also multiple lines of development, including ego and superego development. Do these aesthetic devices have parallels in normal late adolescent development?

As we return to *The Shadow Line* to follow the sequence of characters who act as reflectors or foils to promote the narrator's self-development, particularly his sense of identity, one might keep in mind clinical work with an adolescent. Most interesting, perhaps, and crucial to the young captain's emerging identity are the foils. When the narrator signs off his ship in the beginning, he becomes aware of the contrast between himself and the two engineers, each of whom sees the world through a specific bias. By contrast, then, the captain-to-be is provoked to examine his own identity. Will he follow through with his plans to become a "landsman," or is he a "seaman"? He now refers to himself conflictually as "a man without a ship . . . a mere potential passenger" (p. 8). Hence, the action of the foils on the narrator's identity and self-development is implicit, a kind of catalytic action.

In the period before he gets his command, the captain-to-be encounters a sequence of other foils who facilitate the development of his identity. The steward with his quibbling, pleading, and cowardice provokes, by contrast, the captain's heightened identity as a seaman. A second foil, the arrogant Hamilton, follows. Again, the narrator's interaction with and awareness of Hamilton as a "fraud" seem to act to foster a greater sense of his true identity as a sailor. He now begins to act assertively with the steward and confronts him about the intercepted cable. Other figures act as foils to provoke identity conflict in the young captain. Captain Ellis, for example, a glorified bureaucrat, is seen by the narrator in very ironic terms as a "Deputy Neptune," with a pen that is likened to Neptune's trident. Also, the nameless steamer captain is painted as an insecure master of a boat that serves only for transport. Again, these characters promote by contrast the narrator's growing identity as a seaman who sails, as a man with true authority.

Yet, the captain's development of identity is not one of easy consolidation of identity but—like a real adolescent—one of conflict, anxiety, and gradual integration. After he signs his contract as captain, he uneasily notices a change in Ellis's demeanor toward him; suddenly, he is a captain worthy of respect, and he is not quite ready for it. When the narrator climbs onto his ship and speaks his first words to his crew, he says only, "I am your new captain" (p. 52). This is more than mere introduction; it is as if, in his anxiety, he must immediately affirm for himself and his crew his new identity. Even more so, the scene that follows is full of aspects of the captain's struggle to accept his new identity. He sits down for the first time in the cabin to await the chief mate and becomes exquisitely aware that he sits in "the captain's chair" (p. 52). As if to cinch this focus on identity and self, Conrad next steers the young captain to a mirror. This is a very sensitive moment, for he feels an odd "sympathy" for this "quietly staring man" (p. 53) in the mirror. He struggles against a loneliness that comes of his distance from his former identity. Thus, in assuming command, it is identity conflict and the sense of self that preoccupies the young captain; this theme is also Conrad's major thrust.

Perhaps the most important foil in the young captain's self-development is the chief mate, Mr. Burns. Burns acts in multiple ways to promote the narrator's evolving identity and sense of self. On meeting Burns, the captain experiences a sense of discomfort and realizes that he is reminded of his youth and inexperience. That is, the worn, older Burns somehow evokes for the narrator his identity conflict around being captain. Burns also sets up the dead, former captain as foil for the narrator. Throughout the work, the dead captain is an active presence in the young captain's mind. The contrasts between the self of the dead man and the young captain are obvious: the old man's wish to drift and his death wish are counterposed with the narrator's hopeful aims and struggle to survive. The action of the old man as foil on the young captain's self is implicit in his feeling a "semi-mystical bond" with the dead man: "That man had been in all essentials but his age just such another man as myself . . . in the end his life was a complete act of treason" (p. 62). Significantly, a solidifying of identity follows this sequence, and the young captain makes his first assertive acts of command.

Let us now return to Mr. Burns, as foil. In the course of the novella, Burns becomes progressively more ill with malaria, raving deliriously about the dead captain's curse. The narrator experiences conflict, vacillating between a regressive pull to superstition and a rational view of

209

his fate. At times, he uses the language of animism, like Burns. Yet, somehow, the more he hears Burns rave, the more he turns to rational thinking. Again, it is as if Burns, qua foil, promotes an enhancement of the narrator's rational self.

At other times, Burns seems to confront the narrator with aspects of his self that he must diminish. For instance, when the young captain discovers that the quinine has been replaced, he is shocked and flirts with regressive despair. He smashes the remaining bottles without checking them and then runs to Burns's cabin to tell him. Burns is lying in bed, attempting to clip his bearded neck with scissors. However, the captain, in his regressed state, thinks Burns is trying to cut his throat. After he recovers from his shock, the captain realizes that he had projected an aspect of his despairing self onto Burns, perceiving him as suicidal. Here, then, Burns functions to present the narrator with a negatively valued aspect of himself—his capacity to regress and despair—and ultimately promotes a more consolidated, less regressive self.

The Critical Persona

In addition to foils, *The Shadow Line* also contains a number of characters who act as reflectors to promote a shared feature of the narrator's self. First, we have Ransome, the nurturant steward, who reflects the narrator's benevolence toward the crew. Then, there is the kindly doctor on shore, who acts as a "humane" reflector, supporting the young captain's struggle to assume responsibility and authority.

Foremost, however, stands Captain Giles. Giles acts not only as reflector but as a critical persona for the narrator, promoting multiple lines of development. These include a number of normal transitional steps from late adolescence to early adulthood: a broadening of ego functioning, including an increase in the use of mastery and sublimation, and of the executive function of the ego, turning grandiose fantasy into goal-directed action. Giles also catalyzes a critical change in the narrator's superego, helping to transform his tendency to be vindictive and rigidly moralistic—another developmental task of this phase. Finally, Giles facilitates a "narcissistic decentering" that allows the young captain to see more clearly his adolescent egocentrism (Elkind 1967): that important objects have internal lives independent of him and that their actions do not inevitably relate to him, like planets orbiting his sun.

As a critical persona, Giles acts first to promote an enhancement in the narrator's ego functioning. We recall Giles at the beginning encouraging the young captain to pay attention to the small plot around him, to be aware, to deduce. Giles's style of observing and probing stands the captain in good stead later on when he perceives Burns's envy and stands up to his supernaturalism. Rather than reacting angrily, he "thinks it through," à la Giles.

Giles works an important influence, too, on the narrator's adolescent-like egocentrism and superego functioning. These elements are intimately linked. From the start, the young captain sees others as planets in his universe, to be judged by his own moral code. Therefore, he can look down his nose at the cowardly steward and despise Hamilton for his arrogance. Similarly, he thinks Giles's comments intrusive and boring since they can be of no possible use to him. In time, however, Giles supports a narcissistic decentering within the captain. Through confrontation, Giles makes him aware of the motivations of others and helps to modulate the young captain's narcissistic rage on discovering the steward's plot. Following his interactions with Giles, the narrator's egocentric worldview begins to diminish; he is able to relate to the acid steamer captain and to the feisty Burns without narcissistic injury.

The narrator's superego initially functions much like that of an adolescent. He sees moral issues in "black and white" and is harshly judgmental. Giles, however, responds to the young man's judgments in a benign, neutral manner, "through the ego." This results in critical internalizations that act to modify the young captain's superego. Giles urges the narrator not to punish the steward but rather to use his ego to deal with what he has learned about the available command. Following Giles, the captain's morality changes. He refrains from reporting the steward and from rebuking Mr. Burns. Ultimately, the modulating of his superego allows him to view his crew with benevolence, as they struggle miserably to perform their functions.

Giles's contact with the narrator is also critical in transformations of his narcissism and grandiosity. With adolescent bravado, he compares himself to a king, his ship to a "princess," and his crew to colonials whom he will rule. However, the captain's grandiosity is sanded down by the stuff of experience. His grand voyage is aborted, and his ultimate goal becomes only to get his ship to the nearest port. Reality, then, resonates with Captain Giles's obscure comment to him that he "will have his hands pretty full of tangled up business" (p. 43). The narrator uses this internalized bit of Captain Giles to gradually temper his grandiosity into workable ego aims and ideals.

Clinical and Developmental Implications

I have attempted to demonstrate that Joseph Conrad's novella is especially evocative of aspects of the development of the self in the transition from late adolescence to adulthood. I have traced several facets of the young captain's emerging self: consciousness of the self and others, identity, and narcissistic transformations. I have suggested that these aspects of the developing self are catalyzed by the narrator's interactions with important characters, that is, with reflectors and foils. A single character, Captain Giles, seems critical to multiple lines of development, a critical persona.

For the clinician, *The Shadow Line* will resonate with what we know of late adolescent development. The young captain's evolution of self in all its facets, the shaping of his ego ideal, the transformation of his narcissism—all will provide a helpful backdrop to clinical work with adolescents. Certainly, the line of self-development stands as only one of many aspects of development that scrutiny of the novella will yield.

Conversely, the contributions of clinical authors will inform a reading of *The Shadow Line*. Adatto's (1980) and Ritvo's (1971) reviews, Blos's (1974) and Jacobson's (1964) work regarding late adolescent ego ideal formation, and the contributions of Kohut (1971), Wolf et al. (1972), and others on the development of the self will deepen and add pleasure to the clinician's reading of this work. Several caveats, however, bear restating. First, *The Shadow Line* is not a treatise on development; it is a literary work. As such, we take from the work whatever validly represents human development. Gedo (1970) has argued persuasively against the too-free use of myth and literature to make clinical generalizations. Second, *The Shadow Line*, as a work of art, ought not be viewed reductionistically; what we may learn from the novella about development is but one element among many, including aesthetic, biographical, historical, and structural aspects.

Nevertheless, certain aspects of *The Shadow Line* may provoke us to questions regarding late adolescent development. Most interesting, perhaps, are the characters that function as foils. Do they have analogues in normal and pathological development? Wolf (1986) has discussed the function of "adversarial selfobjects," which "sustain the self by providing the experience of being a center of initiative through permitting non-destructive oppositional self-assertiveness" (p. 492). Perhaps such characters as Burns promote an internal experience (M. Basch, personal communication, 1987) for the captain akin to the experience of an adversarial selfobject. If so, do these objects figure normally in late adolescence? What determines whether a foil like Burns will be used adversarially to promote a positive aspect of the self or as the basis for a self-destructive identification? Might this be used in the treatment of adolescents with pathological identifications?

Similar questions might be raised in regard to the reflectors in *The Shadow Line*. Perhaps reflectors promote internal experiences that share features with what Kohut (1984) has called "alter-ego selfobjects." Do such objects exist in late adolescence, and, if so, is there a psychopathology related to the absence of or the inability to use these objects? Now let us return to Captain Giles as critical persona. Might he, too, have a parallel in normal late adolescent development? If so, are such objects, which promote multiple lines of development, indeed critical?

Beyond these questions, I would like to suggest that Captain Giles and the adolescent therapist have much in common. Giles, with his obscure questioning, gentle prodding, and wholesale confrontations, works as a curious "quasi-therapist" for the young captain. Without rendering much abuse to *The Shadow Line,* one can read Giles's comments as "interventions," ranging from clarifications and confrontations to interpretation and direct advice. Perhaps we can learn something from Captain Giles.

After hearing the story of the aborted voyage, the quinine, and the dying crew at the end, Giles observes: "A man should stand up to his bad luck, to his mistakes, to his conscience, and all that sort of thing. Why—what else would you have to fight against?" (p. 132). In his somewhat ponderous comment, Giles serves a number of functions, very much like a therapist. In a supportive and empathic fashion, he helps the captain to organize his internal experience, to put it into words. Essentially, too, he tells the captain that the world is no nar-

213

cissistic adolescent garden. He confronts the narrator with the actuality of his bad luck and his mistakes. Yet, critically, he implies that this is not something to regress from or despair about. Rather, one should "stand up to"—attempt to master—all these.

The young captain responds that he plans to sail on, as soon as he can get a fresh crew. Giles grunts approvingly: "That's the way. You'll do" (p. 132). Giles reflects this, finally, with the last words he speaks in the novella: "Precious little rest in life for anybody. Better not think of it" (p. 132). Thus, Giles, like a good therapist, facilitates development in the young captain and then puts into words the developmental steps the narrator has taken, with a note of encouragement. The young captain can now recognize that grandiose fantasy must be translated into a goal, that drift must be transformed into concerted action, and that conflict is an inherent part of life—"precious little rest in life for anybody."

Conclusions

Finally, to return briefly to Conrad's work in broader focus, *The Shadow Line* is a representative work in an entire genre of literature, the bildungsroman, or "work of development." This group may be of special interest for the adolescent clinician. It includes relatively short works, descriptive of various phases of development, but particularly of adolescence. Such works as J. D. Salinger's *Catcher in the Rye,* Thomas Mann's *Tonio Kröger,* Herman Hesse's *Narcissus and Goldmund,* and John Knowles's *A Separate Peace* fall into this group. I would invite the adolescent clinician to explore the bildungsroman further. Study of these works will yield rich rewards, both in enhancing our understanding of development and in provoking questions for clinical validation.

NOTE

1. Unless otherwise identified, all quotations from *The Shadow Line* are from Conrad (1927) and are identified in text only by page numbers.

REFERENCES

Adatto, C. 1980. Late adolescence to early adulthood. In S. I. Greenspan and G. H. Pollack, eds. *The Course of Life: Psychoanalytic Contributions toward Understanding Personality Development,* vol. 2, *Latency, Adolescence, and Youth.* Washington, D.C.: National Institute of Mental Health.

Blos, P. 1974. The genealogy of the ego ideal. *Psychoanalytic Study of the Child* 29:43–88.

Conrad, J. 1927. *The Shadow Line.* New York: Doubleday.

Elkind, D. 1967. Egocentrism in adolescence. *Child Development* 38:1025–1034.

Gedo, J. 1970. The psychoanalyst and the literary hero: an interpretation. *Comprehensive Psychiatry* 11:174–181.

Hawthorn, J. 1985. Introduction. In J. Conrad. *The Shadow Line.* New York: Oxford.

Jacobson, E. 1964. *The Self and the Object World.* New York: International Universities Press.

Kohut, H. 1971. *The Analysis of the Self.* New York: International Universities Press.

Kohut, H. 1984. *How Does Analysis Cure?* Chicago: University of Chicago Press.

Ritvo, S. 1971. Late adolescence: developmental and clinical considerations. *Psychoanalytic Study of the Child* 26:241–263.

Wolf, E. 1986. Selfobject transferences: an overview. *Psychiatric Annals* 16:491–493.

Wolf, E.; Gedo, J.; and Terman, D. 1972. On the adolescent process as a transformation of the self. *Journal of Youth and Adolescence* 1:257–272.

15 PERSONALITY, FAMILY RELATIONSHIPS, AND MORAL DEVELOPMENT IN CHICANO AND BLACK ADOLESCENT GANG MEMBERS

ROSA LINDA ESPINOZA AND ANNETTE EHRLICH

Despite more than a half century of research, youth gangs are only partially understood (Johnstone 1983; Klein 1971; Rodman 1978). Several factors have been cited in the literature as playing causative roles in gang membership: poverty and lack of opportunity (Rodman 1978); the positive appeal and structure offered by gangs (Vigil 1983); poor family relationships (Lowney 1984); a deficient sense of right and wrong (Friedman, Mann, and Friedman 1975); and personality problems, specifically in the areas of impulse control and self-esteem (Klein 1971). Unfortunately, however, the data are weak.

Many reports lack objective test measures (see Morales 1982). The interviewer begins with a particular bias and finds, not surprisingly, that informants say what she or he expected to hear. Also, direct comparisons between gang members and nonmembers from the same neighborhood or school rarely are made (for exceptions to the general rule, see Friedman et al. 1975; Johnstone 1983). As a result, it is not clear what, if anything, distinguishes youth gang members from other similarly disadvantaged juveniles.

Finally, whether those factors presently believed to be important determinants of gang membership have equal weight in all ethnic groups is not clear. Heller (1966), Moore, Garcia, Garcia, Cerda, and Valencia (1978), and Vigil (1983) all have argued that members of Chicano (Mexican and Hispanic background) youth gangs, unlike members of youth gangs from other ethnic backgrounds, exhibit no individual psychopathology and share the familial and moral values of the rest of the Chicano community. While provocative, the ideas of these authors have not been tested experimentally. To date, there appear to have been no studies in which direct comparisons between Chicano youth gangs and other youth gangs were made on the basis of objective test data.

The present study was designed to take account of these deficiencies in the literature. Direct comparisons were made between gang members and nonmembers and between blacks and Chicanos. In all cases, subjects lived in the same neighborhood and attended the same high school. Information about family relationships, personality, and moral development was obtained by means of objective test measures.

Method

SUBJECTS

The subjects were male adolescents between the ages of fourteen and eighteen. There were thirty-three subjects in each of the four subgroups: black gang members, black nonmembers, Chicano gang members, and Chicano nonmembers. All came from a single high school in Los Angeles. Subjects were identified as gang members if, on the authors' questionnaire, they answered "yes" to one of the following questions: "Are you a member of a gang now?" "Have you ever been a member of a gang?" Subjects were identified as Chicanos if, on the authors' questionnaire, they checked off, under ethnic background, "Chicano or Hispanic" (other choices were "black," "white," "other").

TEST INSTRUMENTS

Self-esteem was assessed by means of the Piers-Harris Children's Self-Concept Scale (Piers 1984), an eighty-item test that was designed specifically for children and adolescents. On this test, the higher the score, the higher the individual's self-esteem. Family relationships, impulse control, and moral development were assessed by means of three scales designed to measure these variables that were taken from

217

the Offer Self-Image Questionnaire for Adolescents (Offer, Ostrov, and Howard 1982). On this test, the poorer the level of adjustment, the higher the score. There were thirty-eight items in all, and they were separately reproduced. Both tests have been shown by their authors to be reliable and valid measuring instruments.

A questionnaire designed by the authors also was administered. As already noted, it yielded information about whether subjects were in gangs and about ethnic identification. The questionnaire also provided information about demographics (e.g., age, parents' education), composition of the household, amount and kind of delinquent behavior on the part of the subject, jail record of family members, details about gang membership (how long they had been in the gang, the name of the gang or its territory, and the position held within the gang), and supplementary information about family relationships. Subjects were asked to rate the degree of family closeness (on a three-point scale) and the degree to which their parents or step-parents liked them (on a five-point scale).

PROCEDURE

Subjects were tested in groups of seven in a separate room provided by the school. Because some subjects had poor reading comprehension skills and a short attention span, the investigator was present and read questions aloud.

DESIGN AND STATISTICAL ANALYSIS

For the four formal measures, and also for those items on the questionnaire that were continuously distributed, the data were analyzed by means of two-way analyses of variance. The main effects revealed whether gang members differed from nonmembers and whether blacks differed from Chicanos. The interaction term followed, if significant, by post hoc comparisons revealed whether black gang members differed from Chicano gang members and whether the two black groups or the two Chicano groups differed from one another. For those questionnaire data that were dichotomous rather than continuously distributed, the data were analyzed by means of chi-square analyses.

Results

GANG MEMBERS VERSUS NONMEMBERS

Shown in table 1 are the mean scores for gang members and non-members as well as the results of the statistical comparisons on the four formal measures. Gang members and nonmembers did not differ significantly on the family relationships scale, but there were significant differences on the other measures. By comparison with nonmembers, gang members reported themselves as having poorer impulse control, a less developed sense of right and wrong, and lower self-esteem.

Other significant differences between gang members and nonmembers were found when answers to the authors' questionnaire were analyzed (see table 2). The results can be summarized briefly. (1) Both the mothers and the fathers of gang members had had fewer years of education than the parents of nonmembers. (2) By comparison with nonmembers, gang members had been taken to the police station and to juvenile hall more often and had been booked more often. Nonmembers, it should be noted, as well as gang members had been booked for a variety of offenses, ranging from truancy to burglary. The offenses for which gang members had been booked most frequently were theft, burglary, shoplifting, gang fighting, and carrying a weapon.

On the rest of the items from the authors' questionnaire, significant differences between gang members and nonmembers were not found.

TABLE 1

COMPARISON OF GANG MEMBERS AND NONMEMBERS ON MEASURES OF FAMILY
RELATIONSHIPS, IMPULSE CONTROL, MORALS, AND SELF-ESTEEM

Measure	Gang Members' Mean Score	Nonmembers' Mean Score	F
Family relationships...............	53.4	54.0	.06
Impulse control...................	28.5	25.4	6.53**
Morals...........................	31.6	28.8	4.78***
Self-esteem......................	55.0	20.69	20.69*

* $p < .001$.
** $p < .03$.
*** $p < .05$.

TABLE 2

COMPARISON OF GANG MEMBERS AND NONMEMBERS ON ITEMS FROM THE
AUTHORS' QUESTIONNAIRE THAT REVEALED, BY MEANS OF ANALYSIS OF
VARIANCE, SIGNIFICANT DIFFERENCES BETWEEN THE GROUPS

Item	Gang Members' Mean Score	Nonmembers' Mean Score	F
Mother's years of education........	11.2	12.1	4.68***
Father's years of education	10.5	12.0	30.38*
Taken to police station	2.2	.4	7.92**
Booked at police station	.9	.2	10.63**
Taken to juvenile court	1.0	.2	16.35*

* $p < .001$.
** $p < .01$.
*** $p < .05$.

The average subject was 15.8 years old and was in the tenth grade, lived with both parents (54 percent), lived in a household that numbered (besides the subject) 3.8 individuals, and had parents who were employed (64 percent of the mothers and 77 percent of the fathers).

A large percentage of subjects (72 percent) reported that the parents or other family members had been in jail at some time. To questions about relationships with their families, the average subject reported that the family was close knit (81 percent) and that he felt that he was liked a great deal by the parents (77 percent). Two items, income and occupation of the parents, could not be adequately assessed because only a minority of subjects answered these questions.

CHICANOS VERSUS BLACKS

Shown in table 3 are the mean scores for Chicanos and blacks on the four formal measures. The two groups differed significantly on only one of these measures. Black subjects, both gang members and nonmembers, had higher self-esteem scores than Chicano subjects. On the other three measures—family relationships, impulse control, and morals—there were no significant differences between black and Chicano subjects.

A number of significant differences between black and Chicano subjects were found on the authors' questionnaire. In brief, they were as

TABLE 3

Comparison of Blacks and Chicanos on Measures of Family
Relationships, Impulse Control, Morals, and Self-Esteem

Measure	Chicanos' Mean Score	Blacks' Mean Score	F
Family relationships...............	53.7	53.7	.00
Impulse control...................	27.4	26.5	.51
Morals...........................	30.9	29.6	.97
Self-esteem......................	53.6	60.7	20.69*

$* p < .001.$

follows. (1) Both the mothers and the fathers of Chicano subjects had had fewer years of education than the parents of black subjects. The average black mother had had a year or more of college, and the average black father had completed high school; in contrast, the average Chicano parent had not completed high school. (2) More black than Chicano mothers worked. (3) Most Chicano subjects lived in households in which both parents were present, but most black subjects lived in households in which only one parent was present. (4) Besides the subject, there were fewer individuals in the households of black subjects than in the households of Chicano subjects.

Shown in tables 4 and 5 are the results of the statistical analyses that support the above statements. Table 4 contains the supportive data for those items that were continuously distributed and hence could be analyzed by means of analysis of variance. Table 5 contains the supportive data for those items that were discontinuous and hence had to be analyzed by means of chi-square analyses.

Blacks and Chicanos did not differ with respect to age, whether the father was employed, whether anyone in the family had ever been in jail, delinquency record (being taken to the police station, bookings, appearances in juvenile hall, and nature of the truancy), ratings of family closeness, and feelings of being liked by the parents.

INTERACTION BETWEEN GANG MEMBERSHIP AND ETHNICITY

On one of the four formal measures, the Family Relationships Scale, black gang members reported that their relationships were more pos-

TABLE 4

COMPARISON OF CHICANOS AND BLACKS ON ITEMS FROM THE AUTHORS'
QUESTIONNAIRE THAT REVEALED, BY MEANS OF ANALYSIS OF
VARIANCE, SIGNIFICANT DIFFERENCES BETWEEN THE GROUPS

Measure	Chicanos' Mean Score	Blacks' Mean Score	F
Mother's years of education........	10.1	13.3	55.47*
Father's years of education	9.7	12.8	30.38*
Number of individuals in household (besides subject)...............	4.8	3.0	23.79*

* $p < .001$.

TABLE 5

COMPARISON OF CHICANOS AND BLACKS ON ITEMS FROM THE
AUTHORS' QUESTIONNAIRE THAT REVEALED, BY MEANS OF CHI-
SQUARE ANALYSIS, SIGNIFICANT DIFFERENCES BETWEEN THE GROUPS

Item	Chicanos	Blacks	Chi-Square
Percentage of mothers employed ...	48	80	11.87*
Percentage of subjects living with both parents..................	68	32	26.44*

* $p < .001$.

itive than those of black nonmembers ($p < .05$). On the same scale, the difference between black and Chicano gang members just missed significance ($p < .06$). The trend was for black gang members to report more positive family relationships than Chicano gang members. On the questionnaire, it was found that, in spite of being similar in age, both Chicano youth gang members ($p < .004$) and nonmembers ($p < .05$) were at a lower grade level than black youth gang members.

On all other comparisons between black and Chicano gang members, no significant differences were found on either the formal measures or any of the questionnaire items, including the three questions that related specifically to gang activities. The average gang member subject, both black and Chicano, had been in a gang for 3.2 years. About half the gang member subjects reported that their membership was still ongoing. As for the positions they occupied within the gang, one third of the gang member subjects refused to identify their positions; among the rest, the most frequent response was "member" (other choices were "leader," "fighter," "other").

Discussion

GANG MEMBERS VERSUS NONMEMBERS

Some authors (Brown 1978; Copeland 1974; Heller 1966; Moore et al. 1978; Morales 1982; Vigil 1983) characterize gang members as individuals who have made a good adjustment to a bad situation (poverty and lack of opportunity) and argue that self-esteem is raised through interaction, in the gang, with forceful parent surrogates. Other authors, in contrast, argue that gang members are deviant individuals with poor family relationships, personality problems, and inadequate moral development (Cartwright, Howard, and Reuterman 1980; Friedman et al. 1975; Johnstone 1983; Klein 1971; Lowney 1984). The present findings largely support the deviance position. Gang members were found here to be deficient in impulse control, moral development, and self-esteem, as assessed by self-report measures.

Where the present results do not support the deviance position is in the area of family relationships. Previous researchers have reported that gang members do not get along well with their families, are more likely than nonmembers to come from broken homes, and have parents who are relatively uneducated and that both gang members and their relatives are more likely than nonmembers to have been in jail at some time (Copeland 1974; Friedman et al. 1975; Johnstone 1983; Klein 1971; Moore, Vigil, and Garcia 1983; Morales 1982; Vigil 1983). In the present study, only the difference in parental education was found.

The gang members and nonmembers tested here did not differ significantly on a formal test of the perceived quality of family relationships, and they also did not differ in responses to additional items about family relationships that were part of the authors' questionnaire. Subjects rated their families as close knit and said that their parents liked them a great deal. While it is possible that their answers to questions about the quality of family relationships may have represented wish fulfillment on the part of those subjects who were gang members, it is important to note that gang members and nonmembers also did not differ significantly on other measures pertaining to the family.

For example, whether one or both parents were present and the number of individuals living in the household did not distinguish between gang members and nonmembers. Also, although gang members themselves had had more involvement with law enforcement agencies than nonmembers (they had been taken to the police station and to juvenile court more often and had been booked more often), there were no significant differences between gang members and nonmembers with respect to whether the parents or other relatives had ever been in jail. The data, then, did not support the deviance position with respect to family variables. However, the reason for the difference between the present findings and those reported by prior authors is not clear and awaits further research.

BLACKS VERSUS CHICANOS AND THE INTERACTION BETWEEN ETHNICITY AND GANG MEMBERSHIP

On the formal measure of self-esteem and also on several of the questionnaire items that pertained to family, significant differences were found between all Chicanos and all blacks. There also was a significant difference in grade level between all Chicanos and only those blacks who were gang members. What was not found, however, were significant differences that were specific to the comparison between black and Chicano gang members.

On the basis of their delinquency records, it seems reasonable to conclude that the youth gangs studied here were antisocial in nature. For this type of gang, then, the present data provided no support for the view (Heller 1966; Moore et al. 1978; Moore et al. 1983; Vigil 1983) that members of Chicano youth gangs differ from other youth gangs. On the contrary, the data supported the arguments of Klein (1971) and Morales (1982) that members of Chicano youth gangs, like members of other youth gangs, are disturbed.

One surprising finding was that black gang members reported that they had significantly better family relationships than nonmembers. Here, it is important to emphasize the point noted with respect to the lack of differences between gang members and nonmembers on the Family Relations Scale. The test scores represent the adolescent's perception of family relationships. That perception may differ from reality.

224

IMPLICATIONS

The present findings have implications for the design of intervention programs for youth gangs. It is sometimes claimed (Cloward and Ohlin 1960) that the major determining factor in gang membership is poverty. Although income level and parental occupation could not be accurately assessed here, it was found that parents of gang members had had fewer years of education than the parents of nonmembers. Since the parents of gang members had not even graduated from high school, it seems likely that their income level was lower than that of the parents of nonmembers (who, typically, had had a high school education or better).

Poverty, then, probably is a major contributing factor to gang membership, but it is by no means the only factor. Control subjects came from the same neighborhood and attended the same high school as gang members. The general environment, then, was similar for gang members and nonmembers. One conclusion to be drawn from the present data is that the elimination of poverty, while an important humanitarian goal in and of itself, probably should not be the sole aim of an intervention program aimed at gangs.

Some theorists have argued that gang membership is most likely to occur where there is a combination of poverty and family breakdown (Glueck and Glueck 1950; Meissner 1965). Since, as already noted, significant differences between youth gang members and nonmembers in the quality of family relationships were not found, one inference would seem to be that interventions aimed at improving the family relationship are unlikely to be successful in reducing gang activity. Another possible inference is that some better way needs to be found to assess family dynamics than the one used here.

Conclusions

The major differences found between gang members and nonmembers were in the areas of personality and moral development. It would seem, then, that a successful intervention program cannot be geared entirely to such external factors as provision of jobs and help with school difficulties. Such a program would have to include psychotherapy to deal with personality problems. This conclusion, it must be emphasized, applies equally to Chicano and to black gang members. As for what form such psychotherapy should take, that is not clear on the basis of the present findings.

REFERENCES

Brown, W. K. 1978. Black gangs as family extensions. *International Journal of Offender Therapy and Comparative Criminology* 22:39–45.

Cartwright, D. S.; Howard, K. I.; and Reuterman, N. A. 1980. Multivariate analysis of gang delinquency. IV. personality factors in gangs and clubs. *Multivariate Behavioral Research* 15:3–22.

Cloward, R. A., and Ohlin, L. E. 1960. *Delinquency and Opportunity: A Theory of Delinquent Gangs*. Glencoe, Ill.: Free Press.

Copeland, A. D. 1974. Violent black gangs: psycho- and sociodynamics. *Adolescent Psychiatry* 3:340–353.

Friedman, C. J.; Mann, F.; and Friedman, A. S. 1975. A profile of juvenile street gang members. *Adolescence* 10:563–607.

Glueck, S., and Glueck, E. 1950. *Unraveling Juvenile Delinquency*. Cambridge, Mass.: Harvard University Press.

Heller, C. S. 1966. *Mexican-American Youth: Forgotten Youth at the Crossroads*. New York: Random House.

Johnstone, J. W. C. 1983. Recruitment to a youth gang. *Youth and Society* 14:281–300.

Klein, M. W. 1971. *Street Gangs and Street Workers*. Englewood Cliffs, N.J.: Prentice-Hall.

Lowney, J. 1984. The wall gang: a study of interpersonal process and deviance among twenty-three middle-class youth. *Adolescence* 19:527–538.

Meissner, W. W. 1965. Parental interaction of adolescent boys. *Journal of Genetic Psychology* 107:225–233.

Moore, J. W.; Garcia, R.; Garcia, C.; Cerda, L.; and Valencia, F. 1978. *Homeboys: Gangs, Drugs, and Prison in the Barrios of Los Angeles*. Philadelphia: Temple University Press.

Moore, J.; Vigil, D.; and Garcia, R. 1983. Residence and territoriality in Chicano gangs. *Social Problems* 31:182–194.

Morales, A. 1982. The Mexican-American gang member: evaluation and treatment. In R. Becerra, M. Karno, and J. Escobar, eds. *Mental Health and Mexican-Americans*. New York: Grune & Stratton.

Offer, D.; Ostrov, E.; and Howard, K. I. 1982. *The Offer Self-Image Questionnaire for Adolescents.* 3d ed. Chicago: Michael Reese Hospital and Medical Center.

Piers, E. V. 1984. *Piers-Harris Children's Self-Concept Scale.* Los Angeles: Western Psychological Services.

Rodman, H. 1978. *Poverty and Delinquency: A Theoretical Review.* Washington, D.C.: U.S. Department of Health, Education, and Welfare.

Vigil, J. D. 1983. Chicano gangs: one response to Mexican urban adaptation in the Los Angeles area. *Urban Anthropology* 12:45–75.

LLOYD A. WELLS

As the teacher of a first-year medical school course on human psychological growth and development, I observe that some of my students are disgruntled each year when I talk about their developmental position as late adolescents or emerging young adults. After all, they have contracted adult-sized debts, have competed with a large corps of very bright people across the country in the process of being accepted into medical school, and often have outstanding talents and accomplishments. Nevertheless, many medical students are developmentally at an adolescent level, and many who are striving to become young adults are encouraged by the nature of the medical school experience itself to remain immersed in adolescent issues. The following cases are illustrative.

Case Example 1

The patient was a twenty-year-old freshman medical student who asked for an evaluation for psychotherapy "because it might help me to be more happy." One of his first memories was of studying while his siblings were outside playing and thinking that some day he would be rewarded for trying to accomplish things. He had had an exemplary early academic career. He was obsessed with pleasing his father and had decided that his father could understand him better than any other human being. He held his mother in some contempt over this. In fact, his father tyrannized and controlled her, but he felt that, in spite of this, they had a special relationship.

At medical school, he did extremely well academically but made no friends. He felt alienated from those around him and felt that he was "alone in the universe." He thought that in part his alienation was due to the fact that he was more empathic than the other students, but this image received an enormous blow when he realized, midway through his third year, that he often wished his patients would die so that he would not have so much work.

As time went on, it became apparent that he had a borderline personality organization, with no firm sense of identity, and that he was desperately afraid that lack of structure would demonstrate this to the world and to himself. This narcissistic patient impressed others greatly, gained the reputation of being an excellent student and, later, a fine physician, but had enormous and as yet unresolved issues around both identity and intimacy.

Case Example 2

The second patient was a twenty-seven-year-old third-year medical student who came to see me with the chief complaint, "I think I picked a wife that isn't going to work out."

This student was the older of two boys born to an urban, working-class family. His recollection of early years was replete with memories of his father working at all hours and his mother urging his father to work harder. It became clear that, although the family might not have the social status of other families, they would not be lacking for material goods. While the patient's mother urged her husband on to more and more work, she urged him and his brother to "amount to something." From the time the patient was nine or ten, she told several relatives and family friends that he was going to be a doctor and that his brother would be a lawyer.

The patient did well in high school and was accepted into both a well-known college and a small urban college. His father insisted that he attend the latter, telling his son that the larger liberal arts school might get him less interested in medicine and "more interested in one of those things you can't make any money out of." He completed the course work for graduation in only three years and was accepted into two medical schools.

He entered medical school and did well as a freshman, although he became alienated from both parents when they realized that he used

229

drugs recreationally and wanted him to stop immediately. He began to date a young woman of considerable academic accomplishment in a nonmedical field. They were married after about six months. Following the marriage, the patient began to complain of his wife having alienated him from his parents and also started to complain that she was extremely controlling and made him work very hard so that she could enjoy the pursuit of her interests—this in spite of the fact that his spouse was actually working at a fairly menial job in order to help support him in medical school.

He expressed an interest in "doing well" in any branch of medicine and did not think it was important which one he picked. When his wife became pregnant, he thought that this was part of more "control" on her part. When the child was born, he was initially very pleased, but soon began to talk of how much care the child required and how little time there was left for himself. Within a month, he was calling his son "It."

Case Example 3

The third student was a twenty-six-year-old married father of one child, in his fourth year. He presented as part of an evaluation of his wife for bulimia. The son of a physician, two of his brothers were physicians. He had not seriously considered any other career, although at times he had thought of owning a marina or a bicycle shop. He was doing extremely well in medical school and was being recruited for some outstanding residency programs.

The patient's father was alcoholic, by his account, and had a fine reputation for his research, though not for clinical care. The father spent very little time with the patient's mother, and he remembered how she had complained to him and his brothers about their father. He had promised his mother that he would never treat anyone the way his father treated her.

This student married because of his wife's pregnancy. He found himself having overwhelming urges to care for his wife and child, to make them happy, and to protect them from harm. When his wife told him, in various ways, that she did not want that kind of oversolicitous relationship and that he should examine his own dependency needs, he felt crushed and thought that she must want a divorce. He had believed that, if he did not fully cause her to be happy, she would want no part of him. With time, he withdrew somewhat from the marriage and began to take better care of his patients. Then he often slept at the hospital, even when he was not on call, because of patient needs, and he was quick to detect injustice and ethical aberrations in dealing with patients. When his wife protested that he now had too little time for their child and her, he agreed and began to try to be more balanced for his patients and family. He was hospitalized finally for a psycho-physiologic illness.

Case Example 4

The fourth student was twenty-three years old, a first-year student who came to the attention of the entire first-year faculty because of a preoccupation with grades. In spite of the fact that our grades were on a pass-fail basis, this student kept averages to two decimal places and wanted to argue about at least one answer on every test. Seemingly, this preoccupation summed her up; there was little socializing with anyone in her class.

For a time, she did have a romantic relationship with a young man not connected with the medical center. This ended after she had con-fronted him many times for not being sufficiently neat. She admitted that other relationships had ended for this same reason. This student minimized her problems and refused either individual or group psychotherapy.

Case Example 5

The next student was twenty-five, a second-year student with a bril-liant academic record at medical school and college. He found that medicine was a good alternative to his original choice of professions, politics. Later he decided that he would like to be a novelist. In his past were a great many examples of initial mastery of a field followed by rejection of it. He said that he felt born to do something great, but did not yet know what it would be. His relationships were intense, frequent, sexualized early, and of short duration. He left school at the end of the second year.

Developmental Issues

Of course, most medical students are chronologically young adults. Major issues of this phase of development include coming to terms with choice of life-style, early career struggles, and issues involving relationships. In Eriksonian terms (Erikson 1980), this stage has much to do with intimacy versus isolation. Intimacy involves not only the establishment and maintenance of a close relationship but also coming to terms with the degree to which parents and outside authorities will continue to have an effect on the sense of autonomy and even identity.

Preceding stages of development should have been negotiated by the time a person is in medical school. However, one is never really finished with any life stage. It is necessary to rework the tasks of previous stages in the face of new stresses and roles, and such is the situation for many medical students.

Why do the particular people who appear in medical school come there? Martin (1981) has discussed motivation for medicine on the basis of interviews with over 600 future medical students. He found that conscious motivations for medicine were primarily a sense of altruism and an interest in science, often combined in some fashion. Many of the students also discussed childhood fantasies of being physicians as well as a desire to please their parents. Although they did not spontaneously list these as motivations for medicine, many went on to acknowledge that the quest for security was also part of their choice: not only the chance to make money but also the perceived independence and status of the physician's role and position in society. These conscious factors suggest that many medical students use not just altruism but intellectualization and reaction formation as they begin early adult life. In addition, they are often psychologically dependent, especially on their parents, and they may seek the seemingly ready-made identity of a physician.

Martin (1981) thought that there were four common unconscious factors in the choice of medicine: voyeuristic curiosity, the fear of death and counterphobic mechanisms to deal with it, compliance with parental expectations, and, sometimes, identification with a physician or, in my view, with a fantasized physician and his or her role. Certainly, voyeuristic curiosity and the fear of death are found in varying degrees in most medical students with whom I have had significant clinical contact. Many students also struggle with oedipal issues; increasingly, I think, many of them have to deal with preoedipal issues as well.

The premedical time, during which future medical students should be consolidating late adolescent tasks, is often regressive. Pfeiffer (1983) commented that, in the competition to get into medical school and into the medical school of their choice, students are often in a setting of great anxiety about grades. Their achievement orientation may provide protection from anxiety, but the price they pay is that their concept of themselves and of their worth becomes increasingly linked to very specific achievement.

Obviously, such young people are vulnerable. Unfortunately, society invests them with an idealized role as future healers, making it difficult for them to examine their vulnerability except in occasional antiauthoritarian diatribes. They are far less threatening to most adults than many young people who have more thoroughly come to terms with the demands of late adolescence.

In the twelfth century, Maimonides wrote, "May the thirst for gain and the desire for fame be far from my heart" (Kirsner 1986). Martin's interviews suggest that the thirst for gain is very much present in many medical students. The oedipal and preoedipal strivings of the students make the desire for fame very important to many of them. Yet Maimonides was probably correct that these two attributes, taken together, do little to advance the welfare of the individual or the profession. In 1869, Sir James Paget (1902), who anticipated the biopsychosocial model of illness by more than a hundred years, followed up 1,000 of 1,226 former students of his. Referring to the group as, in part, a "melancholy list," he wrote in conclusion, "Nothing appears more certain than that the personal character, the very nature, the will, of each student had far greater force in determining his career than any helps or hindrances whatever." More than fifty years ago, Streker, Appel, Palmer, and Braceland (1936) reported that nearly 50 percent of a large sample of medical students had neurotic problems that were "handicaps of a major character." From literature, Shaw (1905) wrote of physicians' character structure in the preface to The Doctor's Dilemma: "[I wonder] why the impatient doctors do not become savage and unmanageable, and the patient ones imbecile. Perhaps they do to some extent."

In spite of such concerns raised from the twelfth century on, medical students are viewed as paragons by many segments of society. Often idealized projectively by their parents, they may meet with similar reactions from nonstudent peers. They are told by the deans when they begin school what exemplars of every virtue they represent. They often believe that these statements must be true of others in the class, but

233

they know that they are not true about themselves. Many have to invoke a sense of imposture, which, at its worst, reflects a false self.

The students arrive full of anticipation and idealism. Very soon, however, they discover that they may not be able to continue their usual level of accomplishment. Doubting their ability and sense of self, they become anxious and insecure. For many years, for several of the students, worth has been demonstrated and attained only by achievement (Pfeiffer 1983). Performance has been intrinsically linked with identity, and there are now salient questions about both worth and identity. Women students deal with these issues, and, in addition, they struggle with questions of female roles, often in the absence of female role models. All students must make decisions about time with friends and family. Some must make decisions about the timing of marriage and children (Huebner, Roger, and Moore 1981; Lloyd 1983; Pfeiffer 1983).

Prolonged dependence is commonplace. This dependence is not merely psychological. Most students are variably dependent on their parents for financial support; even so, the average debt of our students by graduation is over $40,000. The students are also directly dependent on approval by faculty for eventually acquiring their degree (Pfeiffer 1983). They are forced into the maintenance of dependent roles with ineffectual but strong opposition to such roles.

Psychological dependence on parents is often welcomed. Dependence on a spouse who must also work to support the medical student and must face the unpleasantness of the student's heightened narcissism on a daily basis can create major problems. It is, perhaps, partly on account of this phenomenon that an estimated 60 percent of medical student marriages end in divorce (Marchand, Palmer, Gutmann, and Brogan 1985). For these spouses, and for the students themselves, disillusionment often sets in quickly.

As the student is forced back to questions of identity, his or her quest for intimacy is often placed on hold, and the stresses of the medical school experience itself continue to have adverse effects on the achievement of intimacy. There is an enmeshment of identity, confusion, and isolation. Stress levels are very high. Over the past eight years, I have asked all the freshman students to take the Holmes-Rahe Social Readjustment Rating Scale; the mean score is 306, with tremendous range. The stresses are, indeed, very great. In general, our students find that their greatest and most helpful coping devices are recreation and humor.

These phenomena occur within the first few weeks and months of the medical school experience. Developmental issues continue to interact with the medical school experience to the point that some theorists have suggested creation of a special set of "developmental tasks" for each year of medical school (Gaensbauer and Mizner 1980; Pfeiffer 1983). Thus, in the first year the tasks are the demands of memorization and intellectual work, competition, determining one's personal capabilities, and achieving adequately while maintaining a sense of overall adequacy, setting limits on the amounts to be learned, and coming to terms with the disruption and dispersion of one's social relationships and network. In the first year, too, the students have an exposure to the unacceptable that will continue throughout medical school. The experience of dissecting a cadaver is not a pleasant one, and students face daily contact with death, decay, and the prospect of their own mortality.

In this developmental view, tasks of the second year of medical school include perseverance, commitment, hard work, and dealing with medical students' disease, the hypochondriacal preoccupation that is often associated with the introduction to pathological states, signs, and symptoms. It seems to me that this very common syndrome is found most often in the students who have entered medical school to overcome death and who are using their professional role as a counterphobic measure.

In the third and fourth years, students deal with their identity as physicians and the loss of idealism, as they spend increasing time in clinical encounters. Obsessive defenses and intellectualization allow them to isolate themselves from patients' affective experiences, a process that often will continue through the student's professional life—at great loss to him and to his patients. Students in the third year also have to deal with a pyramidal management structure—the worst possible structure of those studied for young adults. The student receives many orders and many criticisms. These fuel rage, decrease self-esteem, and often increase performance anxiety.

Thus, students have specific challenges in medical school, challenges that are not unparalleled by those of other professional training but that are threats to the most central core of identity and anxiety—life and death, meaning and nothingness, the perception of their own helplessness at times, and the realization that the world is, indeed, unjust and uncontrollable. These are perhaps the lessons of a life well lived;

they are difficult to encapsulate into a four-year period in the lives of young people with certain defined personality structures.

As they start school, medical students tend to be constricted by their personalities and levels of adaptation. They are exposed to the pyramidal structure to which I have alluded as well as to the many other organizational problems of our medical centers. They must do an overwhelming amount of highly threatening work. Some of the students are masochistic, but most must accomplish to keep up the facade they have developed. Then, they learn that their education is really all about uncertainty, even though peoples' lives will be in the balance. There are few truths in medicine and few certainties. A common early response to this realization is regression. Many students then move on to roles of victimization and antiauthoritarianism, seeming to the faculty much like—as Engel (1969) termed them—an oedipal Red Guard. Again, the stresses of the environment highlight the oedipal issues present in many of the students. A transference develops not just to the teachers but often to the entire institution, and it is not always a positive and idealized one. The student has trouble with his or her close relationships, feels robbed of dignity and sensitivity, and ends up relying on tests and numbers rather than sense and observation.

Given all this, it should be no surprise that many medical students develop psychiatric disorders. Often because of the combination of personality organization and work-role stresses, many students do become symptomatic. In one review of the literature on medical school problems, Marchand et al. (1985) found that between 13 and 68 percent of students have been reported to have significant problems and that about 15 percent have an Axis One diagnosis.

Suicide is the second leading cause of death in medical students across the country (Ross 1973). While the suicide rate for male medical students is slightly less than the age-corrected mean for the United States, the suicide rate for female medical students is almost three times the age-corrected mean (Pepitone-Arreola-Rockwell, Rockwell, and Core 1981).

In a study performed by Levin and Franklin (1984), the students' largest problem, by their own perception, was the realization that they could not learn everything they thought they should learn. Only 2 percent were concerned that alcohol was a problem. In a study by Maddux, Hoppe, and Costello (1986), there was a good correlation between substance abuse and depressed mood. Eleven percent of the students studied met DSM-III criteria for a substance abuse disorder, and 12 percent reported daily use. Thirty-five percent of the cocaine users and 40 percent of the benzodiazepine users, as opposed to only 2 percent of the alcohol users, had actually begun their substance use while in medical school. These findings are of concern because of the high psychiatric morbidity of alcohol and drug abuse, depression, marital problems, and personality disorders reported in practicing physicians.

In the late nineteenth century, almost half the physicians graduating from midwestern medical schools were women (D. M. Wells 1987, unpublished data). Numbers dwindled, and only recently has there again been a large percentage of women medical students. There have been many conjectures about their developmental issues and psychiatric status. In a study performed by Lloyd (1983), there were no significant differences among male and female medical students requesting psychiatric intervention in diagnoses, chief complaints, or general problem areas. Males did have more, and more severe, personality disorders; females had more depression and, overall, a greater problem severity. For many of the female medical students in this study, there was a major conflict between working role and feminine identity.

spousal relationships would have fewer such problems, but, in a study by Hoforek and Sarnowski (1981), married women were found to be actually lonelier than single women, who in turn were lonelier than single men, who in turn were lonelier than married men. In the study by Levin and Franklin (1984), married first- and second-year students of both sexes felt that, overall, their needs were met less well than were those of single students. These findings argue that both men and women medical students are having difficulty coping with the task of intimacy. Symonds (1978) has argued strongly that professional women often have considerable confusion about their feminine identity, along with deeply repressed unfulfilled dependency needs, with a facade of self-sufficiency and a chronic depressive stance that often dates from childhood. I have noticed that female medical students are more concerned with being in the right relationship and the right career choice than with being in a good relationship and a good career choice, which is more frequently acceptable by men. This, too, is a frequent finding in middle and late adolescence of both sexes.

237

Therapeutic Approaches

How can medical educators attempt to deal with these complicated issues of autonomy and identity? What can we as adolescent psychiatrists do that might be helpful to these bright young people who will soon be colleagues? Several approaches have been tried.

L. L. Stephens, an orthopedist, felt that there should be open discussion among faculty and students about such issues as the encounters with morbidity and mortality, questions of identity, and the encounter with one's own unconscious. Certainly, a well-timed observation or shared insights about these nearly universal phenomena can be very helpful to some students, but many are very threatened or, frankly, bored when certain teachers keep returning to such topics over and over again (Werner and Korsch 1976).

Another approach is somehow to flood students with humanities in the mistaken belief that this will somehow make them healthier and better-adjusted people. Often humanities courses in medical schools have the same sort of "applied" science connotations as some social sciences courses. The students often plod through them reluctantly and get little gleam of the joy and liberating features of the humanities. Curricular revision is important and must be continued, but there have been curricular revisions for literally thousands of years. We still do not know the best way to train someone to be a member of our demanding profession. John Hunter was able to argue persuasively and show by example that some students, such as Henry Cline and Everard Hume, could master the essentials of good medical and surgical practice by rigorous participation in a fixed curriculum for between three and five years, while others, such as Edward Jenner, needed a much longer, individually tailored program (Wells 1974). Who can argue with his results? Unfortunately, we live in an age dominated more by the Educational Testing Service, National Boards, and institutional rigidity than by flexibility and genius, and we can expect little experimentation in this vein.

Michael Balint was perhaps the first to offer groups for students in the first year (Tredgold 1972). He made these groups patient oriented, but they primarily explored the reactions of the students to the patients and helped the students explore their own reactions and mental mechanisms. Since that time there have been many attempts to help medical students deal with some of the problems I have discussed through the support inherent in group therapy. Dashef, Espey, and Lazarus (1974) have described an excellent program, as have many others.

Another approach has been the use of individual psychotherapy with medical students. Several schools offer this option, but many medical students are reluctant to take advantage of the opportunity because of concerns about confidentiality and the necessary time commitment. The regressive pull of insight-oriented psychotherapy can also create great conflicts for medical students. Once involved in such therapy, they often might find themselves wishing they had opted for a more supportive approach that would have let them get through their years of training before dealing with major structural issues.

Physicians are notoriously reluctant to seek psychiatric help for themselves or their families, and one can see this reluctance in many medical students as well. Many role models for medical students use a great deal of isolation of affect and undoing in their relationships with the world; they ward off intimacy and view acknowledgment of pain and confusion as marks of infamy. Deans' offices are aware of this phenomenon and attempt to combat it. They often urge students to go for psychiatric assessment and treatment. Unfortunately, there is often an implied threat in such invitations. Such threats are not spoken, usually, nor are they intended most of the time, but the countertransferential quality of bureaucrats with power is well known. Another problem with such referrals is that they often promise much more than is reasonable. The administrator implies to the student that something wonderful will happen shortly after he or she begins to see the psychiatrist. Such statements are frequently made to psychiatrists as well. (Administrators generally do not confront psychiatrists directly since it is rare for senior administrative colleagues to think so highly of psychiatrists' abilities—but smugness at such a juncture is almost predictive of failure in the forthcoming treatment effort.)

In my own work, I try to treat patients who are medical students in either group therapy or individual therapy. Keeping in mind the caveats just expressed, I provide individual therapy to those who are significantly depressed, in symptomatic turmoil about major relationships and life issues, and to those with personality disturbances so great as to preclude a capacity for enjoyment. I view these students as disturbed. Some other students who are referred can be viewed as disturbing—to others. Often the dean's office may focus on a student's antiauthoritarian stance and see it as something far worse than, in fact, it is. Such students should be assessed carefully, but often they do not need treatment.

For the past several years, I have offered a group therapy experience to beginning medical students as an outgrowth of their course in human development. This experience is entirely optional. It follows a lecture on medical school in developmental perspective, which considers some of the material in this chapter. The students are told about the group and told to contact me if they are interested. The group then begins shortly after the course ends and meets weekly until the members decide to disband. Groups have ranged in length from four months to two-and-one-half years. There is no credit given, of course, and participation is entirely anonymous and unknown to the administration. Sessions last one-and-one-half hours. I have sometimes used a co-therapist and sometimes not. The basic theme of the group is announced as the interaction of the medical school environment with the personal issues of group members.

These groups have been extremely interesting. Each has been quite different from the others, but there have been some phases that they have had in common. The first of these might be termed introduction and usually lasts for two sessions. In this phase, the therapist is active and discusses the rationale of group process, other similar groups and their outcomes, and some of the things that have been discussed in previous groups. As time goes on, people tentatively share some of their thoughts, and usually by the end of the second session members are speaking quite spontaneously.

The second phase, which can be called exploration, usually starts about the third session. The students begin to share with each other what medical school has really been like for them. The primary discussion is the medical school experience itself, the demands of work, and the high expectations. Often the students bring up very difficult, reality-based problems and then end by saying, "But it isn't really so bad here, of course."

The third phase, which can be called sharing, begins to relate current life stresses with past events and patterns. In this phase, the students show considerable trust of each other and very little doubt or fear. They begin to talk of their fears for the future, the fact that they may not even like medicine as a career, the fact that they are pleasing a parent by their endeavor, and so forth. There is much sharing about perceived bad patterns, usually having to do with parents, siblings—

240

very important to these young people—and romantic relationships or the lack of them. There is a certain formality, as yet, to the presentation of these issues, and the participant/observer may think they are a bit too pat, too dramatic, too well presented; but they are real for all that.

The fourth phase, which can be called pseudomutuality, is perhaps the most interesting phase of the group and the trickiest one for the therapist. Here the myth of the caring medical school and the caring colleagues becomes very prominent. The students review the stresses they have had and the interactions of these stresses with maladaptive patterns in their lives, ending again with the tame statement, "But at least it isn't that bad here," or, alternatively, "At least everybody in the class is so supportive that it doesn't get out of hand." At some point, a brave soul in the group will contradict this closing statement by saying, "I don't think it is very supportive here," or, "I'm sick of the people in the class."

Surprisingly, this statement often opens the floodgates, and member after member of the group begins to talk about how much he or she dislikes many classmates. The therapist's response is often to say, "Well, why should you like them all? That would be unusual." This statement often provokes surprise by the students, but then, as they think it over and realize that it would, indeed, be odd to like all members of any selected group, they begin to wonder where this perception that they should like them all comes from.

Some view it, in a sophisticated way, as a projective phenomenon, an idealization. Others view it as a parental expectation: the student has competed against "the best" for years to get to medical school; the people there must, indeed, be the best; and the student must try to be liked by them. Indeed, there is a fear within the group that being honest will lead to rejection and a sense of lowered self-worth, and this perception is often frankly discussed at this time.

Over the next couple of sessions there is often an abrupt and vociferous denunciation of medical school, society, parents, and authority— much as one sees in an adolescent group. The therapist is usually denigrated as well and should be willing to receive some of this anger and not fight back on the same primitive level. Interpretive work should begin, however, aimed at examination of displacements and issues of identity, autonomy, and intimacy.

With some interpretations, the group begins to advance again. Often the primitive, pseudomutual view of medical school, though given up, returns within the group itself, and the group expresses its pseudo-mutuality by choosing a scapegoat. Often the scapegoat in the group has been a poor participant with some passive-aggressive characteristics, or, on other occasions, she has been an outspoken woman. Once the choice of scapegoat is unconsciously made, the group essentially freezes out the person selected, is rude, and provides very unpleasant and hostile remarks as therapeutic "feedback." At this point, it is important for the therapist to be aware of what is going on and to interpret it. Often the therapist can get caught up in the pseudomutuality as well and can have the same impulse to extrude the "bad" person and have a group that is wonderful. It is very important for the therapist to provide the victim with clarification and support, overtly. Interpretations about the collective purpose of the group are usually met with angry denials by group members, but they seem to have an effect.

Over the years, all but two groups have managed to navigate this most difficult stage successfully. In those two, the scapegoated students ended up withdrawing from the group. In one case, the scapegoat was a young man with few friends who insisted that medical school was, in fact, supportive, that all the people in it were helpful, but that it was "not for him." He felt he was above the realm of medical students, more sensitive and more needy. He pointedly included his peers in the group in these characterizations. When he became the scapegoat, the group gave him pseudosupport, agreeing perfunctorily with his assessments and strongly urging him to leave medical school. In the second case, the scapegoat was a young man who was married to an artist who was unable to pursue her career as she wished to because of his involvement with medical school. He felt guilty about this situation but did not make any effort to help her explore ways to continue her career. He was generally supported by the group until the middle of this phase, when he was quite suddenly attacked by one group member as being cruel and controlling. Other members agreed quickly. The student opted to leave the group, and group members felt very bad about this. Most felt that they were both jealous of his control over a gifted person and identified his control over her with parental control over them.

The fifth phase of the group, which can be termed mutuality, is a real working phase. Here the students explore each others' reactions to them. They have a chance, in Burns's words, to "see ourselves as others see us." This is not always a pleasant experience, but it is done in a caring environment and is often perceived as helpful. This is certainly the most enjoyable part of the group for me as the therapist, and one sees the students interacting in a much more mature way than they had. Issues of intimacy become part of the group process.

In the final segment of the group, termination, there is often some regression, less sharing and mutuality, and a bit more establishment of privacy. There is some review of progress made and some discussion of harm that may have been done. The decision to conclude the group is mutual and, though rarely unanimous, comes from most group members.

Conclusions

The role of the therapist in these groups has been to facilitate discussion, to prevent catastrophe, and to interpret where necessary, although I think the interpretation should be kept to a minimum. While many students would benefit far more from individual psychotherapy than this kind of group experience, many students are unwilling to make the kind of time commitment required by individual psychotherapy, and there is reason to sympathize with them. I would reiterate that these groups are useful only when participation is entirely voluntary, names of participants are unknown to the medical school, and the group is viewed as primarily supportive and exploratory rather than as treatment for sick students. The stresses of medical education combine with developmental issues in many ways. Our awareness of these combinations is potentially important, not just for these young colleagues, but for the future of medicine.

REFERENCES

Dashef, S. S.; Espey, W. M.; and Lazarus, J. A. 1974. Time-limited sensitivity groups for medical students. *American Journal of Psychiatry* 131:287–292.

Engel, G. L. 1969. The care and feeling of the faculty. *New England Journal of Medicine* 281:351–355.

Erikson, E. H. 1980. *Identity and the Life Cycle*. New York: Norton.

Gaensbauer, T. J., and Mizner, G. L. 1980. Developmental stresses in medical education. *Psychiatry* 43:60–70.

Hoforek, M. J., and Sarnowski, A. A. 1981. Feelings of loneliness in women medical students. *Journal of Medical Education* 56:397–403.

Huebner, L. A.; Roger, J. A.; and Moore, J. 1981. The assessment and remediation of dysfunctional stress in medical school. *Journal of Medical Education* 56:547–558.

Kirsner, J. B. 1986. The changing medical scene (1929–1985): a personal perspective. *Perspectives in Biology and Medicine* 29:227–242.

Levin, R. B., and Franklin, A. L. W. 1984. Needs assessment and problem identification of first- and second-year medical students. *Journal of Medical Education* 59:908–910.

Lloyd, C. 1983. Sex differences in medical students requesting psychiatric intervention. 1983. *Journal of Nervous Mental Disease* 171:535–545.

Maddux, J. F.; Hoppe, S. K.; and Costello, R. M. 1986. Psychoactive substance use among medical students. *American Journal of Psychiatry* 143:187–191.

Marchand, W. R.; Palmer, C. A.; Gutmann, L.; and Brogan, W. C., III. 1985. Medical student impairment: a review of the literature. *West Virginia Medical Journal* 81:244–248.

Martin, M. J. 1981. Psychiatric problems of physicians and their families. *Mayo Clinic Proceedings* 56:35–44.

Paget, J. 1902. What becomes of medical students? In S. Paget, ed. *Selected Essays and Addresses by Sir James Paget.* London: Longmans, Green.

Pepitone-Arreola-Rockwell, F.; Rockwell, D.; and Core, N. 1981. Fifty-two medical student suicides. *American Journal of Psychiatry* 138:198–201.

Pfeiffer, R. J. 1983. Early-adult development in the medical student. *Mayo Clinic Proceedings* 58:127–134.

Ross, M. 1973. Suicide among physicians. *Diseases of the Nervous System* 34:145–150.

Shaw, G. B. 1905. *The Doctor's Dilemma.* In *Bernard Shaw: Complete Plays with Prefaces,* vol. 1. New York: Dodd, Mead & Co., 1962.

Streker, E. A.; Appel, K. E.; Palmer, H. D.; and Braceland, F. J. 1936. Psychiatric studies in medical education. II. neurotic trends in senior medical students. *American Journal of Psychiatry* 92:937–958.

Symonds, A. 1978. The psychodynamics of expansiveness in the success-oriented woman. *American Journal of Psychoanalysis* 38:195–205.

Tredgold, R. D. 1972. Michael Balint and medical students. *Psychiatry in Medicine* 3:385–388.

Wells, L. A. 1974. "Why not try the experiment?" the scientific education of Edward Jenner. *Proceedings of the American Philosophical Society* 118:135–145.

Werner, E. R., and Korsch, B. M. 1976. The vulnerability of the medical student: posthumous presentation of L. L. Stephens' ideas. *Pediatrics* 57:321–328.

17 PSYCHOANALYTIC ASSESSMENT OF YOUNG ADULTS

DAVID DEAN BROCKMAN

Assessment of young adults by the psychoanalytic method must, first of all, take into account how well any individual has succeeded in negotiating and working through the phase-specific tasks and conflicts associated with late adolescence (Adatto 1980; Blos 1979; Chused 1987; Emde 1985; Spiegel 1961) and, by inference, all previous phases of development. More specifically, for late adolescence, I am referring to adult sexual object choice, serious commitment to a career, and a firm, harmonious consolidation of the structures that will compose the young adult personality. These structures, for purposes of elaboration, are considered to be enhanced versions of previously formed and enduring or stable aspects of personality functioning, though one must remember that in any young adult there are frequently unresolved residues of previous developmental phases. Clinical vignettes are included where appropriate to amplify the concepts relating to the young adult. In order to proceed in an orderly way to outline and fill out a credible psychoanalytic assessment of young men and women, I will survey those areas of personality functioning that are important for understanding this developmental phase. This is the period of life following college for some, graduate school for others, and, for those entering business directly out of high school, the time for marriage and starting a family, for entering a profession, building a career, and displaying a "settling down" into recognizable patterns of behavior. Longitudinal studies published so far (Block 1971; Levinson, Darrow, Klein, Levinson, and McKee 1978; Offer and Offer 1975; Vaillant 1977) emphasize the psychosocial aspects of these changes.

246

The internal psychological conditions that permit, facilitate, and ensure the dominance of the principles of continuity (Lichtenberg 1984) over discontinuity are part of what I want to emphasize in this chapter. What is meant by dominance of continuity is that development is a dynamic process of progressive and regressive movements that in the optimal sense proceeds among a variety of possibilities toward adult or genital character formation. The genital character as Reich (1949) described it originally is the sum total of various developmental achievements including decathexis of the Oedipus complex, the free capacity for orgastic sexual behavior within which there has been integration of pregenital drives, and the unfettered use of sublimation, which allows for increased capacities for work and play. Reich's concept of the genital character was a good beginning in describing the inner composition of the young adult personality, but it is inadequate in several respects. This chapter attempts to redress those inadequacies.

Resolution of the Oedipus Complex

One of the first areas of assessment is the relative degree of resolution of or reworking of or new solution for the oedipal conflict. In a clinical instance of a twenty-five-year-old man that I observed, a pathological lag had occurred in the relinquishment of infantile sexual claims on the oedipal object so that the entire personality suffered. What was somewhat spared, as is so often the case, was a precocious and uneven development of specialized and outstanding intellectual achievements. Abstract thinking, mathematical and logical problem solving, and an avid interest in the world of mythic literature presented far fewer conflictual opportunities for regression and, thus, were spared significant loss of function. But extensive investments in pregenital fixations were foci for very painful transference reenactments of early object deprivations and traumatic overstimulations. There were repeated neurotic bouts of bulimia and an ineffective impulse control requiring repeated reassurances about fears of abandonment, overwhelming loneliness, and feelings of worthlessness. There was obvious erosion of self-constancy, object constancy, and separation-individuation developmental achievements. In this clinical instance, there was a failure of the processes of continuity. Energies for engagement in loving relationships and in competitive play and for use with creative talents were seriously hampered.

What I am emphasizing in this brief vignette is one way of describing the disruption of growth in the personality of a young adult. This young man was highly motivated to achieve his dream of certain career goals, and a thorough working through of his unconscious conflicts led to greater comfort in intimacy and freed up energies to be used in creative work and putting his intellectual talents to good use.

In another young man, intense murderous, rageful conflicts with his father were reenacted in the transference as coldness and withdrawal. The nature of his conflict was predominantly dyadic, which interfered with a fully phallic investment in the Oedipus complex. Only when this was analyzed could he enter into a regular competitive father transference, which, when worked through in the psychoanalytic relationship, allowed him to begin to realize some of his professional potentials.

A young adult woman's first three diagnostic sessions were filled with a continuous stream of angry diatribe directed at her father. Her anger was unrelenting and unforgiving for his bullying self-centeredness to her and her mother alike. As an example of his brutish, overbearing penuriousness, she described the story of how her father refused to call a cab and made her mother walk several blocks to the hospital when she was in labor. In terms of developing adolescent sexuality and intellectual capacities, she felt unresponded to and unconfirmed. She was only minimally encouraged by him to be a nurse. In late adolescence, she felt strong enough to break away from this imposed career choice to finish at the top of her law school class and enter a prestigious international law firm. Her heterosexual object choice was distorted and pathologically influenced because of unresolved oedipal issues. She was only dimly aware of her rivalry with her mother.

A twenty-four-year-old professional woman was obsessed with men even though she had just gotten married. She was afraid she would turn out like her mother, who had divorced father when the patient was six months old. Her subsequent relationship with her father was limited, but she had very lively fantasies about him, especially after she had paid a visit to his apartment. The major part of her analysis was consumed with working through the defense against the triadic configuration of her personality.

A young adult woman lost her mother at age fourteen, just at a time when she needed her mother to help her negotiate the developmental tasks of adolescence. Instead, she was thrown together with her father, who did his best to help her, but his emphasis was on intellectual, artistic, and cultural pursuits. Her complaints on entering analysis consisted of depression, an inability to finish her dissertation, and a marked failure to form a lasting relationship with a suitable man. Separation issues and unfinished mourning characterized the first period of the analysis, especially in terms of massive resistance against the development of a utilizable transference. When there has been a working through of the major elements of the oedipal complex through successful psychoanalytic therapy, the personality of the young adult is structurally more well defined (Richmond and Sklansky 1984). It is the consensus of the majority of clinicians, however, that there is often some residue of revivable Oedipus complex observable in every individual with or without thorough analysis (Schlessinger and Robbins 1983).

Separation-Individuation

The late adolescent phase of development (Brockman 1984) is characterized by a reworking of those geographic and, most important, psychological efforts at separation from parents (Isay 1980; Mahler 1969; Mahler, Pine, and Bergman 1975)—specifically, separating from those residues of infantile ties and establishing a unique sense of ego identity (Erikson 1959). In Erikson's words, ego identity is "derived from all [his] preadult experience in order to be ready for the tasks of adulthood" (p. 101). Freud (1926) valued his own Jewish identity when he referred to his freedom to use his intellect and "do without agreement with the compact majority" (p. 274). There were within him "many obscure emotional forces which were the more powerful the less they could be expressed in words, as well as a clear consciousness of inner identity, the safe privacy of a common mental construction." He shared in the B'nai B'rith's ethical and humanitarian interests and standards. Identity consists, Erikson says, of a "persistent sameness within oneself (selfsameness) and a persistent sharing of some kind of essential character with others" (1959, p. 102). Then there is the story about a famous analysand of Freud's who asked whether he would be changed by analysis. Freud's answer was that the man's friends would continue to recognize him afterward.

One of the young adult's tasks involves restoring a relationship with his parents and other authority figures, in the sense of adult to adult, where give and take and mutual respect for differing points of view,

249

abilities, talents, and interests abide. Levinson et al. (1978) referred to the mentor role that a senior colleague has with a young adult who is some eight to fifteen years his junior and who is working on establishing his own identity. It is more of a collegial atmosphere where the senior person accepts and acknowledges his junior colleague's talents and competence. He helps define the newly emerging professional identity of the junior person. In the psychiatric and psychoanalytic specialties, we are familiar with the situation of supervisors and supervisees. Here the relationship is primarily a learning or preceptor situation. The novice must be able to regress in the service of the ego (Kris 1962) in order to place himself in the position of the pupil so that he can be exposed to and familiarize himself with the intricate complexities of his chosen field. But, without a stable sense of separateness, the learning alliance is not strong enough to permit the temporary and reversible regressive relationship with the supervisor-teacher. There is ample opportunity to learn the supervisor's technique and, what is no less important, to imitate and later identify with the supervisor through internalization of those values, ideals, and standards the supervisor and supervisee together consider important.

Internalization and identification are taken up in the next section, but in this context I want to mention that it is often instructional if male supervisees learn about the psychology of their female patients from a female supervisor.

The transferences and countertransferences as well as identifications and counteridentifications have been elaborated by Fleming and Benedek (1966) in their classic monograph. Levinson et al. (1978) correctly interpret the mentor relationship as a loving or libidinally charged one with a predictable course of beginning and middle phases culminating in a natural ending phase and a gradual diminution of the intensity that existed before. In the best of circumstances, ambivalences and competitive rivalries are avoided through analysis since in the psychoanalytic training program the candidate is required to be in analysis himself during a significant part of his supervisory work, and the supervisor must do his "homework" to provide the best possible environment for learning. As a case in point, the Freud-Jung relationship suffered because of unanalyzed problems, notably unconscious homosexual conflicts and power struggles in the relationship.

The supervisor shares in the analytic candidate's ambitions, believes in him, and helps him to define his newly emerging analytic identity.

In a way, as Levinson writes, the supervisor-mentor is like a transitional figure who provides a constructive holding environment (Modell 1976), within which the student's evolving analytic credentials, unique therapeutic style, and consummation of identificatory processes develops and provides a comforting construction of the professional world.

Chekov, the great Russian writer and playwright, praised the young writer Gorky, who as an unknown had idealized Chekov in his letters. Chekov wrote back with helpful suggestions about the writing craft, criticizing Gorky's facile overwriting. He suggested that Gorky exercise restraint because he found Gorky's prose monotonous. He admonished Gorky to be more parsimonious and less verbose in his descriptions. From the very first there was an open advisory literary relationship corresponding to a mentor relationship between the two men (Troyat 1986). As is clear from the foregoing discussion, the young adult is involved in relating to other young adults, and they learn much from each other about separation issues, identifications, and intimacy.

Identification

Freud (1917) writes in "Mourning and Melancholia" that the process of identification follows the abandonment of object cathexes. In metaphorical language, he says the "shadow" of the abandoned object "falls on the ego," which is transformed or altered by the taking in or introjection of the object into the ego. Schafer (1968) describes this process somewhat differently and in clear phenomenological language as the internalization of qualities and characteristics of another person. What is also implied here is that a stable ego ideal must have been established in an enduring way in the personality of the young adult, whose standards, ideals, and values are uniformly adhered to by the group he is joining. These structures, then, are the basic ingredients of the ego ideal and, when the ego ideal is merged with the categorical imperatives, together become the essence of the superego (Hartmann and Loewenstein 1962).

Another form of identification is more like imitation or copying of the supervisor's or personal analyst's style in language, vocal tones, and other attitudinal characteristics. These are more or less superficial experiments in adopting the senior person's technique, style, and personality. Both these types of identification also occur in our work with young adult patients. However, in those cases in which the imitative

251

form of identification is dominant throughout, our diagnostic assessment would suggest serious psychopathology of an inner, empty, object relatedness, which would give rise to archaic transferences arising out of a need for narcissistic merger. The first type of identification makes its appearance in the analytic alliance (Schlessinger and Robbins 1983) as well as in the more important self-analytic function, which in a successful analysis is more prominent in the terminal phase.

Therapeutic Split

For the clinician, it is imperative to ascertain how well developed the capacity for a therapeutic split (Sterba 1934) has been laid down. By "therapeutic split" I mean the concept of a constructive dissociation within the ego of a patient, whereby the observing function is encouraged to separate off from the experiencing function. A therapeutic split is created by the joint efforts of the therapist and the patient within a therapeutic relationship. The therapist encourages the patient to observe what he (the patient) is experiencing and, more particularly, to identify with the therapist's empathic observing capacity. The technique by which this construct and process is created is through the liberal but judicious use of the plural pronouns. For example, the therapist might say, Let us see what is going on in your relationship with your wife, boss, friends, and so on, or, We can understand you better if we look more closely at what is going on here in our relationship. In other words, the patient is alerted to the presence of transferences that can be appropriately interpreted.

Young adults are more likely to have this capacity than their more junior adolescents, though some adolescents may already possess this function (Brockman 1984), thus making analytic work possible at an earlier age than was considered possible (Adatto 1958). Self-constancy, object constancy, self-observation, and self-criticism, together with the therapeutic split, provide the foundation for the young adult's self-analytic function (Schlessinger and Robbins 1983).[1]

Intimacy

What is meant by Erikson's concept of the normative developmental crisis of intimacy versus isolation is not limited to a physical sexual relationship alone; rather, it refers to the clinically based observations of the capacity of young adults for emotional closeness, mutual respect, lessening ambivalence for the loved object, giving the loved object room to develop his or her potentials to the fullest, sharing each other's joys and sorrows, and not engaging in destructive draining of the loved person's sharing of themselves—in short, a mutually loving and being loved relationship. Clinical experience of over thirty years leads me to concur with Erikson (1959) that achieving intimacy is a developmental task that young adult people are greatly concerned with.

There are different forms and aspects of intimacy. Included in experiences of intimacy are tenderness, caring, kindness, respect, friendship, collaboration, dependency, nurturing, affection, romantic love, and sexuality. Both partners learn about the other's inner resources and vulnerabilities and what is offered, demanded, and withheld, all of which implies resolution of ambivalences about the loved object as well as transformations of narcissism. The loving wife helps her husband realize his dream by believing in him and confirming his evolving image of himself and his dream. She acts as "teacher, guide, host, critic, [and] sponsor" (Levinson et al. 1978, p. 109). The loving husband reciprocates. There are many instances recently of the husband staying home with the children while the wife goes back to school to get her degree. In fact, both partners have dreams that are heroic in nature, and the husband must nurture and promote his wife's dreams. As the young adult man learns to accept the feminine in himself and in others, he relaxes and learns to integrate a variety of feminine identifications. He learns that sharing household tasks and caring for children do not make him any less masculine. Instead, his marriage is strengthened, and he feels more committed. In addition, in this greater exposure of the young father to his children they thrive because of a more balanced environment.

Overall, young women seem to be somewhat more ready for and competent with this developmental step than are young adult men, and they achieve the capacity for intimacy a few years earlier. Furthermore, gender differences seem to be connected to readiness for parenthood. Intimacy is integrally connected to procreative aims. Some, but not all, young adult men are regularly concerned with fears of entrapment and of being dominated or controlled by women, who are experienced as the phallic, castrating, or intrusive mother. There may be some holdover of guilt, anxiety, and mystification about the partner from previous phases of adolescence. This complicates settling down with

253

one partner. In fact, some young men experience commitment to another person as too restraining and clearly are not ready for marriage. An example of this problem of intimacy was a young-adult man's rise in business. It was meteoric, but he resisted making a marriage commitment to a young woman with whom he was deeply in love. What restrained him were unconscious resentments toward his mother for divorcing his father and, much earlier, for replacing him with his two younger siblings. Competitive strivings with his father were only a small part of the dynamics of this difficulty.

Moreover, in heterosexual men wishes for closeness become confused with fears of being homosexual, especially when there has been a history of open conflicts with father and frustrated regressive wishes for passive reconciliation. A case in point was Robert, a twenty-six-year-old lawyer, whose physician father had died two years earlier. He started drinking at age fourteen and graduated to drugs soon thereafter in angry rebellion against the loss of his loving grandfather and the fact that his father was always too busy taking care of his patients to devote any time to him. Robert sought help first from Alcoholics Anonymous, through which he gained control over his addictions, but his rage persisted. When he came to analysis he was still actively mourning his father. Another theme, which intermingled with the mourning process, was his wish to transform his marriage into one with a greater emphasis on emotional intimacy. He, too, was greatly concerned with fears of being homosexual that were based on his unconscious wishes for closeness with his father.

It did not take long for him to realize that his rage toward his father was what was interfering with his relationship with his wife. In other words, he had displaced his rage onto her.

One young adult continued a pattern into young adulthood that had begun much earlier in adolescence. He would launch a project to gain his father's approval, but the father would unempathically criticize and humiliate his son. This set up a rageful enmity that could be resolved only by the son tearfully retreating to his room and the father being made to feel guilty enough to come and console the injured son. Often the father would ignore the imposition of guilt, but when he succumbed to it there was a mutually heart-wrenching attempt at reconciliation. Most often, however, reconciliation misfired because neither father nor son was capable at that time of much emotional intimacy. Much analytic work and the acquisition of insight into the oedipal meaning of the son's conflict with his father led to a more cordial nonconflictual relationship with the father and his tentative venture into a more intimate relationship with a young woman.

Career Choice

Levinson et al. (1978) indicated that the young adult struggles with what they call the "novice phase" to establish himself in an occupation by sorting out multiple interests and matching them up with what corresponds best with his conscious and unconscious hopes and dreams. Once the choice is made, he must acquire the skill, values, and credentials for that career. This process is not always a straight line, and for all categories that Levinson studied (the novelist, the biologist, the executive, and the hourly worker) a stable career was achieved only after a circuitous route of several provisional career choices, including entering some blind alleys. The young man who was unsuccessful in achieving reconciliation with his father had great difficulty finding a suitable career. He dreamed of become an entrepreneur and running his own business. At first he was a home builder's assistant; then he was a cab driver while he went to night school to get his college degree. After that he was a manufacturer's representative like his father. But he failed at each venture. He returned to driving a cab. It was only after significant analytic work that he could lift himself out of the twists and turns of a dead-end career. He found his niche in the insurance brokerage business, becoming reasonably successful in this highly competitive field.

Jerome portrayed another example of problems in settling on a career. He was delayed in finishing college because he was asked to take a year off when he did not perform up to his academic potentials. After college he worked in the oil fields and then ended up as a stockbroker, but he found his place in an entrepreneurial business that he created and in which he was extraordinarily successful. He entered analysis considering the very unpleasant possibility of changing careers yet again. Acting out some destructive unconscious conflicts almost destroyed everything he had worked so hard to achieve. He was quite depressed and contemplated suicide. When the analysis uncovered and worked through his rivalrous competitiveness, he was able to decide rationally what was the best plan for him and his business.

Conclusions

The pathway to adulthood is not an easy, straightway course. For many, if not all, a circuitous, complicated, and conflicted route is the rule. What is left out in all prior studies of young adults are data of a depth psychological nature. Clinical vignettes are condensed in this presentation to round out the picture of those areas of interest most often encountered in clinical practice with young adults. Resolution of the oedipal conflict, experiments in separation-individuation, successful adaptations, development of a capacity for self-observation, accomplishment of intimacy with others, and consolidation of the personality as a whole permit the young adult to settle down to a firm commitment to a career, marriage, and the creative use of energies for work and play. Implied in the consolidation of the personality is a firm integration of the ego, ego ideal, and superego structures, which function harmoniously within a meaningful psychobiosocial framework (Schwartz and Wiggins 1986).

NOTE

1. The ego functions Schlessinger and Robbins (1983) list are basic trust; object constancy; self-constancy; dyadic object relationship; dyadic reality processing; tolerance for frustration, anxiety, and depression; triadic object relationship; triadic reality processing; potential for mastery of frustration, anxiety, and depression; regression in the service of the ego; therapeutic split; self-analytic function; self-soothing function; transformation of narcissism; and, finally, the analyst's contribution to the analytic situation.

REFERENCES

Adatto, C. 1958. Ego reintegration observed in analysis of late adolescents. *International Journal of Psycho-Analysis* 39:172–177.

Adatto, C. 1980. Late adolescence to early adulthood. In S. I. Greenspan and G. H. Pollock, eds. *The Course of Life: Psychoanalytic Contributions toward Understanding Personality Development,* vol. 2, *Latency, Adolescence and Youth.* Washington, D.C.: National Institute of Mental Health.

Block, J., in collaboration with N. Haan. 1971. *Lives through Time.* Berkeley, Calif.: Bancroft.

Blos, P. 1979. *Adolescent Passage.* New York: International Universities Press.

Brockman, D. D. 1984. *Late Adolescence: Psychoanalytic Studies.* New York: International Universities Press.

Chused, J. F. 1987. Psychoanalysis of the young adult: theory and technique. *Journal of the American Psychoanalytic Association* 35:175–187.

Emde, R. N. 1985. From adolescence to midlife: remodeling the structure of adult development. *Journal of the American Psychoanalytic Association* 33:59–112.

Erikson, E. H. 1959. *Identity and the Life Cycle.* Psychological Issues Monograph Series, no. 1. New York: International Universities Press.

Fleming, J., and Benedek, T. 1966. *Psychoanalytic Supervision.* New York: International Universities Press.

Freud, S. 1917. Mourning and melancholia. *Standard Edition* 14:243–258. London: Hogarth, 1957.

Freud, S. 1926. Address to the society of B'nai B'rith. *Standard Edition* 20:273–274. London: Hogarth, 1959.

Hartmann, H., and Loewenstein, R. M. 1962. Notes on the superego. *Psychoanalytic Study of the Child* 17:42–81.

Isay, R. A. 1980. Late adolescence: the second separation stage of adolescence. In S. I. Greenspan and G. H. Pollock, eds. *The Course of Life: Psychoanalytic Contributions toward Understanding Personality Development,* vol. 2, *Latency, Adolescence, and Youth.* Washington, D.C.: National Institute of Mental Health.

Kris, E. 1962. *Psychoanalytic Expressions in Art.* New York: International Universities Press.

Levinson, D. J.; Darrow, C. N.; Klein, E. B.; Levinson, M. H.; and McKee, B. 1978. *The Seasons of a Man's Life.* New York: Ballantine.

Lichtenberg, J. 1984. Continuities and transformations between infancy and adolescence. In D. D. Brockman, ed. *Late Adolescence: Psychoanalytic Studies.* New York: International Universities Press.

Mahler, M. 1969. *On Human Symbiosis and the Vicissitudes of Individuation,* vol. 1. New York: International Universities Press.

Mahler, M.; Pine, F.; and Bergman, A. 1975. *The Psychological Birth of the Human Infant.* New York: Basic.

257

Modell, A. 1976. The "holding environment" and the therapeutic action of psychoanalysis. *Journal of the American Psychoanalytic Association* 24:285–307.

Offer, D., and Offer, J. B. 1975. *From Teenage to Young Manhood.* New York: Basic.

Reich, W. 1949. *Character Analysis.* New York: Orgone Institute Press.

Richmond, M. B., and Sklansky, M. A. 1984. Structural change in adolescence. In D. D. Brockman, ed. *Late Adolescence: Psychoanalytic Studies.* New York: International Universities Press.

Schafer, R. 1968. *Aspects of Internalization.* New York: International Universities Press.

Schlessinger, N., and Robbins, F. P. 1983. *A Developmental View of the Psychoanalytic Process.* New York: International Universities Press.

Schwartz, M. A., and Wiggins, O. P. 1986. Systems and the structuring of meaning: contributions to a biopsychosocial medicine. *American Journal of Psychiatry* 143:1213–1221.

Spiegel, L. 1961. Disorder and consolidation in adolescence. *Journal of the American Psychoanalytic Association* 9:406–416.

Sterba, R. 1934. The fate of the ego in analytic therapy. *International Journal of Psycho-Analysis* 15:117–126.

Troyat, H. 1986. *Chekhov.* Translated by Michael Henry Heim. New York: Dutton.

Vaillant, G. E. 1977. *Adaptation to Life.* Boston: Little, Brown.

18 CAREER CHANGE IN EARLY ADULTHOOD: DEVELOPMENTAL CONSIDERATIONS

EUGENE H. KAPLAN

In a fanciful version of turning against the self, the very principles of psychoanalytic theories of development might be applied to a study of their evolution. A history of the development of these theories reveals their expansion in scope and sophistication, in the face of interruptions, arrests, and deviations associated with early experience.

Freud (1905) launched the developmental point of view with formulations about psychosexual stages set in a framework of libido (drive) theory. These hypotheses about stages spanning the first years of life were derived from his self-analysis and work with adult patients. From this vantage point emerged the emphasis on the centrality of the Oedipus complex (Leavy 1985). Stimulated by these conceptualizations to treat and observe children and adolescents, analysts began to uncover the preceding and succeeding phases, significantly reducing oedipal centrality.

As psychoanalytic theory elaborated the structural and adaptive points of view, developmental concepts expanded to encompass infancy through the end of adolescence. This point in theoretical evolution conferred on adolescence a degree of centrality for subsequent adult development reminiscent of that given originally to the oedipal phase. Early analytic formulations regarded adolescence as little more than a later version of the Oedipus complex (Jones 1948). Subsequent notions assigning consolidations of psychic structure to the end of adolescence confer a false sense of fixity and finality (Kaplan 1980). Similarly, Escoll (1987) states that, while consolidation is considered the hallmark of late adolescence, the process may occur more gradually and unevenly,

259

sometimes into the later young adult or adult years. Emde (1985) identified the significant obstacle to the advance of developmental theory in terms of a conceptual model based on gross aspects of physical growth. This model assumes progress to maturity to be more or less complete at the end of adolescence. Emde particularly cites Erikson (1945, 1950, 1956, 1968) as expanding Hartmann's (1939) adaptive point of view and concept of "average expectable environments" beyond infancy to the entire life cycle and conceptualizing a series of phase-related crises and goals and a continuing, lifelong separation and individuation.

A review of the longitudinal studies of Block and Haan (1971), Eichorn, Clausen, Haan, Honzik, and Mussen (1981), Emde (1985), Levinson, Darrow, Klein, Levinson, and McKee (1978), Offer and Offer (1975), and Vaillant (1977) finds evidence for continued development and restructuring during adulthood in two major areas: self-organization and defensive organization. Emde suggests that the favorable reorganization of the unconscious and the reorganization, restructuring, and more adaptive coherence of the self-system in psychoanalysis may be a special case of what happens more generally as a function of adult experience under favorable environmental circumstances.

Early adulthood, from the late teens to the early thirties, is demarcated by the two Eriksonian polarities of identity versus identity diffusion and intimacy versus isolation. In Levinson et al.'s (1978) schema, the novice phase of adulthood (late teens to early thirties) presents four salient developmental tasks: (1) forming the dream, (2) forming mentoring relationships, (3) forming a marriage and family, and (4) forming an occupation. The first task, "forming the dream," is analogized to Winnicott's transitional phenomenon. Testing out the newly emerging self is facilitated by adults approximating Winnicott's "good enough mother" of early childhood. The second task is "forming mentoring relationships" with adults who support this "vague sense of self-in-the-adult-world." Serving also as teacher, sponsor, host, model for identification, adviser, and source of moral support, the mentor's primary function is to support realization of the dream and affirmation of the emerging self. Mentoring is a form of love relationship lasting from two to ten years, often ending in strong conflicts and bad feelings. Its loss promotes further internalization. The third task, "forming a marriage and family," requires acceptance of parenthood, of sharing a dream with the spouse, and of both the masculine and the feminine parts of the self.

The work of Offer and Offer (1975) provides a valuable developmental bridge from adolescence to early adulthood. Their longitudinal study describes three routes through normal male adolescence: continuous, surgent, and tumultuous growth.

1. *Continuous growth group.*   From excellent genetic and environmental backgrounds and stable families, these young men had no serious illness or object loss in childhood. Their parents encouraged independence and seemed to grow themselves with their adolescent's growth, with a reciprocal sense of gratification. This group went from fourteen to twenty-two smoothly and with self-assurance; at age twenty-two they showed optimal functioning and the absence of clinical psychiatric syndromes.

2. *Surgent growth group.*   Here development occurred in spurts. These young men's families were more likely to have experienced separations, deaths, or severe illnesses. More prone to depression, anxiety, and self-esteem problems, they relied more on parents and peers. There were value conflicts between these adolescents and their parents and between the parents themselves.

3. *Tumultuous growth group.*   Less stable backgrounds and more lower-middle-class members characterized this group compared to the other two. Strong family bonds distinguished the young men from delinquents. They traversed adolescence with inner turmoil often manifest as overt behavioral problems at home and at school. They had recurrent self-doubts, escalating conflicts with parents, and debilitating inhibitions.

While the surgent group had the same percentage of clinical psychiatric syndromes as would be expected by the normal group distribution, the tumultuous group had twice as many and the continuous group none.

Emde (1985) finds the validity of the Offers' categories enhanced by their correspondence with both male and female samples in the Berkeley-Oakland study (Block and Haan 1971). By implication, the trajectory for completion of developmental tasks is extended for the surgent and tumultuous groups. We should expect an overrepresentation from these two groups among those who make a career change in early adulthood, reflecting a protracted struggle to achieve a satisfactory intrapsychic compromise formation permitting career commitment.

For normative adolescents, especially males, the future is frequently conceived and organized around an occupational choice conferring identity (Offer 1969). The transition from supportive parental and school relationships to impersonal bosses may provoke a postadolescent identity crisis with an intersystemic conflict between the ego ideal and the superego (Marcus 1980). The outcome is more severe with a rigid and harsh superego that demands fulfillment of unrealistic ego ideals; depression may result (Bemporad, Ratey, and Hallowell 1986). While the focus of media coverage is on adolescent suicide, the problem is significantly worse for young adults aged twenty to twenty-four. The 1984 suicide rate for the age groups fifteen to nineteen and twenty to twenty-four was, respectively, 9.0 and 15.6 per 100,000 (Mercy 1987).

Dewald (1980) lists a variety of unconscious factors significantly influencing conscious adult decisions about occupation and profession. These include positive or negative identifications with important childhood objects, fears and/or needs for competitive struggle, narcissistic needs, the expression of otherwise unacceptable instinctual drive derivatives, parental and internalized superego values and demands, unconscious guilt and/or shame, and reversals from passive to active.

Like all behaviors, career choice results from the interaction of psychodynamic factors with environmental circumstances. Headlee and Kalogjera (1987) give a systematic account of the process of general choice: choice, forcing the surrender of alternatives, creates conflict and mobilizes defenses against change. The defenses include repression of the awareness of choice, obsessions/compulsions, procrastination, distortion of alternatives, displacement of responsibility for choice, and regression to dysfunctional loss of control. The process of resolution may involve the reaction of past separation-individuation experiences, repetition-compulsion, mourning of unfulfilled expectations, and narcissistic injuries. The desirable outcome of the choice conflict is establishment of identity cohesion and developmental synchrony; failure of the process results in psychopathology.

Career change may both reflect and facilitate the reworking of unconscious conflicts, furthering progression through adulthood. This developmental advance may be impeded if conflicts are sufficiently severe; in this instance, career change would signify a neurotic pattern persisting unchanged. The subjective phenomenology of vocational decision is highly variable. An attraction or dissatisfaction may burgeon gradually or crystallize with unexpected suddenness. The conscious experience may feel as if it were an act of will or, in the literal denotation of vocation, heeding a call. Bouts of inexplicable boredom, depression, or anxiety may initiate the process, the reasons for these moods becoming apparent later.

Moreover, choices are made predominantly on the basis of imagining. Imagination, no matter how realistic, can never apprehend fully the anticipated reality. We do not know what a profession is really like until we are in it, and then it is too late. From the perspective of the historical past and multiple unconscious motivations, that reality is different for each of us (Spruiell 1983). Therefore, the realization of the aspiration may prove a distressing confirmation or reassuring corrective of anticipatory dread. The actuality, not the aspirant, may be found wanting, resulting in disillusionment. Furthermore, other unanticipated latent conflicts may be mobilized.

The specific examples of career change studied concern mostly older medical students and physicians who changed specialty. We expect the shared common fantasies about the profession to contribute, in their individual versions, to motivations and conflicts. Society grants medicine social prestige and economic status and waives the taboos surrounding the body. The physician may uncover and probe the body's orifices and cavities and delve into patients' innermost secrets. These pertain to the fundamentals of human existence, procreation, birth, and death. In response, conflicts over childhood sexual curiosity, aggression and fears of death, sadomasochism, narcissism, and wishes for omnipotence are mobilized.

Clinical Observations and Inferences

The clinical data are drawn from thirty patients treated with psychoanalysis (four), extended psychotherapy (twelve), and consultation and brief psychotherapy (fourteen). Their ages ranged from twenty-two to thirty-seven. The forces of social change have opened the gates to groups for whom the medical career exceeded cultural expectations and strivings. This series includes nine women whose delayed choice of medicine evinced conflicts stemming from traditional ideals of femininity incorporated in the superego and the ego ideal. Most reports in the literature describe potential obstacles to women's professional achievement in terms of sex-role stereotyping, traditions within the medical hierarchy, and strains arising from balancing professional and

263

family obligations (Fenton, Robinowitz, and Leaf 1987). Five came from ancillary professions (nursing, pharmacy, medical technology); for them, medicine had been psychologically out of reach initially. Several clearly derived momentum from identification with their professional, albeit nonmedical, fathers. By contrast, physicians' daughters do not usually manifest this pattern of delay.

Two women lacking such parental identificatory impetus had found their way to medicine through a lover-mentor relationship with an older physician. Both had escaped first from their families of origin through very early marriage and motherhood. Interestingly, the one who discarded the relationship after becoming established in her new profession had followed a surgent pattern in adolescence; the other, who remained enmeshed, described a tumultuous adolescent growth pattern. Some women showed inner conflicts over competition and assertiveness at odds with the traditional ego ideal of female docility and compliance to authority. For several others, the conflict was over the competing demands of their love relationships. Superego-dictated compliance to family insistence that they personally fulfill, rather than delegate, homemaking and caretaking duties, led two married women to serious neglect of their medical studies.

An unmarried student under no such external pressure showed a variation on this pattern. With each new love affair, she lost interest in her studies. Before medical school she had rationalized this reaction, blaming the inherently boring nature of her highly paid job. Now she was puzzled because medicine was far from boring. While identified with her professional father, she had also unconsciously internalized the family ideal that a woman worked to keep busy until she found a man, to whom she was to devote herself entirely.

The detour to a less prestigious profession is found also among men from working-class backgrounds, for psychological reasons similar to women raised traditionally. In addition, the blue-collar archetype of going to work and getting married right after high school is associated with early identity closure and constriction of flexibility and autonomy (Trent and Medsker 1968). Ambition sufficient to overcome such forces also raises the intensity of the resultant inner conflict.

This sociocultural correlation was absent in three medical students whose career detours were linked to fears of humiliating public exposure of failure. All were middle-class males. A traumatic origin was identified in one case. An elementary school teacher had tormented him as the class scapegoat for months before overt psychosis led to the teacher's removal. Consequences were evident immediately in peer relationships and later career choice. He dropped out of engineering school to take menial jobs, first in a factory and then a hospital. (Father was an engineer, mother a nurse.) Eventually, he became a technician. Success and recognition built his confidence over the next few years until he could return to college for premedical studies.

In a second case, the fear of failure covered unconscious guilt over success. Despite outstanding grades and family encouragement to pursue medicine, the young man rationalized his choice of an ancillary profession; the easier course of study enabled him to work to support his wife and child. However, before completing this program, he was persuaded to apply to medical school. The letter of acceptance provoked exhilaration so intense as to be indistinguishable from anxiety. A moderate depression, punctuated by anxiety attacks, set in. Psychotherapy elicited the fantasy underlying the anxiety episodes—humiliating public exposure of his ignorance to his classmates. They represented his beloved ne'er-do-well brother. The patient considered himself just as irresponsible with time and money as his brother was, making his own success intolerable in the face of the brother's failure. Here, unconscious guilt was responsible for the career detour and the anxiety attacks.

Contact with the third student was insufficient to elucidate his fear of humiliating failure. In two other cases, conflicts over rivalry with an older brother figured significantly in the psychodynamics of career choice and change.

In recognition of excellent performance on a tertiary care unit, a resident was to be appointed attending physician in charge on completion of training. As the date drew near, anxious self-doubts effloresced into certainty that patients under his care would die from his incompetence. The anxiety became disabling and suicidal thoughts reached the planning stage. We learned that his older brother had almost succumbed in childhood to the very category of life-threatening illness treated in the unit. Although the brother had recovered fully, near fulfillment of his death wishes had caused symptoms in the highly competitive youngster. This link to the past mobilized a dormant conflict and transformed the present. As a resident, he could rely on the power of his superiors as the protective buffer against his death wishes. After six months of torment, he resigned the position, and the anxiety and depression quickly dissipated. He has functioned well since, including life-and-death situations, demonstrating Spruiell's point that reality differs for each of us.

For another young man, the guilty triumph over his older brother was interwoven with old conflicts in the relationships with both parents. His neurotic inhibition was so severe that analysis was required. Mark, a tall, soft-spoken, personable twenty-three-year-old, entered analysis complaining of paralyzing indecision, intense feelings of worthlessness, chronic anxiety, and insomnia. For eighteen months since his college graduation he had been drifting, visiting school friends. Childhood rivalry with his only sibling, a twenty-month-older brother, had posed a particular problem because of the brother's small stature and lesser intellectual endowment. Surpassing his brother in height at age seven, Mark felt inhibited to compete by parental disapproval. His mother had marked difficulty in setting limits, inducing guilt in Mark for forcing her to say no. The mother was a psychotherapist, and a knotty problem arose in analysis from her having substituted "psychoanalytic" interpretations of Mark's behavior in lieu of more conventional limit setting. As a result, interpretations offered in the analysis invariably stirred up resistance based on the maternal transference. Father had a pronounced self-esteem problem with much self-deprecation; the repository of his narcissism was in idealization of Mark. After perennial complaints, father sold his successful manufacturing firm, retiring in his early fifties while Mark was in college. In the course of the analysis, we came to understand many facets of his paralyzed inaction. Mark could never be sure whether a wish or an action was authentically his own or motivated by a wish to please. Unconsciously, pleasing his mother meant sacrificing his autonomy. Moreover, pleasing his father posed the dilemma of fulfilling the father's failed aspirations and thus surpassing him when he had been schooled not to surpass the older brother. Inaction not only avoided these conflictual dangers but also had the unconscious meaning of a self-affirming anal negativism. In that paralyzed state, he accepted whatever jobs and women came his way, inevitably inferior to his capacities. When his parents moved to the country, Mark was galvanized into action. After two years of analysis, his actions had a different quality than before. He found an apartment in the city and a job commensurate with his capacities and terminated. In a chance encounter seven years later, Mark approached me, introducing his wife and little toddler. He reported that, after several successful years in real estate, he had returned to school and was now a senior medical student. Mark volunteered smilingly that none of my interpretations had sunk in until after he had left analysis. He intimated further that identification with me had influenced his choice of medicine.

Identification with parental psychopathology may be implicated in career change. Wes, a married lawyer in his late twenties, sought consultation before leaving his prestigious firm to become a golf pro. He described a warm and friendly relationship with his parents. They had respected his independence, both in marrying a woman of different background and in moving to another city. It became clear that his original career choice was based on identification with his parents and their unfulfilled aspirations. Both parents had law degrees but had never practiced. Moreover, Wes had identified with many of his mother's phobic tendencies. He felt increasingly anxious and trapped in his present position, with the urge to get outside to breathe. Wes had ended the consultation firm in his decision. Follow-up some eight years later elicited a highly positive outcome. With his wife's support, Wes had worked as a golf pro for several years, with special satisfaction in teaching. Then, with trepidation, he was persuaded to enter the management of a large, sports-related business. Now, in his late thirties, Wes is like his father, a successful businessman with a law degree. He is now identified with his father rather than with his father's aspirations.

A married engineer who had followed compliantly in his father's footsteps provides another example of identification with parental psychopathology. He was in his late twenties when his father suffered a major depression. Shaken and disillusioned, he began to question his choice of engineering and eventually switched to medicine. This implied both a move away from compliance to greater autonomy and the initiation of a process of disidentification. He spontaneously attributed his own low self-esteem and depressed moods to failure to fulfill his father's impossible perfectionistic expectations. He reasoned further that his father had fallen victim to these very expectations himself. Engineering had been settling for less on both their parts. It was too late for the older generation but not for the younger.

Conflicts over parental demands and expectations are a common factor in change of career. Peter, an unmarried family practitioner in his late twenties, entered psychoanalysis shortly after leaving his father's office to establish his own practice. He had a twinlike relationship with his next younger brother, Jack, barely a year his junior. In the

267

face of their father's tormenting controllingness, Peter was overtly compliant and Jack the rebellious one. However, both expressed the opposite ambivalent polarity covertly. Peter had followed the straight and narrow—college, medical school, and residency into his father's office. Jack had gone into advertising, dropping out to join a commune after a big promotion. Then Jack went to medical school, with plans to join a medical mission sponsored by his father's denomination. However, the father would not be pleased; he raised loud objections, on trivial grounds, to Jack's impending marriage. Peter defied his father through relationships with women unacceptable on religious grounds. With analysis, Peter transcended the compliance/defiance bind to autonomy, ultimately falling in love with a woman despite her acceptability to his father and moving some sixty miles away. Meanwhile, Jack reluctantly returned from the overseas mission when his wife became pregnant and soon sought another foreign assignment. Without treatment, Jack remains locked in the compliance/defiance dilemma.

Identity Problems in Older Medical Students

In the anachronistic classroom situation of the preclinical years, older medical students are more likely to suffer a significant identity crisis marked by depression, confusion, and an impaired sense of continuity of the self. Rakoff (1981) defines identity as the continuing sense of self experienced by the individual and recognized by society. The previous career identity often loses its prestigious currency in medical school, and the older student feels regressively like a grade school pupil. Moreover, the heavy study schedule encroaches on those facets of identity fed by hobby, sports, and avocations.

Those least affected by identity disturbances seemed capable of fulfilling their study obligations with time to spare. That time was devoted to activities and relationships sustaining the continuity of their established identities, mostly at the expense of relationships with classmates. Consequently, a large number of older students in a class tends to erode its cohesiveness.

As defined, identity crisis results from the loss of correspondence between the inner sense of identity and the confirmation from societal recognition. Identity crisis is to be distinguished from the graver condition to which narcissistic, borderline, and psychotic patients are prone—identity diffusion, in which discrepant and contradictory self-representations are implicated. If identity crisis arises when others do not see us as we see ourselves, identity diffusion occurs when what we see is a collection of irreconcilable, antithetical selves.

The three students in my series with the most pronounced identity disturbances all had antecedent problems in this area. Two, a man and a woman, had achieved counterculture renown after assuming negative identities in rejection of their families of origin. Both had turned to medicine later in a more positive reworking of these issues.

In psychotherapy, the young man learned that he blamed his workaholic father's neglect for his mother's premature death from complications of alcoholism. Underlying this medical student's complaint, that school took away the activities that made him feel himself, was a conflicted unconscious identification with father. In his singleminded devotion to studies, to the neglect of his own wife, he was a replica of father. Exclusive devotion to study also constituted self-neglect, his somatic symptoms manifesting identification with his neglected cirrhotic mother.

The young woman's negative identity was complicated by unresolved oedipal conflicts. In medical school, it took new form as a contentious exception whose seductive defiance sorely vexed the administration. The authorities unconsciously represented both parents: the overly rigid establishment mother discomfited by the daughter's misbehavior and an outwardly respectable father whose delight in the mother's discomfiture was subtle but discernible.

Another young man, the vehicle of his mother's grandiose expectations since his father's death in the young man's childhood, had achieved recognizable success in business. These internalized maternal demands made submergence in the regressive classroom atmosphere narcissistically intolerable to this thirty-five-year-old. Renewing his business involvement to shore up his self-esteem encroached increasingly on study time, eventually placing him in academic jeopardy.

In the treatment of a former seminarian, the psychodynamic themes of inner and outer control of bodily processes, emotions, and relationships traversed three generations. The father's serious adolescent delinquency had come to an end through military service and religious conversion. To the upper-class grandparents, the cure was almost as offensive as the disease. Reared in an atmosphere of joyless severity, the son followed the designated path to the seminary unhappily but with faithful obedience. Over time, the unquestioning faith with which he had entered the seminary was increasingly clouded over by doubt. Then a scholarship plum in advanced theological studies became his apple in the Genesis garden. Exposure to novel and contradictory theological debates catalyzed his loss of faith. He left the prestigious institute, eventually finding his way to medicine. This may be termed a deconversion or anticonversion because it shares the salient attributes of the conversion experience; he left religious life with the sense of transformation into a new person, disavowing his past. The parallels to father's descriptions of his religious rebirth are obvious. Meanwhile, the actions of the ex-seminarian's younger brother showed identification with father and counteridentification with his sibling, my patient. For, after serious adolescent delinquency, the brother underwent conversion, devoting himself to a religious life thereafter. With psychotherapy, the patient uncovered repressed emotions, notably rage as well as the disavowed past. Working through led to their acceptance and integration. The presenting hypochondriacal preoccupation with hypertension evolved gradually to the awareness that this was anxiety, then to the surfacing of anger so intense as to threaten loss of control. This is what had made him anxious. Once able to tolerate the conscious awareness of anger, he soon added the capacity to figure out what was making him angry. At the beginning of treatment, he had constantly monitored his blood pressure; at the end, he was monitoring moods and thoughts instead. While the patient was vulnerable during his crisis of faith, the strength and celerity with which the discrepant religious self-representation was disavowed averted identity diffusion. Instead, the consequence was a truncated and impoverished sense of identity. Owning up to his past became a reconciliation with the disavowed part of himself, reinforcing the sense of continuity and otherwise enriching the sense of identity.

Change of Medical Specialty

Change of medical specialty is determined by the same unconscious factors enumerated by Dewald (1980). For two psychiatrists who began in obstetrics, that first choice posed a frightening threat to defenses against unconscious, hostile, sadistic impulses toward mother. In the first case, we reconstructed the erosion of the early warm closeness to the mother when his father's business failed and both parents became depressed. This was exacerbated by the birth of a sibling. In the second case, both parents were unavailable for narcissistic rather than depressive reasons. I surmised that the child's autonomous strivings had dispelled the mother's earlier closeness.

Both became child psychiatrists, choosing intervention on behalf of the child rather than the mother as a more satisfactory compromise solution for their unconscious conflicts, furthering their adult developmental progression. With greater severity of conflict, career changes may fail to advance their reworking toward better resolution. In the face of external change, the unchanging neurotic pattern is repeated. Tom, a senior family practice resident, entered psychotherapy in a frenzy of indecision about his next career move. At first, he seemed a postadolescent example of powerful wishes for omnipotentiality (Pumpian-Mindlin 1965). Medicine had appealed to him because of the wide range of specialty choices. This was gratifying initially but agonizing ultimately when he had to choose a specialty. Every choice involved a renunciation; for Tom, choosing was losing. It became clear that his indecisiveness stemmed from intense separation anxiety since childhood, culminating in an immobilizing depression in his freshman year of college. Tom's indecisiveness also represented a fear of being swallowed up by a controlling, intrusive mother against whom identification with a fearful, compliant father rendered him powerless. The scenario of indecisiveness was played out in two marriages ending in divorce. Once free of their stifling entrapment, Tom sought to maintain contact with both ex-wives to keep open the option to remarry. Initially drawn to pediatrics, Tom could not bear giving up adults and had chosen family practice. Loss was intolerable; he wished time would stand still so that no one close to him would die. His mother's contempt of his father for the timidity that chained him to one inferior position all his working life spurred Tom's struggle to be different. This was reinforced by the mother's shift of her aspirations from his father to him. Tom's fantasy ideal was the Renaissance man, and he wished to go through life acquiring ever more expertise and knowledge while giving up nothing. Tom's evasive solution of his presenting problem at this point was to apply to law school, using the prospect of a combined career in the future to postpone a definite choice in the present.

271

Relationships and the Mentor

Relatively few patients reported mentor relationships. Some may have been missed since they were not inquired about systematically. Speculatively, individuals who change careers may be less likely to form mentor relationships. A gender difference may also be construed. Beyond the practical need of professional women for the support of a mentor in advancing in male-dominated preserves (Collins 1983), women in general assign greater importance to relationships than men do. Women seem more likely to find their career through a relationship; conceivably, men might have to choose their career before finding a mentor.

Vaillant's (1977) longitudinal study, which emphasizes the importance of current relationships, concludes that the best predictor of healthy adult functioning in men is a stable marriage. In the subtle, reciprocal influence of personality and environment, the fortuitous availability of good spouses and mentors interacts with individual differences in finding, forming, and sustaining these relationships. Combined together, they constitute fate; either spouse or mentor may become a tormentor.

How the spouse "supports the dream" is obviously a significant influence. In the course of her transition from an ancillary profession to medicine, a young woman divorced her husband, who opposed the change, and subsequently married a physician highly supportive of her career. She had already formed her dream and went on to obtain the support for its implementation. The man whose acceptance to medical school triggered depression and anxiety attacks came from the same ancillary profession as this woman. In addition to the unconscious quiet over besting his older brother, he had to contend with conscious guilt engendered by his wife's disapproval.

Women's mentors are more likely to be or become lovers and spouses. One-fifth of Collins's 400 respondents reported a sexual relationship with their mentors. Marie Bonaparte, the princess who became psychoanalyst, found many mentors to support her intellectual and scientific interests; several were her lovers. Her family had exerted fierce opposition to these interests (Bertin 1986).

A gifted classical musician in psychotherapy for anxiety in rehearsal and performance attributed her difficulties to parental opposition to a concert career. She was still a child when the teacher who had convinced her parents of her great talent died. Their half-hearted support cost valuable time. Once in high school, she took control of realizing her ambitions, but she was forlorn in the belief that she could never catch up. These inferiority feelings were reinforced by internalized parental disapproval. The parents approved her first marriage (while at the conservatory) as socially and financially advantageous. Her reasons for divorce included her husband's indifference to her career. A liaison with a much older virtuoso led not only to marriage but also to a mentorship in which she changed her instrument to his.

My impression is that, the more troubled the man, the more easily discernible are connections between difficulties in relationships and career; Tom had to retain and acquire ever more professions and women. Another married male resident's similar but less severe separation problems affected both areas. Simultaneously dissatisfied with his wife and fearful of losing her, his serial affairs both courted her loss and provided for that contingency. He was apparently committed to his specialty; yet his ambition would dissipate without a show of special interest from his attendings. Another physician resorted to change in order to evade hostile confrontations. He would quit a position to avoid a showdown with his chief or move to another city to escape the fallout from a broken engagement.

Emde's (1985) characterization of psychoanalysis as a special type of facilitator of adult development is a restatement, in a more sophisticated developmental framework, of Freud (1937, p. 225): "What analysis achieves for neurotics is nothing other than what normal people bring about for themselves without help." Viewing the analyst as a special kind of mentor, we might reword Freud's statement, Normal people secure their developmental advance with help in the form of a mentor relationship; they do not require professional help.

To some degree, every patient in analysis or psychotherapy harbors wishes both for personal closeness and to become a therapist as well. In training analysis and in the psychotherapy of psychiatric residents, the latter wish is realized and the mentor function more prominent. This component is enhanced as well in medical students and young adults like Mark whose career objectives have not yet crystallized. Wishes for self-healing or healing one's family may motivate the choice of psychiatry as a career (Frank and Paris 1987). Identification with the therapist in his or her professional role in the course of the psychotherapeutic experience potentiates these motives.

In the psychoanalysis of children and adolescents, the established criterion for termination is the analytically facilitated advance to the next developmental phase. Our improved perspective on adult development converges with Freud's (1937) remonstrance against prophylactic attempts to mobilize and analyze latent conflicts. We must await future vicissitudes in the course of life for their activation. In other words, the criterion for termination of analysis of adults is essentially the same as for preceding phases. The Freud work cited is "Analysis, Terminable and Interminable." A complete analysis is an impossible ideal. What we accomplish in reality are pieces of analysis.

Conclusions

Psychoanalytic developmental theory encompasses the entire life cycle. Contemporary conceptualizations emphasize continuing development of the self-organization and the defense organization in adulthood.

Psychodynamic and environmental factors interact in career choice. Since every choice simultaneously forces a renunciation, the process automatically mobilizes conflict and defenses against change. Superego demands, narcissistic and instinctual needs, and identifications are among the unconscious constituents affecting choice. Career change may either reflect and facilitate reworking of core conflicts, furthering developmental progression through adulthood, or express an unchanging repetition of a psychopathological pattern.

The clinical observations and inferences are based on thirty patients, mostly older medical students and physicians who changed specialty. Entry into medicine was delayed as initially beyond the aspirations of women reared with traditional ideals of femininity and of men from working-class backgrounds. Some of the conflicts affecting career change in middle-class individuals included competitive rivalry with siblings and parents, parental demands and expectations, and identification with parental psychopathology. Older medical students are more likely to suffer significant identity crisis during the preclinical years. Women appeared more likely to form mentor relationships. The more troubled the men, the more evident the links between difficulties in relationships and career.

Psychoanalysis may be reviewed as a special form of facilitation of adult development provided by ordinary relationships in normals. As a corollary, the analyst or therapist may be regarded as a version of the mentor.

NOTE

This chapter has been presented previously at the Medical University of South Carolina Department of Psychiatry Grand Rounds, Charleston, S.C., April 28, 1987, and to the annual meeting of the American Society for Adolescent Psychiatry, Chicago, May 8, 1987.

REFERENCES

Bemporad, J.; Ratey, J.; and Hallowell, E. 1986. Loss and depression in young adults. *Journal of the American Academy of Psychoanalysis* 14:167–179.

Bertin, C. 1986. *Marie Bonaparte*. New Haven, Conn.: Yale University Press.

Block, J., and Haan, N. 1971. *Lives through Time*. Berkeley, Calif.: Bancroft.

Collins, J. 1983. *Professional Women and Their Mentors*. New York: Prentice-Hall.

Dewald, P. 1980. Adult phases of the life cycle. In S. Greenspan and G. Pollock, eds. *The Course of Life: Psychoanalytic Contributions toward Understanding Personality Development,* vol. 3, *Adulthood and the Aging Process*. Adelphi, Md.: National Institute of Mental Health.

Eichorn, D. A.; Clausen, J. A.; Haan, H.; Honzik, M. P.; and Mussen, P. H. 1981. *Present and Past in Middle Life*. New York: Academic.

Emde, R. 1985. From adolescence to midlife: remodeling the structure of adult development. *Journal of the American Psychoanalytic Association* 33(suppl.): 59–112.

Erikson, E. 1945. Childhood and tradition in two American Indian tribes. *Psychoanalytic Study of the Child* 1:319–350.

Erikson, E. 1950. *Childhood and Society.* New York: Norton.

Erikson, E. 1956. The problem of ego identity. *Journal of the American Psychoanalytic Association* 4:56–122.

Erikson, E. 1968. *Identity Youth and Crisis*. New York: Norton.

Escoll, P. 1987. Psychoanalysis of young adults: an overview. *Psychoanalytic Inquiry* 7(1): 5–30.

Fenton, W.; Robinowitz, C.; and Leaf, P. 1987. Male and female psychiatrists and their patients. *American Journal of Psychiatry* 144(3): 358–361.

Frank, H., and Paris, J. 1987. Psychological factors in the choice of psychiatry as a career. *Canadian Journal of Psychiatry* 32:118–122.

Freud, S. 1905. Three essays on the theory of sexuality. *Standard Edition* 7:125–245. London: Hogarth, 1953.

Freud, S. 1937. Analysis, terminable and interminable. *Standard Edition* 23:211–253. London: Hogarth, 1964.

Hartmann, H. 1939. *Ego Psychology and the Problem of Adaptation.* New York: International Universities Press, 1958.

Headlee, R., and Kalogjera, I. 1987. A critical analysis of the process of human choice. *Psychiatric Journal of the University of Ottawa* 12(1): 16–20.

Jones, E. 1948. *Papers on Psycho-Analysis.* London: Bailliere, Tindall, & Cox.

Kaplan, E. 1980. Adolescents, age fifteen to eighteen: a psychoanalytic developmental view. In S. Greenspan and G. Pollock, eds. *The Course of Life: Psychoanalytic Contributions toward Understanding Personality Development,* vol. 2, *Latency, Adolescence and Youth.* Adelphi, Md.: National Institute of Mental Health.

Leavy, S. 1985. Demythologizing Oedipus. *Psychoanalytic Quarterly* 54(3):444–454.

Levinson, D. J.; Darrow, C. N.; Klein, E. B.; Levinson, K. W.; and McKee, B. 1978. *The Seasons of a Man's Life.* New York: Ballantine.

Marcus, I. 1980. The influence of development upon career achievement. In S. Greenspan and G. Pollock, eds. *The Course of Life: Psychoanalytic Contributions toward Understanding Personality Development,* vol. 2, *Latency, Adolescence and Youth.* Adelphi, Md.: National Institute of Mental Health.

Mercy, J. 1987. Young adults greater suicide risk than teens. *Medical World News* (April 10), p. 38.

Offer, D. 1969. *The Psychological World of the Teenager.* New York: Basic.

Offer, D., and Offer, J. 1975. *From Teenage to Young Manhood.* New York: Basic.

Pumpian-Mindlin, E. 1965. Omnipotentiality, youth and commitment. *Journal of the American Academy of Child Psychiatry* 4:1–18.

Rakoff, V. 1981. A reconsideration of identity. *Adolescent Psychiatry* 9:24–32.

Spruiell, V. 1983. The rules and frames of the psychoanalytic situation. *Psychoanalytic Quarterly* 52:1–33.

Trent, J., and Medsker, L. 1968. *Beyond High School*. San Francisco: Jossey-Bass.

Vaillant, G. E. 1977. *Adaptation to Life*. Boston: Little, Brown.

19   COMPROMISED DEVELOPMENT:
THE COMPLEX PLIGHT OF YOUNG ADULTS
WITH MENTAL/EMOTIONAL DISORDERS

HILARY RYGLEWICZ AND BERT PEPPER

The unifying topic of this special section is "Transition to Young Adult-hood." Yet the focus of this chapter is a large, heterogeneous population of young people for whom that transition is imperfect at best, impossible at worst. This is the population of young adults in the age group sixteen to forty years old who live and struggle with serious, ongoing mental and emotional disorders. For these young people, the developmental process has been complicated, compromised, arrested, or foreshortened by the effect of severe disorder and its many consequences. By the time they reach the delicate, treacherous channel to adulthood, these chronological young adults are unable to brave or to navigate its waters.

Increasing evidence of a biogenetic basis for the major mental disorders does not relieve us of the need to explore the developmental history of these young people. On the contrary, we need to look carefully at the developmental process—in part normal, in part atypical—that has been the compromise such a young adult has made between his or her capacities and the demands and resources of the environment. We need also to be concerned with the young person's developmental process as it extends into the older young adult years—well beyond the usual time span of childhood and adolescence. And we need to ask what further developmental progress is possible for a young person whose serious, ongoing mental disorder has arrested or compromised other aspects of development, resulting in a failed or flawed transition into true, autonomous adulthood.

This chapter will take a retrospective view of the complexities and problems of social and psychological development for the person who has grown up in the community with a mental disorder and will raise some concerns of community psychiatry and the mental health service delivery system about this large and very diverse population of young adults, many of them dual-problem and multiproblem patients.

Compromised Development and Its Side Effects

Of course, the developmental phases of adolescence and young adulthood, while they can be clearly differentiated conceptually, are two adjacent parts of one continuum—that is, life. In psychological terms, we know that the developmental tasks of adolescence—like the tasks of earlier stages of development—if not adequately mastered at the age-appropriate time, remain to hamper or even prevent the achievement of autonomous adulthood. In terms of social development, we know that a person with an impairment of any kind, whether physical or mental, is hindered in the normal developmental process. From the point at which that impairment becomes a handicap—a barrier to whatever skill development or form of personal/social functioning is called for—that person's developmental course becomes problematic or atypical. That is, a child who is physically unable to use his or her legs is unable, therefore, to learn to walk; and, even if the physical impairment is temporary, not learning to walk at the age-appropriate time has a decisive effect, not only on development of the skill of walking, but on a host of related physical, psychological, and social developments and interactions that are related to physical mobility. Similarly, the impairment of a mental disorder—a brain or chemical disorder, such as schizophrenia, learning disability, or substance addiction—has both direct and indirect effects on the developmental process from the earliest age of onset, that age at which the person's impairment begins to have an identifiable effect on the experience of the self in the social environment.

By the time a young adult is identified as having serious, ongoing mental or emotional disorders, that person's course of development has been affected in multiple and complex ways by the entire process of growing up with (or into) a problem. We are looking, then, not merely at a schizophrenic or a manic-depressive or a substance abuser but at a person who has both a major disorder and an individual and complex developmental history. This history consists in part of efforts to function in the social environment in spite of a specific vulnerability or impairment. For each such person, these efforts have resulted in certain expectations and coping strategies and, for many, in dysfunctional patterns such as a personality disorder and/or the habitual use of alcohol and drugs. Thus, we meet young adult patients with layers of impairments and distortions in personal and social development—bipolar disorder superimposed on passive-aggressive personality and complicated by substance dependence, to name one possible combination of labels.

Mainstreaming and Noninstitutionalization

These complications are in part a product of our present era in psychiatric treatment, in which the policies of mainstreaming in the educational system and deinstitutionalization/noninstitutionalization in the mental health system have both resulted in maintaining children and adults with special vulnerabilities and needs in what we regard as a normal environment. Our policy and effort is to keep such persons in the community, to live, develop, and function as best they can, side by side with their age-mates, in the demanding, stimulating, and sometimes hazardous community environment. We have, to be sure, some supports and accommodations for people with specific handicaps—ramps for those impaired in their ability to walk, special classes for children impaired in their ability to learn, residential treatment centers for some children and adolescents who are impaired in their ability to live in what would be their natural settings, psychiatric emergency services for people in acute episodes of mental illness, and even, in some fortunate communities, reasonably adequate treatment and support programs for persons with serious, ongoing mental disorders, who are impaired in their ability to fend for themselves.

But our basic message to the vulnerable person in our society is, Try to live like everybody else—even as the subtext of that message is, You are, however, not as good as others, nor will you have the same chances. The positive part of the message is its offer of the opportunity to approximate, as nearly as possible, a normal life in a normal environment rather than a severely constricted life in an institution. The negative aspect lies in the gap between this expectation and what the vulnerable person can actually do and in the related gap between the supports that person needs for full development and functioning and the relative lack of supports actually available.

The new generation of young adults who have grown up in the community with serious mental/emotional disorders is one of the populations most heavily affected by these gaps and mixed messages. The common characteristics of these young people clearly differentiate them from the earlier generations of mentally ill persons who became long-stay institutional patients. These differences are related to their spending most of their lives, both before and after the development of a chronic psychiatric disorder, in the community mainstream.

Characteristics of Younger versus Older Patients

What are the characteristics that have set this new generation apart from their predecessors? In our work at Rockland County Community Mental Health Center, we have taken, for the past decade, a very broad perspective on this large and diverse population, viewing the characteristics that many hold in common as more noteworthy than the more familiar differences suggested by their diagnoses. In the present era of mental health treatment, and for purposes of delivering effective programs and services, we find young adults with diverse disorders—schizophrenia, bipolar disorder, personality disorders—to have more in common with each other than with older members of their respective diagnostic groups. In contrast to the older patient, the young adult is likely to have high expectations combined with low self-esteem, use/abuse of alcohol and other drugs and/or hypersensitivity to their effects, high risk of problems with the law and/or family violence, continued involvement and dependency issues with parents, high risk of suicide and suicidal ideation, unstable relationships combined with sexual activity and sometimes parenthood, and treatment resistance/treatment rejection. With regard to their ongoing conflicts and continuing dependence on parents, we have noted that, in a functional sense, such young adults seem to be stuck in the transition from childhood dependence to adult independence, from parental or quasi-parental support to self-supporting work, adult autonomy, and an expanding network of relationships.

While these young adults may or may not be correctly described as stuck in an adolescent stage of psychological development, they commonly present some of the behaviors and quandaries that are familiar characteristics of adolescents—in particular, the ambivalent struggle with dependency, whether on families, therapists, or treatment and support systems. This is not surprising if we make, again, the analogy with the child who is unable to learn to walk because of impairment in the use of his or her legs. Many young adults with chronic mental disorders want to "walk"—away from parents, therapists, and the status of psychiatric patient—but are impaired by being unable to stand on their own two feet. Therefore, their dependency persists, with increasing anxiety and ambivalence, both for them and for their parents and parent figures.

Diagnoses and the Dual- or Multiple-Disorder Patient

What are the disorders that hamper such young adults in making the transition to autonomous adulthood? Despite our unifying perspective, we can identify subgroups in terms of diagnosis, age of onset, and relationship with the treatment system. In Rockland County Mental Health Center's samples of the young adult long-term patient population, a sizable subgroup of patients carries diagnoses of schizophrenia or bipolar disorder, while another, overlapping subgroup shows personality disorders, with or without major mental illness. A high proportion of these young adult patients in psychiatric programs also shows alcohol or drug use/abuse as a socially disabling condition and also as a factor inhibiting personality development. We know both from our own patient cohorts and from data reported in other treatment systems that there is a large proportion of "dually diagnosed" (psychiatric and substance abuse) persons among patients diagnosed with major mental disorders. Most young people today—with or without mental/emotional disorders—make at least some experimental or chronic use of alcohol, marijuana, or other drugs. Such experimental use now occurs at alarmingly early ages—reported as eight to ten years of age—and impinges disastrously both on children whose brains are still in the process of development and on those already impaired by mental and emotional disorders, mild mental retardation, learning disability, or other conditions.

Thus, we must now consider substance use and abuse to be expectable factors complicating evaluation, diagnosis, and the course of treatment for young adults with serious, ongoing mental disorders. For all the various subgroups of young adults, including those with major mental illness, an important task for clinicians, treatment systems, families, and other concerned persons is to determine which of their problems in functioning result from the truly chronic limitations imposed by a brain or chemical disorder and which result from overlays acquired in the process of development and interaction with the social environment. The latter may include flawed or arrested personality development, family stress, use of drugs and alcohol as a dysfunctional coping strategy, excessive stimulation and demands of the community environment, expectations of normal success, expectations of failure, and so on.

The advent of DSM-III has been a truly important step in helping us to look at people through multiple lenses rather than only through the lens of a specific diagnosis of mental illness. DSM-III encourages clinicians to think along multiple axes. It can lead us to reflect on the interaction of a brain or chemical disorder with the environment in the process of social development. It invites us to recognize that what we actually see in the functioning of many young adults with mental/emotional disorders is not only or necessarily a result of mental illness but may also reflect development that has not yet taken place or a personality disorder formed to mediate between a brain impairment and the demands of the outside world.

The Normal and the Impaired Child

One way of thinking about this developmental process for the person with a major mental disorder is to think of that person as born into the world with the normal needs and strivings of all human beings: the need for food, shelter, protection, and nurturing; the need for relationships in which basic trust can be developed; the need for friends, as companions as well as sources of feedback and support in the long process of social development; the need for a set of values and attitudes, a coherent way of perceiving life; the need for some measure of control over oneself and over life events; and the need to be recognized and treated as a normal person with the rights and dignity owed to every human being.

What is the situation of a person with a mental disorder or impairment in trying to fulfill these ordinary human needs? The chid whose behavior deviates from the norm or who is seen as different is at a severe disadvantage in almost every life situation; for some such children, even the most basic needs are not adequately met. The responses and social interactions that are readily available to most children—the average expectable environment—are more or less unavailable or distorted for the child whose atypical behavior and developmental process is in some fashion disturbing to parents, siblings, teachers, peers, and others. Whether the quality of attention given is supportive or rejecting, it nearly always feeds back to the child a sense of being "different," and this awareness cannot fail to have pervasive effects on the developmental process. The degree, extent, and forms of the effects depend on when the disorder or impairment shows itself and on how severely it impairs age-expected functioning. For many children whose "difference" shows up early and affects many aspects of functioning, the disorder that is visible on the surface consumes the attention of others, and the normal person within goes unnoticed.

This is a problem that has attended implementation of both the policy of mainstreaming in education and the policy of deinstitutionalization in mental health. It is a problem shared by the child or adult with a mental disorder and the people in his or her social environment, whether family or strangers. Difference cannot fail to attract attention, especially if its manifestations require constraint, restraint, or any other specialized response. The child in a normal environment cannot fail to know his or her difference; the disorder stands out, whether subtly or in bold relief, both in the child's own attempts to function and in the reactions of others. On the other hand, in the social environment that is designed around the disorder—the hospital, the special class, the family whose life has become focused on an illness—what the child fails to know and experience is his or her normality, those respects in which he or she is truly "just like everybody else." Both mainstreaming and deinstitutionalization can be seen as efforts to downplay the consequences of disorders that set children or adults apart from the general population. As such, they hold out possibilities that are hopeful in concept but more problematic in their implementation. We cannot really provide a normal environment for a child or an adult with a serious, ongoing mental disorder; that is, we cannot create a world in which handicap has no consequences. What we can hope to do is to provide as nearly normal an environment as possible, accompanied by whatever special supports the person needs to function in that environment.

Implications for Assessment and Treatment

The import of this thought for our purposes is that both assessments of and responses to the adolescent or young adult with mental disorders must address not only the primary diagnosis or presenting problems in the here and now but also the complications and skill deficits that have developed in the course of that young person's development. For most young adult patients, a complex interplay of deficits and dysfunctional patterns has developed over time. These include severe deficits in social, learning, and coping skills as well as efforts to compensate for these skill deficits or to evade those situations in which the absent skills are required. For the young person who will later develop schizophrenia, the problems in development may include avoidance of social contact, complex or overstimulating situations, and close relationships as well as extreme sensitivity to life changes and other sources of stress. These avoidances may take the form of social withdrawal, learning or behavioral problems, or other overt difficulties in age-appropriate functioning. They may also take the form of retreat into behaviors that appear more typical of adolescents—for example, frequent use of marijuana, mood swings, and/or acting-out behavior—and only later show up as serious pathology. The young adult who is easily diagnosed with borderline personality disorder in his or her twenties may have appeared in adolescence to have been merely overreacting to family crisis or to first love by acting out or threatening suicide.

Whatever the forms in which these earlier signs of trouble have appeared, an important consequence is that the dysfunctional efforts at coping themselves complicate and compromise the developmental process. The young person with an impairment that interferes with learning not only is affected in the capacity to do school work but also is likely to avoid a broad range of learning and social situations as well as challenges and demands of other kinds. That person then becomes still further impaired in the entire process of intellectual and social development, through not engaging in the multiple experiences involved in the developmental process. The young person who takes refuge in substance use or abuse because he or she is paralyzed by anxiety not only runs the risk of developing an addiction but also develops a pattern of evasion as a means of coping with pressure and

285

conflict. Yet it is through conflict and its resolution that the growth and development of the self take place. Five years later, that young person may overcome his or her addiction through specific treatment, but those five years also represent lost opportunity—the loss of multiple and complex experiences that could have contributed to the process of personal and social development. This loss may be compensated for in further development during the young adult years; yet such compensation may never be complete once the synchronization and fine-tuning of the developmental process along its various developmental lines suffer a major disruption. There is a time to learn in school, to play games, to run with a group of peers, to have a close friend; later, one may make up some ground, but the years of childhood are already gone, and the deprivations of these earlier years have left their mark.

Discussion

The developmental history of the young adult with a serious mental/emotional disorder can be seen as a complex compromise among the normal efforts to grow, the handicap of an organic or psychological disorder, and the mixed messages, offerings, and demands of the social environment. The young adult with a disorder who is living in the community today is in a more complex and less protected environment than that of the institutionalized psychiatric patient of yesteryear, as he or she struggles to cope with life despite ongoing and serious impairments. We are accustomed to seeing in the older chronic patient the devastation of a long, destructive process of psychotic illness plus a long conditioning to the passivity of institutional life—both of these blurring beyond recognition the earlier developmental issues or personality adaptations. But the younger patient, living side by side with age-mates in the community, stands out as a mixed picture or functional profile—a person whose normally expected course of development can be traced even though it has been slowed, flawed, or distorted by a psychiatric disorder or a substance abuse problem and by the interaction of these disorders with the entire process of socialization in the community environment.

This compromised development shows itself in everyday life as a lack—or, rather, an uneven development—of essential personal and social (interpersonal) capacities and skills, depending on the specific disorders and the age at which the person's difficulty became an overt handicap in personal functioning and social interaction. Since every relationship and life activity requires the exercise of such skills on an age-appropriate level, and since most activities and roles require a number of such capabilities in complex interaction, it becomes crucial to distinguish the deficits that result from ongoing major mental disorders from those that reflect a compromised psychological and social developmental process. A young adult with schizophrenia, another recovering from an addiction, a third with borderline personality disorder, and a fourth who has made habitual use of marijuana each have had to cope with different organic and personality factors that have limited and distorted the normal processes of maturation and skill building. Yet all may share the kinds of deficits that prevent a person from holding a job. Similarly, each may have different reactions to the stress of trying to work—paranoid thoughts, a temptation to use drugs, a suicide attempt, an anxiety attack—but each will fall back on that stress reaction more or less quickly depending on the compensating skills and ego strengths he or she has been able to develop before the age of onset of the diagnosed disorders.

Conclusions

The major implication of these concepts when we consider treatment and program planning for young people with serious long-term mental disorders in the community is that we must think not only of rehabilitation—the process of recovery or adaptation to an illness—but of habilitation or development. In treatment planning and activities, not only the problem of major mental disorder but the adaptations, dysfunctional coping efforts, and missed developmental opportunities that have attended its development must be addressed. Through attending to all aspects of a young adult's present functioning, we may be able to separate that part of the person's disorder that is truly chronic—the organic component—from that which can be modified through work that is essentially developmental and remedial in its nature.

20   TREATMENT OF CHRONIC MENTALLY ILL
YOUNG ADULTS WITH SUBSTANCE ABUSE
PROBLEMS: EMERGING NATIONAL TRENDS

M. SUSAN RIDGELY, HOWARD H. GOLDMAN,
AND JOHN A. TALBOTT

The state of the art in treating chronic mentally ill young adults is not
well advanced (Adler, Drake, Berlant, Ellison, and Carson 1987). When
one considers the additional problem of addressing substance abuse
(programmatically) among chronic mentally ill young adults, it would
be more accurate to describe the development of treatment as in its
infancy, characterized more by trial and error than by implementation
of established treatment protocols. There are virtually no data on concurrent treatment of coexisting disorders (Kofoed, Kania, Walsh, and
Atkinson 1986). Yet we do know something about the characteristic
way these patients approach treatment systems and about their needs
and motivations, which gives us something to work from in our development of programs. As Bachrach reminds us, however, it is necessary to focus beyond the development of "technology" to the reasons
why we do not already incorporate what we know into our programs,
whether these be attitudinal (the stigma against young patients as "difficult") or simply a response to the inertia of the mental health and
substance abuse systems of care (and the lack of reward for going
beyond the boundaries of one's system) (Bachrach 1982b; Jeffrey 1979).
In fact, it is germane to question whether the focus of new programming
will be on the most sensible approach to the problem or on the more
political question of what the existing order will permit.

This review of the "state of the art" in treatment and training represents a continuation of the collaborative effort of the federal Alcohol, Drug Abuse and Mental Health Administration (ADAMHA) and the University of Maryland Task Force on Chronic Mentally Ill Young Adults with Substance Abuse Problems. In 1985–1986, under the leadership of Dr. John A. Talbott, chairman of the Department of Psychiatry at the University of Maryland School of Medicine, the university undertook the development of a report to investigate, analyze, and present information on the state of the art in research and data collection on chronic mentally ill young adults with substance abuse problems and to create a research agenda for the component institutes of ADAMHA (the National Institute on Drug Abuse, the National Institute on Alcohol Abuse and Alcoholism, and the National Institute of Mental Health [NIMH]). That report, representing phase 1 of the project, is entitled "Chronic Mentally Ill Young Adults (18–40) with Substance Abuse Problems: A Review of Relevant Literature and Creation of a Research Agenda" and is available from the Mental Health Policy Studies Program of the University of Maryland School of Medicine. This chapter represents an interim report on phase 2 of the project, describing the state of the art in treatment programming and training.

Five Broad Questions concerning Programming for Chronic Mentally Ill Young Adults with Substance Abuse Problems

A review of treatment approaches aimed toward the development of programming principles for this population should attend to five broad questions. (1) What constitutes mental health treatment for chronic mentally ill persons (i.e., what "technology" do we have at our disposal)? How has this treatment been modified to address the special needs and patterns of service utilization of chronic mentally ill young adults? (2) In the "generic" sense, what constitutes substance abuse treatment? What "technology" is available? (3) What constitutes a "hybrid" program? Are hybrid programs necessary, or is the answer a better matching of patients to primarily mental health or primarily substance abuse facilities? If "matching" is the answer, how do we do it more effectively than in the past? (4) If hybrid programs are the answer, how do we produce a hybrid, and where do we place it (mental health or substance abuse system)? Does it matter? (5) Beyond specific program development, what do we do to make our mental health and substance abuse systems more "user friendly" for chronic mentally ill young adults? What is necessary in terms of system-wide change? Addressing these broad questions will bring us to a discussion of specific program principles involved in engaging and treating this very needy population.

QUESTION 1: WHAT CONSTITUTES MENTAL HEALTH TREATMENT FOR CHRONIC MENTALLY ILL YOUNG ADULTS?

The focus of mental health treatment for chronic mentally ill persons has moved from the more traditional goal of reducing the symptoms of serious psychiatric illness (with its attendant focus on specific diagnosis) to increasing the person's functional capacity and quality of life (with a focus on disability rather than diagnosis) (Bachrach 1983). This is to say not that treatment of symptomatology (such as the use of neuroleptics to control hallucinations and delusions) is no longer practiced but rather that the focus has shifted and more special attention is given to other areas of support. Not only has traditional psychopharmacology and, in some cases, psychotherapy not been abandoned, but it is considered by many to be a necessary component to maintaining a level of functioning necessary for community living and, thereby, participation in other therapeutic activities. But, clearly, the emphasis in the 1970s was toward the recognition that traditional outpatient mental health care was not sufficient to enable many, if not most, chronic mentally ill persons to maintain and enhance their lives in the community (Test, Knoedler, Allness, and Burke 1985). The NIMH's Community Support Program most clearly articulated the necessity of other supports, focusing on housing, rehabilitative and supported-work activities, income maintenance, case management, and the like (Goldstrom and Manderscheid 1983). In many ways, this came as recognition that the community mental health center movement, though positive for many patients, had not addressed the multiple needs of chronic mentally ill persons because it had left unaddressed the multiple functions that state mental hospitals previously had performed in these patients' lives (Goldman and Taube 1986). Programming was needed that stretched beyond the core community mental health services model.

The promulgation of the Community Support Program's principles clearly fostered the development of a new technology in community-based care. This model, known generally as the psychosocial rehabilitation program, began to address the multiple needs of patients, including the need to have someplace to congregate and to establish a supportive network. Many more traditional mental health programs began to address the broader "social welfare" needs of their patients and also began to make their systems more accessible and better able to respond to crises.

Questions have been raised, however, about the participation of chronic mentally ill young adults in community support programs. We know that at least some young adult patients will not attend programs frequented by older, "deinstitutionalized" patients. What is not so clear is whether they object to socializing with older patients, whether the programming does not really address their needs, or both. We do know that many "vote with their feet" at any kind of structured program and turn up in emergency rooms and other crisis facilities. In times of increasingly limited health care resources, minimizing the risk of relapse and the utilization of expensive hospital resources should be a high priority (Damron and Simpson 1985).

In general then, it is necessary to determine if advances in the treatment of chronic mentally ill persons generalize well to the treatment of chronic mentally ill young adults and, if they do not, what modifications are necessary to these programs. While this more general question is beyond the scope of this study, it should be helpful to identify those features of mental health programs that attract and engage chronic mentally ill young adults. Because chronic mentally ill young adults show little motivation to engage in treatment, it seems likely that programs that are able to tap into some of their other motivations—such as the motivation to avoid being labeled mentally ill or the motivation to have as normal a life as possible (i.e., to live in an apartment and not a "mental health facility," to aspire to and obtain competitive employment, etc.)—may have an edge (Adler et al. 1987; Bender 1982; Lamb 1982). Offering patients opportunities in exchange for accepting help may be one approach that works.

QUESTION 2: WHAT CONSTITUTES SUBSTANCE ABUSE
TREATMENT (OR, MORE SPECIFICALLY, WHAT ARE
WE LOOKING FOR SUBSTANCE ABUSE TREATMENT
TO DO FOR THESE PATIENTS)?

Although the approach may be different and may focus on the consumption of a particular substance, substance abuse programs generally have one goal: to get the person to stop abusing substances. Depending on the need of the individual patient, the program may address detoxification from the physical effects of the substance (alcohol or drugs), interrupting the physical or belief system that maintains the drug use, or substituting other activities/relationships for those that tend to reinforce the old habits/abuse. These programs have different formats, including whether they physically remove patients from their environment (hospitalization or residential community), but almost all of them involve drug/alcohol education, the use of peer groups for both confrontation about substance abuse behavior and peer support in the change process, as well as individualized treatment (such as individual or group psychotherapy). Covert substance abuse is usually monitored by use of urinalysis or breathalyzer tests. Additionally, there are a number of pharmacological treatments used in connection with substance abuse programs. These include, for example, the use of disulfiram (Antabuse) to interfere with the consumption of alcohol and the use of methadone as a substitute for heroin, in the case of opiate addiction.

The question of whether patients need residential or hospital-based treatment to learn to abstain from substances is of particular interest in treating chronic mentally ill young adults. Some believe that removing abusers from an environment that supports substance abuse into a nonnormalized, often medical, setting is the only way to terminate substance abuse. Others feel that the "downside" to this approach is that such programs may lack the necessary ingredients to foster the generalization of new behavior and the maintenance of change to the community environment in which the patient ultimately must function. This debate within the substance abuse field is of critical interest to clinicians who recognize that many chronic mentally ill people have problems with generalizing and are particularly apt to discontinue contact and neglect follow-through once outside the inpatient setting (Caton 1981; Geller 1986; McCarrick, Manderscheid, and Bertolucci 1985).

Alcoholics Anonymous (AA) and other self-help groups modeled on its principles continue to play a key role in most substance abuse programs. Even many rigorous, time-limited inpatient programs encourage or require attendance at additional self-help meetings outside the confines of the program. Others introduce AA as a form of continued "aftercare."

It should be mentioned at this point that one of the commonest complaints among mental health providers is that their patients are not welcome in these groups. Some mental health providers have started their own chapters of AA and NA (Narcotics Anonymous) for psychiatric patients. The pressure toward abstinence from all mind-altering substances has been a problem for psychiatric patients in many AA programs. Many AA members frown on (and often actively discourage) the use of psychotropic medications. It becomes difficult, then, to separate the needed and, therefore, "good" drug from those to be avoided.

QUESTION 3: WHAT IS A "HYBRID" PROGRAM? IS THE DEVELOPMENT OF HYBRID PROGRAMS THE ANSWER, OR IS THE ANSWER A BETTER "MATCHING" OF PATIENTS TO PRIMARILY MENTAL HEALTH OR PRIMARILY SUBSTANCE ABUSE TREATMENT FACILITIES?

It seems reasonable to assume that the answer to the problem of addressing both the need for mental health treatment and the need to help young psychiatric patients abstain from the use of alcohol and drugs is to combine the features of mental health and substance abuse treatment (especially since referrals across the system lines have been notoriously bad in the past). Yet this is an assumption that has to be addressed. It is clear that there are systems problems (i.e., arbitrary service divisions and a lack of sensitivity for and expertise in each other's fields) that prevent easy passage across boundaries. What is not so clear is whether a successful approach to the problem must address the two "illnesses" concurrently or whether fixing the systems problems could provide for a continuum of care for patients with dual disorders. If there were to be a gatekeeping function or facility that would assess the overall need of the individual and refer to facilities/programs in both systems (and if those programs were familiar with both mental illness and substance abuse), could these chronic mentally ill young adults be appropriately treated in existing programs, even more "traditional" programs? It is likely that there are identifiable subgroups of chronic mentally ill young adults with specific needs (Hall et al. 1979). More traditional programs with a single focus on substance abuse or mental health services may provide a component within a continuum of care for these patients.

QUESTION 4: IF A HYBRID IS THE ANSWER, HOW DO WE PRODUCE ONE, AND WHERE DO WE PLACE IT? DOES IT MATTER?

Because the goals of mental health intervention and substance abuse intervention for chronic mentally ill young adults are complementary, it should be possible to create a hybrid program that addresses both of these "illnesses" concurrently. As mentioned, both approaches seek to achieve recognition and control of the manifestation of the problems, to educate the young adults about their illness and thus the necessity for taking responsibility for their behavior, and to provide opportunities for positive (i.e., educational, vocational, or recreational) community activities and relationships.

Producing such a program is not an easy task. In many localities, boundaries of the mental health and substance abuse systems are not permeable. Funding for such dual-focus programs is hard to find. Yet patients present themselves to treatment settings as whole individuals, not according to the neat boundaries of our service systems (Bachrach, Talbott, and Meyerson 1986; Crowley, Chesluk, Dilts, and Hart 1974).

Should hybrid programs be placed within the mental health system or within the substance abuse system? Some would argue that chronic mentally ill young adults are, by definition, a psychiatric population and, thus, that the primary focus of program development should be in the mental health system. Others argue that staff at substance abuse facilities are more familiar with manipulative and disengaged patients and thus are equipped to handle a population that the mental health system has trouble handling (Hall et al. 1977). It is interesting to note that programs currently focused on the chronic mentally ill young adult with substance abuse problems operate in both the mental health and the substance abuse systems. Is that a function of preference or of the fact that one of the two systems was willing to tackle the problem?

QUESTION 5: BEYOND SPECIFIC PROGRAM
DEVELOPMENT, WHAT DO WE DO TO MAKE OUR
MENTAL HEALTH AND SUBSTANCE ABUSE SYSTEMS
MORE "USER FRIENDLY"? WHAT IS NECESSARY IN
TERMS OF SYSTEM-WIDE CHANGE?

As was well documented in our earlier report, the problem of patients refusing to participate in programs and becoming noncompliant with treatment planning is not simply a problem of the patients. It is also a problem with caregivers and our systems of care (Bachrach et al. 1986; Crowley et al. 1974; Glass 1982; Goldfinger, Hopkin, and Suber 1984; Talbott, Bachrach, and Ross 1986). The mental health and substance abuse systems cling to arbitrary service divisions and categorical boundaries (with attendant funding policies) because it is administratively efficient. Because there are mutually exclusive programs, patients must present only one problem at the door, or they are turned away. Such problems exist even within the substance abuse field, as many programs address the abuse of alcohol or the abuse of other drugs but not both (Crowley et al. 1974). If patients do not or cannot adapt to the way we organize services, the system defines them as "bad patients" and, in turn, reinforces their "bad habits," that is, the over-utilization of costly inpatient and emergency services (Goldfinger et al. 1984).

Within the description of these problems is the agenda for change. As Talbott and colleagues have noted, systems can fail in one of two ways: with structural deficits (the lack of a sufficient array of services addressed to need) and with process failures (the lack of continuity of care). Recommendations focus on developing some "resiliency" of the system and, in this case, permeability across the boundaries of two separate systems (Talbott et al. 1986).

Principles of Programming for Chronic Mentally Ill Young Adults with Substance Abuse Problems

As mentioned, development of treatment protocols for chronic mentally ill young adults with substance abuse problems that attend to both mental health and substance abuse issues is rudimentary at best. Yet review of the literature on treatment issues and review of programs serving chronic mentally ill young adults indicates similarities among these programs that begin to emerge as principles for treatment programming. These are identified as important issues to be addressed in the development of programs: engagement; assessment; concurrent treatment; outcome; and systems change.

ENGAGEMENT

The literature on nonpsychotic, chronic mentally ill adults describes their contacts with health professionals as "erratic, dramatic, and emotionally intense" (Adler et al. 1987, p. 1). The same tone is taken in the majority of references to the erratic, crisis-oriented patterns of service utilization among chronic mentally ill young adults in general (Bachrach et al. 1986; Bender 1986; Diamond 1984; Lamb 1982; Stein and Test 1982). Commentators and program staff stress the difficulty associated with establishing the necessary trust relationship that will get chronic mentally ill young adults into treatment. Stein and Test (1982) also emphasize that engagement is not a one-time process, highlighting the necessity to retain patients in treatment as well as to attract them into treatment in the first place.

Concerns about engagement tend to focus on one of two issues: developing an ongoing relationship with patients who are known to have difficulty developing and maintaining stable relationships and motivating young patients to enter treatment under which the ultimate goal is abstinence from alcohol and drugs.

First, developing relationships that will engage and retain patients in treatment is a difficult proposition. Because autonomy is a "most cherished possession" for many chronic mentally ill young adults, attempting to lure them into a relationship that will abridge their autonomy or that is perceived by them to be abridging their autonomy is a treatment issue that must be addressed (Bender 1986). These young adults struggle with authority and must be convinced that the treatment team has something worth listening to before they will be ready to listen. Developing trust relationships occurs over time and is enhanced if program staff are able to help with crises in a concrete fashion (Lamb 1982). Engagement is typically characterized by a lot of "approach/avoidance" behavior, and programs that succeed may have to be willing to tolerate the stresses associated with this type of crisis management (within the confines of their program), foregoing, for the moment, what they may deem is "best for the patient." Segal and Baumohl (1980), in their discussion of programming for the homeless/vagrant chronic mentally ill young adult, have addressed the fact that the intake procedures in many programs may be contributing to "avoidance." The intake process often requires the early detailing of much personal information. They suggest that these procedures be modified to require a minimum of information at the outset, with more information to be obtained during the process of engagement through "gradual disclosure settings." Such settings, "coffee houses" and "community living rooms," allow informal interaction between staff and potential patients, creating social interaction and not the social distance involved in more encumbered intake and assessment procedures.

Several programs for chronic mentally ill young adults with substance abuse problems have used just such models for engagement. For instance, one substance abuse treatment unit provides a coffee house program for chronic mentally ill young adults. The program is open, and potential patients can come when they feel like talking, as opposed to "therapy sessions" by appointment. Patients can talk in a group or see a counselor on a one-to-one basis. The "down side" is that they may see different counselors each time they walk in, but continuity of counselor may be less important than engagement in these initial stages. These coffee houses, as well as the social club atmosphere at psychosocial rehabilitation programs, may be perceived as less threatening and less stigmatizing by some patients.

A related problem has to do with the issue of motivation for treatment. Some chronic mentally ill young adults simply prefer to see themselves as "victims" of society and not as mentally ill (Lamb 1982). They do not seek out treatment because they do not define themselves as needing treatment, either for mental illness or for substance abuse. They do not fully understand the effect of recreational use or polydrug abuse on their course of community life or, in the case of those who willingly (or begrudgingly) accept mental health treatment, the fact that substance use/abuse may result in additional psychiatric hospitalizations that are purely substance abuse related and not a result of the mental illness per se (Crowley et al. 1974; Safer 1986). Denial of substance abuse problems is particularly difficult to manage without the prior establishment of a trusting, therapeutic relationship. Thus, it is especially difficult to conceive of a program that can demand abstinence at the door and still hope to engage a majority of chronic mentally ill young adults in treatment. The issue of abstinence becomes especially tanglesome, though, by the very fact that substance use/abuse tends to complicate a clear assessment and development of an appropriate course of treatment. Programs must achieve a balance regarding these two necessities. (Some have chosen to do that by not requiring total abstinence during the engagement phase and proceeding with drug education and peer support activities while giving potential patients time to make their own decision about when abstinence is a real likelihood. Rules are enforced, though, about use on the premises of the program facilities in order to maintain the integrity of the program for use by the other patients.)

Some psychosocial rehabilitation programs do not address the issue of motivation for treatment head-on but rather use other motivations to try to engage young adults in their programs. Recognizing the fact that many chronic mentally ill young adults would like to establish as normal a life as possible, day-treatment programs offer young adults the opportunity to live in subsidized apartments and make use of vocational opportunities. These "rewards" are tied, however, to staying in the program and working toward abstinence. Another program focuses on the desire for recreational activity by having their own version of the "athletic club" and getting potential patients into their programs through peer groups established by playing team sports. Peer group influence is particularly strong in reinforcing substance abuse and can be used in the opposite way to support abstinence.

ASSESSMENT

As was clear in the earlier report of the Task Force, assessment is an area of continuing concern with regard to patients involved with both mental illness and substance abuse. As was documented, substance abuse can complicate diagnosis both by masking symptoms of underlying disorders and by contributing to dysfunction (Egri and Caton 1982; Freed 1975; Lieberman, Goodbar, Grant, Grottole, Holmberg, Lenoci, Levine, and Moras 1984; Pepper 1985; Tsuang, Simpson, and Kronfol 1982). What is also clear is that, while a significant proportion of psychiatric patients is involved in substance abuse, these patients are not a reliable source of information on their own substance use (Hall et al. 1977, 1979; Pepper 1985; Rockwell and Ostwald 1968; Shern, Bartsch, Coen, Ellis, and Wilson 1985). In fact, in one study of drug and alcohol abuse among psychiatric patients of a university psychiatric hospital, toxicological examinations at admission revealed psychoactive drugs in nearly half the patients at admission, and many tests were positive for drugs that the patients denied using (Crowley et al. 1974).

Though clear assessment of both mental disorder and substance abuse is needed, most commentators have focused their attention on the lack of good information about substance abuse among the chronic mentally ill young adult patients because that is what is most lacking or inaccurate. Good substance abuse assessment procedures should include (1) using routine urinalysis or breathalyzer tests (Richardson, Craig, and Haugland 1985; Rockwell and Ostwald 1968); (2) taking comprehensive drug histories, including types, duration, frequency of use, and pattern of use of each substance (Westermeyer and Walzer 1975); (3) interviewing family members to elicit additional information on current substance abuse and history as well as the family history of mental illness and substance abuse (Tsuang et al. 1982); (4) interviewing significant others (Safer 1986); (5) reviewing medical records (Safer 1986); (6) reviewing court records (Safer 1986); and (7) making repeated clinical observations (Safer 1986).

Possibly the most controversial issue in the assessment area is the issue, again, of abstinence. Pepper and colleagues, for example, call for a significant period of abstinence (six to eight months) prior to diagnosis to make clear that the toxic effects of substances are not interfering with the proper diagnosis: "Anything less than total abstinence is insufficient for this purpose" (Pepper and Ryglewicz 1984). Others believe that this might be the method of choice but is simply not an option with most of these patients and that initial diagnostic impressions will eventually be modified by information gathered through clinical observation over time.

While total abstinence may not be possible in the early stages of contact with a patient, it is clear that a lack of sufficient attention to the issue of substance abuse is a formula for treatment failure. Hall and colleagues, in their study of community mental health center outpatients, found that therapist recognition of drug involvement was limited, absent patient reporting. Of great concern is the fact that, if drug abuse was not initially included in the differential diagnosis, it was unlikely to emerge later as a factor explaining the patient's behavior unless the patient subsequently reported it (Hall et al. 1977).

Programs involved in serving this population have faced the tension between the need to engage the patients and the need to apply a whole array of intrusive assessment procedures (or at the least procedures perceived as being intrusive) in order to diagnose correctly and plan for treatment. Perhaps it is necessary to address the tension by choosing to focus on one as the most critical initial problem, tackling the other issue at a later time.

CONCURRENT TREATMENT

Programs that are attempting to address the needs of chronic mentally ill young adults with substance abuse problems have been developed under a variety of auspices. Regardless of auspice, however, these programs seem to involve a core set of mental health services and a core set of substance abuse services provided either within the actual structure of the program or in direct relationship to the program. (It should be noted from the outset that many traditional programs include only the first set of the mental health services.)

The core set of mental health services includes the following.

Stabilizing symptomatology. Most programs that attempt to serve chronic mentally ill young adults in the community either provide medication management and therapeutic activities as part of their protocol or see that their patients are involved in various treatment activities and settings as part of their overall treatment planning.

Medication management. Medication management is a particular concern as it has been shown that noncompliance with prescribed medication is associated with increased behavior problems, particularly acting out in the community, and a direct cause of relapse and rehospitalization (Damron and Simpson 1985; Diamond 1984; McCarrick et al. 1985; Talbott et al. 1986). Beyond the problem with noncompliance is the additional issue of the possible negative interactive effects of psychotropic drugs with street drugs and alcohol. Treffert, for instance, has stressed the need for careful monitoring of psychotropic medication when it is known that the patient uses marijuana (Treffert 1978). Knudesen and Vilmar (1984), in their review of the clinical cases of ten schizophrenic patients in treatment with neuroleptics, found that cannabis could cause acute psychotic exacerbation even in patients receiving otherwise adequate treatment with neuroleptics.

Medication management is especially critical in connection with the use of disulfiram (Antabuse) to control the intake of alcohol. Some commentators discourage the use of Antabuse because of the possibility of psychiatric side effects, while other programs have found it to be a necessary part of the protocol for alcohol-abusing patients. (Kofoed et al. [1986] present a cogent discussion of the pros and cons.)

Therapeutic supports. Beyond medication management, patients have individualized need for other therapeutic supports. Some are involved in individual or group therapy. Psychotherapy for chronic mentally ill (nonpsychotic) persons is usually time limited and focused on problem solving rather than on insight into psychological conflict and behavior change motivated by that insight (Green and Koprowski 1981).

Crisis management. Acute hospitalization is used on an intermittent basis if stabilization/maintenance is not possible in a community program. It is critical that a program have or have access to a crisis management component, for a number of reasons. First, applying the best technology available to patients at the time of an acute episode may help prevent chronic disability (Gruenberg 1982). This is especially true for patients without a long history of psychiatric hospitalizations. Second, as mentioned previously, a program that has the capacity to respond to a potential patient's crisis in a concrete way may have a better chance to engage that patient in their program and thus follow through with a longer-term treatment plan (Lamb 1982). Third, if there is any hope of interrupting the service utilization patterns of chronic mentally ill young adults, a program (or system) must have the capacity to divert them from the use of expensive emergency room services, which, besides being expensive, do not provide the most appropriate treatment for these patients (Egri and Caton 1982). For example, one day-treatment program provides its own twenty-four hour crisis service for the patients within the psychosocial rehabilitation program. Because the staff are so familiar with the patients and their histories (mental illness and substance abuse) and also know what prescribed medications they are currently using, their experience has been that their crisis service is both efficient and effective. Because they focus on substance abuse as well as mental illness as possible causes of acute exacerbation of symptoms, they have been able to identify the problem correctly and intervene, preventing psychiatric rehospitalization for many of their patients.

301

Early intervention in crisis situations is important, but equally important is a focus beyond medication management and traditional therapeutic techniques. Social interaction and coping skills (evidenced by independent living and employment) are also compromised by chronic mental illness and substance abuse. Some commentators believe that simply using traditional office psychotherapy and medication management not only goes beyond being insufficient as a treatment plan but also actually allows significant role dysfunction to develop (Test et al. 1985). Rather than "managing" the patient, focus on active intervention in these two broad areas is necessary (Geller 1986).

Development of social network. Establishment of a positive social network is regarded by commentators and program staff alike as a critical function of any program that wishes to engage and treat chronic mentally ill young adults. "Isolation" is a description often used to characterize the existence of chronic mentally ill young adults. Some relate poorly to their families or are overly dependent, but many others have isolated themselves from family and have difficulty in establishing and maintaining social relationships. Still others have developed peer relationships within the urban drug subculture, and these peers reinforce substance-abusing behavior (Bergman and Harris 1985; Lamb 1982). Having opportunities to socialize, having access to positive recreational activities, and having a supportive peer group are stabilizing influences on patients who otherwise may drift from program to program (or out of the treatment system altogether). Some commentators believe that the development of a social network for patients with disrupted natural social networks is so important that without it other conventional treatments will fail (Segal and Baumohl 1980).

Residential opportunities. Appropriate, supportive housing for chronic mentally ill young adults is high on the priority list of needs detailed by most commentators and program staff (Adler et al. 1987; Glass 1982; Hoff et al. 1983; Pepper, Kirshner, and Ryglewicz 1981; Shern et al. 1985; Towber and Ladner 1985; Woy and Goldstrom 1982). In most localities, there are simply not enough housing slots to come close to meeting the demand. Opportunities should be available for special residential treatment programs, for supportive housing such as group homes, and for more "normative" housing opportunities such as cooperative apartments. As mentioned, the opportunity of an apartment in a "normal" setting may be so attractive to some patients that it will motivate them to stay with the treatment program.

Vocational/prevocational activities. The desire for and expectation of employment may be one of the characteristics that differentiate chronic mentally ill young adults from their older chronic mentally ill counterparts. While some patients may not have realistic expectations, the desire for employment can nevertheless be a significant motivator and thus can be a significant component in a service program (Egri and Caton 1982; Test et al. 1985). Sheltered workshops can be used for some patients, but occasionally programs fail by attempting to use the same structure as used with older "institutionalized" patients, ignoring young patients' desires to be working with age peers and on productive activities that will lead to competitive employment. Although a spectrum of rehabilitative activities must be available within the treatment system, not all activities need to be on site or within the confines of the program. The vocational area provides a clear example of the need for an individualized approach to programming for chronic mentally ill young adults. Not all patients will "fit" a certain intervention, and, if they do not "fit," they will not participate.

Case management. Most programs serving the chronic mentally ill, especially those developed on the principles of the federal Community Support Program initiative, recognize a separate intervention called "case management." In addition to other therapeutic and maintenance efforts, case managers help the patients tie together the various pieces of support available to them. Such services include obtaining entitlements, obtaining housing and rehabilitation opportunities, and obtaining mental health interventions as well as the day-to-day activities that make all these possible. Case management typically is not an office-bound activity, and assertive, ongoing case management may be a key to engaging and keeping patients involved in the treatment system.

Family support and education. Beyond helping patients understand and accommodate their illness and its implications for living, families need similar education and support. The focus of family support groups such as those under the auspices of the National Alliance for the Mentally Ill has been both to educate and to help the family cope with a mentally ill relative. Al-Anon takes a similar approach with respect to substance abuse and focuses on helping the family member to be confrontative (pushing the abusing family members toward taking responsibility for their own abuse) and yet supportive of steps toward treatment.

The core set of substance abuse services includes the following.

Drug education. Programming for chronic mentally ill young adults with substance abuse problems attempts to provide very basic information on both the physiological effects of alcohol and drugs and the specialized effect these substances might have on persons already suffering from chronic mental illness (Bergman and Harris 1985). Drug education involves both the simple imparting of information and attempts to persuade chronic mentally ill young adults to look at their own lives for evidence of substance abuse–related impairment. Some programs use disease models, for example, likening the effect of alcohol and drug use on chronic mentally ill persons to the effect of sugar on persons with diabetes and state, "Your friends may not have real problems with smoking pot, but you are vulnerable by the nature of your disease." If patients lack motivation for abstinence but are sufficiently motivated to stay out of the psychiatric hospital (especially state mental hospitals), knowing about relapse rates among users may have a positive effect.

For those patients who are using alcohol and drugs to self-medicate, attempts to persuade may be focused on convincing the patient that self-medication may be working for now but is not an effective long-term solution (Khantzian 1985).

Group therapy.   Since peer support seems to be such an important factor in substance abuse behavior and to adolescents and young adults because of their developmental phase, many programs have attempted to turn peer support into a tool to support abstinence (or at least control of recreational use). In their survey of patients in the Community Connections Program, Bergman and Harris (1985) found that two-thirds of the patients who used drugs reported that they did so to be part of their peer group and were encouraged in drug use by their peers. Cohen and Klein (1970) drew a similar conclusion from their work with a young psychiatrically hospitalized population.

Most programs reviewed used the technology of group work to begin to construct for the patient a more positive peer reference group, with the goal of influencing their substance use/abuse. Groups were focused either on patients entering the program and still struggling with identifying themselves as abusers or on groups of patients committed to achieving abstinence. (In a sense, the AA model incorporates both levels of patient into one larger group, but some programs felt that there should be two levels, with patients moving to a new level when they were ready to make a commitment to treatment and attempting abstinence.)

The use of "confrontation" in group work with chronic mentally ill young adults remains somewhat controversial. Many substance abuse programs employ intensive confrontation, especially peer confrontation, as an integral part of their group method. Even mental health clinicians have seen confrontation as useful to groups in promoting group cohesiveness, with patients beginning to take responsibility for one another (Bergman and Harris 1985). Unfortunately, other clinicians warn of the problem of more fragile chronic mentally ill patients being unable to withstand such techniques, with the result being decompensation rather than insight.

Self-help groups. Alcoholics Anonymous is the model for most self-help efforts in programs that serve chronic mentally ill young adults. Either patients are encouraged to attend "generic" groups in the community (AA, NA, or "On Our Own" groups [self-help groups for psychiatric patients]), or specialized groups are developed within the program. Rather than being time limited, as are some therapy groups, these groups provide continuing support to patients as they leave programs or move from one phase of a program to another.

Individualized treatment planning. Before leaving the issue of concurrent treatment, it is necessary to restate the importance of individualized treatment planning. As is clear, not all programs include all the components described above. To the extent that they do not conform to this concurrent treatment model, where do the more traditional inpatient/outpatient programs belong within a system of care? One answer may be found in the recognition that chronic mentally ill young adults with substance abuse problems are not, in fact, a homogeneous group with one set of needs. It has been proposed that there are identifiable subgroups of chronic mentally ill young adults with specific needs (or special needs at special times) that may not match the protocol described above. These patients may need more traditional programs for a limited period of time within a broader context of care. Identification of these subgroups should suggest different hospital and follow-up treatment approaches (Perkins, Simpson, and Tsuang 1986).

OUTCOME

One of the key questions in program development (and subsequent evaluation) is, What is success? How will we know if the program is working? Most of the programs serving chronic mentally ill young adults with substance abuse problems have not undergone formal evaluations, and this is clearly an important area for future efforts. In many ways, our research has pointed up just how woeful our current data are. The consideration of all such indicators is important since we are still in the trial-and-error stage of program development.

Because failure in compliance with treatment programming, resulting in premature termination by the patient or by the staff for disciplinary reasons, is such a problem for chronic mentally ill young adults, some program staff have used retention in treatment as an "outcome" measure (Talbott et al. 1986). For example, Kofoed and colleagues use treatment retention as a measure of program success because it reflects (within their program structure) both abstinence and compliance with ongoing treatment of major mental illness.

Additionally, some program staff regard engagement in productive activity (either leisure or work related) to be an important indicator of success in the program.

Efforts at more formal treatment assessment have been suggested in our earlier report.

SYSTEMS CHANGE

Most commentators who have written on principles of programming for chronic mentally ill young adults have focused their discussion as much on systems issues as on specific proposals for programming, indicating the importance they place on systems change in addressing the needs of this population. Many of these "laundry lists" have similar features and reflect a similar train of thought regarding solutions to systems problems (Bachrach 1982a, 1983; Glass 1982; Goldfinger et al. 1984; Hall et al. 1977; Lamb 1982; Sheets, Prevost, and Reihman 1982; Stein and Test 1982; Talbott et al. 1987).

Interestingly, many of these commentators find enough discouraging news about problems inherent within the mental health care system (to the extent that a system can be said to exist in some localities) without even touching on the additional problems inherent in trying to bridge two systems—the mental health care system and the substance abuse care system. (It should be noted that in some localities to cause system change may actually mean bridging three systems, where alcohol and drug abuse treatment and mental health are all handled under different auspices.)

Talbott and colleagues and the Group for Advancement of Psychiatry have conceptualized systems problems as a dilemma of "interactive fit" between the patient, the caregiver, and the system of care. There is also an interactive fit problem between the mental health and the substance abuse systems. Taking their principles a bit farther, adjusting the resiliency between the two (or three) systems becomes the key factor. This may mean breaking down the categorical boundaries between the mental health and substance abuse systems (and, likewise, the program boundaries within these systems) to allow patients to move freely and have access to a variety of programs. Individual programs have helped break down the barriers between systems by several methods: (1) cooperative agreements, (2) shared staffing, and (3) staff training one another across systems.

Cooperative agreements. These are usually somewhat formalized agreements between programs that set up referral procedures and detail any cooperative programming. What is key in the area of cooperative agreements is that they be real agreements and not "paper" agreements.

Shared staffing. Hybrid programs have been developed in a number of sites by, for example, having substance abuse treatment personnel detailed to a mental health program for a regular portion of their time. They may participate in a number of program activities, including treatment planning, running treatment groups (as an individual therapist or together with a mental health staff member), and consulting with treatment personnel on assessment of substance abuse problems.

Staff training. As a way of opening up communication and breaking down the barriers between the two fields, some mental health programs, for example, have detailed their staff to the local substance abuse facility to provide in-service training on assessment of mental illness and received in-service training from the staff of the local substance abuse facility on assessment of substance abuse problems. This has not only resulted in the transfer of useful information but also promoted contact and mutual respect among the treatment personnel. Program staff believe that this promotes group cohesiveness among treatment personnel, regardless of their initial identification with one field or the other, and forestalls some of the usual "dumping" of patients from system to system.

Training Issues

There is consensus that additional training is needed for those who are to provide services for chronic mentally ill young adults with substance abuse problems. This training can take the form of curriculum development for professional schools as well as productive in-service training options for current treatment personnel. One of the biggest issues in training continues to be the lack of knowledge about mental illness characteristic of substance abuse treatment personnel and the lack of knowledge about substance abuse characteristic of mental health treatment personnel. Few clinicians have training in both fields. This is partly attributable to the differences between the fields in education and philosophy.

Mental health personnel are primarily professionally trained with degrees in medicine (psychiatrists and nurses) or in psychology, social work, or allied professions. Substance abuse workers are often paraprofessionals and often are, themselves, recovering alcoholics or abusers. Many in the mental health field believe that professional training is necessary to work with chronic mentally ill persons. Many in the substance abuse field feel that personal experience is the best training for working with substance abusers.

For substance abuse treatment personnel, mental illness is an unknown, and there is an unpredictability to the behavior of psychiatric patients that is not present with their other patients. This unpredictability may mean that they may get "conned" by behavior that would never have fooled them in another patient (Damron and Simpson 1985). Mental health treatment personnel, on the other hand, often regard substance abuse treatment as some sort of "magic" that is beyond their capability. Alternatively, they may just be frustrated with being manipulated by substance-abusing patients and wish to be rid of them.

Training, then, may involve sharing information about the illnesses (mental illness and substance abuse) and sharing clinical experience in assessment/diagnosis and treatment principles. Other training may involve realigning the expectations caregivers have about their patients. Finally, training may involve determinations about which patients are proper referrals across program lines.

Curriculum development is a critical concern but not one that has been sufficiently addressed by either the professions, the professional schools, or their organizations. Within the medical field there has been some development of residency programs, including work in public-sector psychiatry programs through which psychiatric residents are exposed to (and supervised in the treatment of) dual diagnosis patients. These programs seem to be predominately related to medical training and seem to be the exception rather than the rule.

Conclusions

This chapter represents a synthesis of available information on the state of the art in the treatment of chronic mentally ill young adults with substance abuse problems and the training of clinicians to work in programs designed for this population. This interim report will be revised and supplemented. What is clear at this point, however, is that in the last ten years there has been significant development in technology for treating chronic mentally ill persons and for treating persons who abuse alcohol and drugs. It is not necessarily the development of new technology that is key but rather a refinement and adaptation of existing treatment strategies to this special population.

NOTE

This chapter was originally presented at the annual meeting of the Society for Adolescent Psychiatry, May 10, 1987, Chicago. This research was funded through a cooperative agreement between the University of Maryland School of Medicine, the Mental Hygiene Administration of the State of Maryland, and the Alcohol, Drug Abuse and Mental Health Administration of the U.S. Department of Health and Human Services. Opinions expressed in this paper are those of the authors and do not necessarily represent the views of the sponsoring agencies.

REFERENCES

Adler, D.; Drake, R.; Berlant, J.; Ellison, J.; and Carson, D. 1987. *Interactive Fit: A Guide to Non-psychotic Chronic Patients*. Group for Advancement of Psychiatry, no. 121. New York: Brunner/Mazel.

Bachrach, L. L. 1982a. Program planning for young adult chronic patients. In B. Pepper and H. Ryglewicz, eds. *The Young Adult Chronic Patient*. New Directions for Mental Health Services, no. 14. San Francisco: Jossey-Bass.

Bachrach, L. L. 1982b. Young adult chronic patients: an analytical review of the literature. *Hospital and Community Psychiatry* 33:189–197.

Bachrach, L. L. 1983. Planning services for chronically mentally ill patients. *Bulletin of the Menninger Clinic* 47:63–188.

Bachrach, L. L.; Talbott, J. A.; and Meyerson, A. 1986. The chronic psychiatric patient as a "difficult patient": a conceptual analysis. In A. Meyerson, ed. *Barriers to Treating the Chronic Mentally Ill.* New Directions for Mental Health Services, no. 33. San Francisco: Jossey-Bass.

Bender, M. G. 1986. Young adult chronic patients: visibility and style of interaction in treatment. *Hospital and Community Psychiatry* 37:265–268.

Bergman, H. C., and Harris, M. 1985. Substance abuse among young adult chronic patients. *Psychosocial Rehabilitation Journal* 9:49–54.

Caton, C. 1981. The new chronic patient and the system of community care. *Hospital and Community Psychiatry* 32:475–488.

Cohen, M., and Klein, D. 1970. Drug abuse in a young psychiatric population. *American Journal of Orthopsychiatry* 40:448–455.

Crowley, T. J.; Chesluk, D.; Dilts, S.; and Hart, R. 1974. Drug and alcohol abuse among psychiatric admissions. A multidrug clinical-toxicologic study. *Achives of General Psychiatry* 30:13–20.

Damron, S. W., and Simpson, W. R. 1985. Substance abuse and schizophrenia: a health maintenance perspective. Paper presented at the ninety-third annual meeting of the American Psychological Association.

Diamond, J. R. 1984. Increasing medical compliance in young adult chronic psychiatric patients. In B. Pepper and H. Ryglewicz, eds. *Advances in Treating the Young Adult Chronic Patient.* New Directions for Mental Health Services, no. 21. San Francisco: Jossey-Bass.

Egri, G., and Caton, C. L. 1982. Serving the young adult chronic patient in the 1980's: challenge to the general hospital. In B. Pepper and H. Ryglewicz, eds. *The Young Adult Chronic Patient.* New Directions for Mental Health Services, no. 13. San Francisco: Jossey-Bass.

Freed, E. 1975. Alcoholism and schizophrenia: the search for perspectives: a review. *Journal of Studies on Alcohol* 36:853–881.

Geller, J. 1986. In again, out again: preliminary evaluation of a state hospital's worst recidivists. *Hospital and Community Psychiatry* 37:386–390.

Glass, J. 1982. Summary of proceedings: The young adult chronic patient: ADM working conference. Paper presented to the National Institute on Drug Abuse, October 21–22.

Goldfinger, S. M.; Hopkin, J. T.; and Suber, R. W. 1984. Treatment resisters or system resisters? toward a better service system for acute care recidivists. In B. Pepper and H. Ryglewicz, eds. *Advances in Treating the Young Adult Chronic Patient.* New Directions for Mental Health Services, no. 21. San Francisco: Jossey-Bass.

Goldman, H. H., and Taube, C. 1986. Mental health financing and the future of the state hospital. *American Journal of Social Psychiatry* 5:26–30.

Goldstrom, I. D., and Manderscheid, R. W. 1983. A descriptive analysis of community support program case managers serving the chronically mentally ill. *Community Mental Health Journal* 19(1): 17–26.

Green, R. S., and Koprowski, P. F. 1981. The chronic patient with a non-psychotic diagnosis. *Hospital and Community Psychiatry* 32:479–481.

Gruenberg, E. 1982. Social breakdown in young adults: keeping crises from becoming chronic. In B. Pepper and H. Ryglewicz, eds. *The Young Adult Chronic Patient.* New Directions for Mental Health Services, no. 14. San Francisco: Jossey-Bass.

Hall, R., et al. 1977. The effect of unrecognized drug abuse on diagnosis and therapeutic outcome. *American Journal of Drug and Alcohol Abuse* 4:455–465.

Hall, R., et al. 1979. Relationship of psychiatric illness to drug abuse. *Journal of Psychedelic Drugs* 11:337–342.

Hoff, M. K., et al. 1983. The chronically mentally ill: a descriptive analysis. *Administration in Mental Health* 10:171–180.

Jeffrey, R. 1979. Rubbish: deviant patients in casualty departments. *Sociology of Health and Illness* 1:142–155.

Khantzian, E. J. 1985. The self medication hypothesis of addictive disorders: focus on heroin and cocaine dependence. *American Journal of Psychiatry* 142:1259–1264.

Knudesen, P., and Vilmar, T. 1984. Cannabis and neuroleptic agents in schizophrenia. *Acta Psychiatrica Scandänavia* 69:162–174.

311

Kofoed, L.; Kania, J.; Walsh, T.; and Atkinson, R. 1986. Outpatient treatment of substance abusers with other co-existing psychiatric disorders. *American Journal of Psychiatry* 143:867–872.

Lamb, H. R. 1982. Young adult chronic patients: the new drifters. *Hospital and Community Psychiatry* 33:465–468.

Lieberman, P. B.; Goodbar, N.; Grant, T.; Grottole, E.; Holmberg, S.; Lenoci, B.; Levine, M.; and Moras, K. 1984. The treatment of patients with substance abuse and other axis-I disorders in a general psychiatric facility. Connecticut Mental Health Center. Typescript.

McCarrick, A. K.; Manderscheid, R.; and Bertolucci, D. 1985. Correlates of acting-out behaviors among young adult chronic patients. *Hospital and Community Psychiatry* 36:848–853.

Ottenberg, D. J. 1978. Clinical and programmatic perspectives. In E. Gottheil, A. T. McLellan, and K. A. Druley, eds. *Substance Abuse and Psychiatric Illness*. New York: Pergamon.

Pepper, B. 1985. The young adult chronic patient: population overview. *Journal of Clinical Psychopharmacology* 5:3.

Pepper, B.; Kirshner, M.; and Ryglewicz, H. 1981. The young chronic patient: overview of a population. *Hospital and Community Psychiatry* 32:463–467.

Pepper, B., and Ryglewicz, H. 1984. The young adult chronic patient: a new focus. In J. A. Talbott, ed. *The Chronic Mental Patient: Five Years Later*. New York: Grune & Stratton.

Perkins, A.; Simpson, J.; and Tsuang, M. 1986. Ten year follow-up of drug abusers with psychoses. *Hospital and Community Psychiatry* 37:481–484.

Richardson, M. A.; Craig, T.; and Haugland, G. 1985. Treatment patterns of young chronic schizophrenic patients in the era of deinstitutionalization. *Psychiatric Quarterly* 57:243–249.

Rockwell, D. A., and Ostwald, P. 1968. Amphetamine use and abuse in psychiatric patients. *Archives of General Psychiatry* 18:612–616.

Safer, D. 1987. Substance abuse by young adult chronic patients. *Hospital and Community Psychiatry* 38:511–514.

Segal, S., and Baumohl, J. 1980. Engaging the disengaged: proposals on madness and vagrancy. *Social Work* 25:358–365.

Sheets, J.; Prevost, J.; and Reihman, J. 1982. Young adult chronic patients: three hypothesized subgroups. *Hospital and Community Psychiatry* 33:197–203.

Shern, D. L.; Bartsch, D.; Coen, A.; Ellis, R.; and Wilson, N. 1985. A model for estimating optimal residential/service settings for types of chronically mentally ill individuals—project summary. Denver, Colo.: Department of Institutions, Division of Mental Health, May 23.

Stein, L. L., and Test, M. A. 1982. Community treatment of the young adult patient. In B. Pepper and H. Ryglewicz, eds. *The Young Adult Chronic Patient*. New Directions for Mental Health Services, no. 14. San Francisco: Jossey-Ross.

Talbott, J. A.; Bachrach, L.; and Ross, L. 1986. Noncompliance and mental health systems. *Psychiatric Annals* 16:596–599.

Talbott, J. A., et al. 1987. The chronically mentally ill: what do we know, and why aren't we implementing what we know? In W. W. Menninger and G. T. Hannah, eds. *The Chronic Mental Patient/II*. Washington, D.C.: American Psychiatric Press.

Test, M. A.; Knoedler, W.; Allness, D.; and Burke, S. 1985. Characteristics of young adults with schizophrenic disorders treated in the community. *Hospital and Community Psychiatry* 36:853–858.

Towber, R., and Ladner, S. 1985. Psychiatric indication and alcohol abuse among public shelter clients. Paper presented at MSIS ninth annual National Users Conference, National Institute of Mental Health, Washington, D.C., November 22.

Treffert, D. 1978. Marijuana use in schizophrenia: a clear hazard. *American Journal of Psychiatry* 135:1214–1215.

Tsuang, M. T.; Simpson, J.; and Kronfol, Z. 1982. Subtypes of drug abuse with psychosis: demographic characteristics, clinical features and family history. *Archives of General Psychiatry* 39:141–147.

Westermeyer, J., and Walzer, V. 1975. Sociopathy and drug use in a young psychiatric population. *Diseases of the Nervous System* 36:673–677.

Woy, R. G., and Goldstrom, I. D. 1982. The young chronic mental patient: report of a national survey. Rockville, Md.: National Institute of Mental Health.

313

PART III

PSYCHOPATHOLOGICAL ISSUES IN ADOLESCENT PSYCHIATRY

EDITORS' INTRODUCTION

Changing concepts pose a fundamental dilemma, the acquisition of new perspectives usually leads to the abandonment of old definitions, and this may result in conflicts around conceptualization. The understanding of adolescence and adolescent process is an example of this ambivalence as the phenomenological views of the early twentieth century have changed to a developmental perspective. The following chapters present a dynamic view of adolescent pathology that illustrates this principle.

Aaron Esman reviews current concepts in borderline personality disorder in adolescents. Stemming from the effects of developmental defect during childhood and adolescence, the clinical picture that Esman describes of a personality organization characterized by identity diffusion, affective instability, maladaptive behaviors, social ineptitude, shallowness of object relations, and the use of primitive defenses traces the pathogenesis and psychodynamics attributed to this syndrome by a number of adolescent psychiatrists. Esman discusses a number of treatment modalities but concludes that little agreement exists and that much that is still unknown dominates understanding this disorder.

Lewis A. Kirschner reexamines the developmental function of acting out. He views the adolescent as expressing, in dramatic form, a particular developmental issue and attempting to evoke responses that are necessary for progression to a higher or more integrated level. A review of Loevinger's theories describes the developing ego as continuously striving to construct a cohesive sense of self. Adolescent behavior suggests that acting out can be placed on a continuum of levels of ego development, preconformist, conformist, and postconformist. The author concludes from case examples that an episode of acting out can draw attention to a break in a subject's sense of continuity of self while the level of ego development dictates the form, structure, and kind of object needs.

Charles Jaffe and Peter Barglow examine insights obtained from adult psychoanalytic reconstructions and adolescent psychotherapy from multiple perspectives and attempt to apply these ideas to infant observational research. A collaboration between the two authors treating a mother and her now-adolescent son provided a special opportunity to view the infant-mother interaction retrospectively and to shed new light on the research findings. The authors discuss the continuity present through the caretakers' empathic availability, adjustment in infancy, and the presence of pathology in adolescence by examining in detail the reciprocal contributions of psychoanalysis and research to the validity of psychoanalytic reconstruction.

Vivian M. Rakoff examines the emergence of adolescence as a separate stage of development, a condition apart from the preceding stages. He sees the adolescent not as a new human type but as reflecting a new emphasis on "some perennial human capacities" and adolescence as a period characterized by "dilemmas and opportunities of choice" and, consequently, expressing individual personality formation. As a emerging psychiatric patient, particular syndromes, such as suicide and depression, anorexia nervosa and bulimia, substance and drug abuse, and forms of religious malaise and anomic rootlessness, reflect the "epoch-dependent" adolescence. Rakoff sees these problems as disorders of aspiration, reactions to the sense of inadequate achievement, constant self-doubt, and restless yearning and searching. Robert W. Buchanan presents a discussion of Rakoff's chapter.

318

21   BORDERLINE PERSONALITY DISORDER IN ADOLESCENTS: CURRENT CONCEPTS

AARON H. ESMAN

There is an inherent paradox in the contrast between psychiatry's current pursuit of greater specificity and "scientific" precision and the increasing popularity of so nonspecific and apparently imprecise a term as "borderline" disorder. Originally conceived as denoting a condition transitional between neurosis and psychosis, it has come to have more definable referents as spelled out in such systems as DSM-III as well as in the formulations of such students as Otto Kernberg, Grinker, Gunderson, and others. There is fairly general agreement among all that, at least with adult patients, a particular clinical syndrome is being designated, although the precise descriptive features of the syndrome and its place in the spectrum of psychiatric disorder remain open for discussion.

With respect to children and adolescents, however, the picture is somewhat less defined, although here too descriptions, explanations of etiology and pathogenesis, and therapeutic prescriptions are abundant. My aim in this chapter is to review this growing literature in an effort to represent the views of English-language students of this field as accurately and as comprehensively as possible. It should be noted that the bulk of the literature on the borderline disorder, at least in English, is to be found in American publications. Indeed, a survey of the two major British journals—the *British Journal of Medical Psychology* and the *British Journal of Psychiatry*—from 1980 through 1986 yielded only five papers dealing with this subject, two of which were by the same author (Bird 1980; Holm and Hundevatt 1981; Macaskill 1982; Macaskill and Macaskill 1981; Tarnopolsky and Berelowitz 1984). None deals with borderline adolescents. Further, virtually all the references in these papers are from the American literature. Tarnopolsky and Berelowitz (1984) point out that only about 25 percent of psychiatrists at the Maudsley Hospital use this diagnosis; Macaskill and Macaskill (1981) report a similar proportion among Scottish psychiatrists. As the latter state, "In total contrast to the position in North America, British psychiatry has had very little to say about the borderline patient" (p. 97). It appears that the greater influence of psychoanalysis in American psychiatry is at least partly responsible for this situation since the borderline concept has, as will be seen, emerged largely from psychoanalytically oriented studies.

Description of the Syndrome

Perhaps the earliest account of "borderline" disorders in children and adolescents is that of Ekstein and Wallerstein (1954), who described fluctuating "ego states" and ineffective regulatory mechanisms in such patients. Their report was soon followed by that of Geleerd (1958), who, elaborating on the recent descriptions of childhood psychosis by Mahler and others, defined a group of children and adolescents who, though not overtly psychotic, were characterized by "disturbances in the ego and its development . . . manifested in the pathological development of object relations with the mother" (pp. 293–294). These children are dominated by fantasies of and longings for omnipotence, and they experience anxiety not as signal anxiety, as does the neurotic, but as traumatic anxiety. Rosenfeld and Sprince (1963) arrived at similar views from their studies of borderline children at Hampstead.

In a similar vein, Pine (1974) attempted to sharpen and codify the phenomenology and metapsychology of borderline disorders in children and adolescents, building on Mahler's conceptual foundation. Arguing against the notion of a unitary syndrome, Pine accepted the "spatial metaphor" inherent in the term—that of a spectrum of disorders occupying a boundary zone between neurosis and psychosis: "What unites these children is the presence of severe developmental failure or deviation in the realm of ego functioning and object relationship . . . , chronic ego deviance, shifting levels of ego organization, internal disorganization reactive to external disorganization" (pp. 366–367). The "upper border" of this range of pathology, he said, merged with the neuroses and the "lower border" with clearly defined psychotic conditions in such a way as to make sharp definition difficult if not impossible.

The most substantial body of contributions to the delineation of the syndrome (and, as we shall see later, other aspects as well) is that of Masterson. In his early reports of the Payne Whitney follow-up study (Masterson 1967), he demonstrated stability of character pathology in psychiatric illness in adolescence and helped destroy the stereotype of "normal adolescent turmoil." Subsequently, on the basis of his own work and that of others (e.g., Rinsley 1968, 1978), he defined the borderline syndrome as one of a "developmental arrest," incorporating "maladaptive defenses," "maladaptive object relations," and "maturational lags." He delineated the clinical picture in 1973 as consisting of (1) acting out behaviors (antisocial activity, drug abuse, etc.); (2) difficulties in separating from parents; (3) a history of "narcissistic, orally fixated character structure"; (4) parents with borderline personality structures; and (5) deviant communication patterns in the family.

At about the same period, Grinker (1978; Grinker, Werble, and Drye 1968) defined the borderline syndrome in adults on the basis of empirical study. The criteria he and his colleagues evolved from factor analysis were (1) the prevalence of anger in the person's affect expression; (2) defects in affectionate relationships; (3) absence of indications of self-identity formation; and (4) prominent depressive loneliness. Further, O. Kernberg (1967) offered the initial statement of his extensive work on the syndrome of "borderline personality organization," defining a clinical picture in adults that more recently (O. Kernberg 1978) he has indicated applies equally to adolescents—a picture consisting of "identity diffusion," the predominance of primitive defenses such as splitting and projective identification, and the preservation of reality testing.

Kernberg's description was based on what he calls "structural" rather than clinical-descriptive criteria. At the same time, he acknowledges that the application of these criteria in adolescents is complicated by the developmental flux that characterizes this period. Thus, the common and normally occurring increase in narcissism, the frequent emergence of perverse sexual fantasy, and the frequently subtle and gradual emergence of overt schizophrenic symptoms may at times cloud the picture. Kernberg maintains, however, that the issue of identity diffusion can be seen as central to the diagnosis and that the retention of some measure of reality testing can serve to distinguish "borderline personality organization" from more advanced psychotic states.

In a more extended description, P. Kernberg (1979, 1983) offers a detailed "profile" of the borderline adolescent. Such patients, she says, have failed to achieve object constancy or a sense of autonomy. Their reality testing is spotty, often dependent on borrowing such judgments from others. Their affects are unstable, characterized principally by fear, distrust, and rage, and they lack an expectation of gratification from others. Frustration tolerance is low, and there is little capacity to deal adaptively with loss or depressive affect. Superego integration is defective owing to the pervasive use of splitting and projection. Object relations are arrested and pathological in nature and social skills characteristically limited. Relationships with parents are characterized by idealization or devaluation, and sibling rivalry is unusually intense. The oedipal conflicts are overlaid by primitive preoedipal issues, and sexual fantasies thus tend to be sadistic or perverse. Transient psychotic episodes may occur under stress.

In an interesting variant, Slavin and Slavin (1976) described two styles of adaptation in late adolescent borderline college students—one group that chose to enter an "experimental" unstructured program and another group that remained in the regular curriculum. Of the former, 67 percent withdrew from college, while, of the latter, only 25 percent did so. The "experimental" group was more rebellious and felt oppressed by the "rigidity" of the regular curriculum, but it could not tolerate the lack of structure of the new one. The "regulars" were detached and academically conforming, but they were engaged in persistent and intense separation-individuation struggles with their parents, consistent with Masterson's formulations.

Finally, the framers of DSM-III-R (American Psychiatric Association 1987), building on the studies already described as well as those of Gunderson and Kolb (1978) and others, formulated as the official criteria a pervasive pattern of instability of mood, interpersonal relationships, and self-image, beginning by early adulthood and present in a variety of contexts, as indicated by at least five of the following: (1) a pattern of unstable and intense interpersonal relationships characterized by alternating between extremes of overidealization and devaluation; (2) impulsiveness in at least two areas that are potentially self-damaging (e.g., spending, sex, substance abuse, shoplifting, reckless driving, or binge eating); (3) affective instability, that is, marked shifts from baseline mood to depression, irritability, or anxiety, usually lasting a few hours and only rarely more than a few days; (4) inappropriate, intense anger or lack of control of anger (e.g., frequent displays of temper, constant anger, or recurrent physical fights); (5) recurrent suicidal threats, gestures, or behavior or self-mutilating behavior; (6) marked and persistent identity disturbance manifested by uncertainty about at least two of the following: self-image, sexual orientation, long-term goals or career choice, type of friends desired, or preferred values; (7) chronic feelings of emptiness or boredom; and (8) frantic efforts to avoid real or imagined abandonment.

In essence, then, the past three decades of clinical work have led to widespread consensus that the clinical picture of the borderline adolescent is of one who, though not psychotic, has a personality organization more primitive than that of the normal or neurotic adolescent—one characterized by what has been termed "stable instability." Prominent features are identity diffusion, affective instability and impulsivity, maladaptive and often self-destructive behaviors, social ineptitude, shallowness of object relations, and predominant use of so-called primitive defenses such as splitting and projection.

Shapiro (1983) cautions about the uncritical application of adult criteria to the behavior of children and adolescents. There is danger of misdiagnosis, he suggests, with attendant consequences for proper therapeutic management. At the least, he concludes, we should be certain that this presumed childhood disorder is continuous with borderline personality disorder in adults and use rigorously defined criteria to avoid premature diagnostic closure. These admonitions are sound, but they seem intended to apply primarily to the use of this terminology for latency-age and preadolescent children. Whether clinical descriptive criteria such as those of Masterson and DSM-III or "structural" (metapsychological) criteria such as O. Kernberg's are used, it appears that a group of patients showing this level of personality organization and function can be defined and, even in childhood and adolescence, understood and treated in ways specific to their clinical characteristics.

Pathogenesis and Psychodynamics

There is widespread agreement that the clinical picture described reflects a disturbance in personality development, whether understood as a developmental arrest or fixation or as a defensive regression from more advanced positions. Further, most investigators believe that particular qualities of family interaction are, if not totally responsible for the disorder, at least significant contributors to it.

The most categorical formulation of the psychogenesis of adolescent borderline disorders is that of Masterson (1972, 1973), Masterson and Rinsley (1975), and Rinsley (1978). In this view, a specific fixation occurs at the rapprochement substage of separation individuation as defined by Mahler—that is, the "rapprochement" crisis is never satisfactorily resolved. This arrest of development is induced in the child by a mother who, herself suffering from borderline pathology, encourages and rewards clinging attachment behaviors and discourages or punishes separation or gestures toward autonomy. Thus, in Masterson and Rinsley's view, "split object relations units" are established intrapsychically, with maternal introjects maintaining the persistence of the original maternal attitudes.

It should be noted that Mahler herself (Mahler and Kaplan 1977) took exception to this position. Though acknowledging the likelihood of some relation between borderline disorders and the rapprochement crisis, Mahler and Kaplan emphasized the importance of "subphase adequacy," maintaining that the influence of earlier subphases must be taken into account as well as the crucial organizing importance of the oedipal conflict as shaped by earlier phase and subphase deviation. The intent of their statement was clearly to downplay the pathogenic specificity of disturbances in rapprochement as advanced by Masterson and by Masterson and Rinsley. In a related communication (Esman 1980), I expressed similar reservations while agreeing that, at least in certain cases, issues related to rapprochement appear to have a central role.

In a related vein, Giovacchini (1979, 1985) has sought to account for borderline pathology in adolescents as a consequence of maternal failure to provide consistent competent caretaking. The mother's inconsistency, he suggests, generates a "primal confusion" between frustration and gratification and interferes with the establishment of object constancy. In the service of their own narcissistic and symbiotic needs, many such mothers treat their children as "transitional objects," dehumanizing and controlling them while failing to soothe them so as to permit the establishment in them of internalized self-soothing functions.

Similar conclusions are derived by Zinner (1978) and Zinner and Shapiro (1975) from the concurrent study of borderline adolescents and their families. They see the critical psychological dysfunction in such cases as the predominant defensive role of "splitting," a consequence of the imposition on the child of "split parental images" by parents who oppose efforts at achievement of autonomy. "Unconscious family assumptions and fantasies" serve to inhibit and restrict the child's growth; the "second individuation phase" of adolescence triggers regression to earlier points of fixation and/or generates intense interpersonal as well as intrapsychic conflict.

This attention to the etiological role of maternal failures is complemented by Anderson's (1978) reflections on the critical importance of fathering and of "paternal empathy" in the child's development. Borderline adolescents have suffered from lack, loss, or deprivation of such experience, he says. "Good enough fathering is a coordinated initiative essential to creation of the depersonified superego ideal which affords illusory protection" (pp. 393–394). One might note here the concurrence of this formula with that of Winnicott's "good enough mothering," which, in Giovacchini's terms, allows for the establishment of an internalized soothing function.

In contrast to this emphasis on the parental contribution to the structural disorder of the borderline, O. Kernberg (1979) tends to highlight the intrinsic aspect of the patient's own pathological organization in engendering family dysfunction: "The predominance of primitive defensive operations . . . may permit the adolescent borderline patient to induce complementary pathology in key family members with whom he lives. . . . It is important for the therapist to evaluate the extent to which the patient is responding to pathological pressures from his parents and to what extent he is inducing such pressures in them" (p. 305). Kernberg's emphasis on what he considers the unusual constitutional intensity of aggressive drive pressure in borderline pathology stands in considerable distinction to the more usual attribution of such aggression to the child's reaction to parental insult or deprivation.

Certain of the apparent contradictions in these formulations of etiology and psychodynamics are addressed by Michels (1986) in his discussion of Gunderson's contributions in the 1983 panel "Research in Borderline Personality Disorders." As Michels points out, one trend in the literature "describes families that are close bonding, intrusive, smothering . . . [while] the other describes families that abandon, withdraw or are abusive or absent." He suggests that this difference rests on the difference between genetic/reconstructive and developmental/

325

observational approaches to data; the developmental approach might well highlight patterns of distance, neglect, and remoteness, while the reconstructed experience of the patient in treatment might emphasize painful moments of intrusiveness and overinvolvement. "The world of childhood reconstructed in the inner experience of patients is not likely to be a valid replica of the world of childhood constructed from observations of children and parents. It is likely to emphasize the painful and conflictual experience they suffer rather than the totality of their experience" (p. 188).

The reader will have noted the absence thus far of reference to biological considerations in the etiology and pathogenesis of borderline disorders in adolescents. In fact, the literature in this area is sparse indeed. A number of authors have considered possible biological factors in adult borderlines, though as yet little of a conclusive nature has been defined. For example, and of possible relevance here, Andrulonis, Glueck, Stroebel, and Vogel (1982) have proposed three subtypes of adult borderlines, in one of which there is a history of head traumas, epilepsy, or encephalitis and in another a history of attention-deficit disorder or learning disability.[1] Akiskal (1981) has explored the boundary between adult borderline disorder and depressive illness and suggests that in many cases the former is a subtype of the latter. Stone (1980) cites a number of studies that support the association between borderline disorder and affective illness both in adults and in children.

Nevertheless, the research in biological contributions to or determinants of borderline disorders in adolescence remains to be done. One study that offers some clues is that of Fard, Hudgens, and Welner (1978), in which a group of twenty-four "undiagnosable" hospitalized adolescent patients was followed over a seven-year period. On follow-up, fifteen had been ill in the interim or were still ill; each of them had shown overtly psychotic symptoms at the time of hospitalization. Of the nine who were well at follow-up, none had such symptoms initially; they had been predominantly depressed and shown reactive conflicts with their parents. Thus, it appears from this study that the borderline adolescent with psychotic symptoms, however transient, may have a poorer prognosis than and be biologically vulnerable in different ways than is the more depressed antagonistic adolescent.

The studies of Cohen et al. (1983) cast some light on the nature of this vulnerability, at least in a certain group of cases. In their view, certain biochemical deviations—particularly in the catecholamine systems—may predispose the child toward attention-deficit disorder, which is marked by impulsivity, poor attention span, and hyperirritability. "In this progression," they state, "a child who has difficulty in muting inner tensions and habituating to stimulation experiences recurrent anxieties and is irritable with care givers; this tension generates troubles in parenting, and that interaction leads to distortions in the child's creation of the internal representation of the mother as caring and good, in the establishment of transitional objects, the maturation of methods for modulation of anxiety . . . difficulties in self-control, narcissistic balance and sublimation" (p. 215). It may well be that at least some adolescent and adult "borderlines" are grown-up ADDs. Clearly, however, these findings and speculations require further studies with more precise diagnostic criteria and more sensitive assessments of chemical markers than have been carried out thus far.

Therapy

However great the challenge that borderline adolescents pose to the diagnostician and to the theoretician, that which they offer to the therapist exceeds it by far. Impulsive, affectively unstable, mistrustful, and given to the use of externalization, splitting, and projection as principal defenses, they present those who seek to care for them with monumental tasks and with unremitting stimulation of countertransference responses (Greenberg, Haiman, and Esman 1987). It is of course precisely these difficulties that lend to them a substantial measure of fascination.

As with most clinical conditions whose boundaries and whose etiology are unclear, many therapeutic prescriptions compete for the clinician's favor. Perhaps the most controversial of these is that advanced by Laufer and Laufer (1984), whose discussion of the psychoanalytic treatment of what they call "developmental breakdown" in adolescents includes accounts of such work with patients who appear clearly to be "borderline" cases. Laufer and Laufer attempt to carry on "classical" analyses, deviating only when necessary to protect the welfare of the patient and the continuity of the treatment. Unfortunately, it appears from their description that a number of their patients have suffered severe psychotic episodes in the course of treatment or have terminated prematurely. Cahn (1988) and Esman (1988) have questioned, as does O. Kernberg (1979), the use of "classical" psychoanalytic technique in the presence of the grave structural defects and fragility that characterize the borderline adolescent.

Kernberg's views of the therapeutic approach to the borderline adolescent are essentially identical to those he advances for adults. That is, he recommends the use of "psychoanalytic psychotherapy" as opposed both to classical psychoanalysis and to "supportive" psychotherapy. This implies a face-to-face setup with appointments scheduled at least two and preferably three times a week. Interpretations should, he suggests, be addressed from the outset to the patient's "primitive transference" manifestations and his use of "primitive" defenses, with emphasis on the "here and now" of the patient-therapist interaction. Genetic reconstructions should be reserved for later phases in treatment when the therapeutic alliance is secure, when the patient has a sustained capacity for reflection, and when less primitive defenses are in evidence. Throughout, the therapist should maintain a position of "therapeutic neutrality," using "supportive" measures including hospitalization sparingly but firmly as needed to maintain clear boundaries and to prevent and control self-destructive behaviors. Kernberg reminds the reader of the necessity for distinguishing "normal" adolescent behaviors from borderline psychopathology.

It is, however, Masterson who has most systematically articulated a treatment approach to the borderline adolescent. In a series of communications (Masterson 1972, 1973, 1975), he described a mode of therapy based increasingly on his previously mentioned developmental hypotheses. Since in his view the borderline adolescent is fixated at the rapprochement subphase of separation-individuation, therapy must be designed to advance the separation-individuation process while protecting the patient from self-destructive actions that are aimed at maintaining pathological symbiosis. Accordingly, the patient should be hospitalized in a structured, closed unit with clear behavioral expectations. Separation from parents should be strict and categorical, at least during the early phase of the treatment process (see also Rinsley 1968). The "acting out" should be strictly controlled by clear limit setting, and confrontations should be explicit so as to reduce splitting and projection and to elicit over time what Masterson calls "abandonment depression." This can in turn be psychotherapeutically treated, allowing for a mourning process and new, presumably healthier introjections to occur that are based on the relationship with a therapist who encourages individuation. Parents are treated separately from the adolescent patient. Simon (1984), whose views parallel those of Masterson, advances the value of day-treatment programs that emphasize acquisition of social skills, group therapeutic interactions, and well-designed program structure.

In contrast, Zinner (1978) and Shapiro, Shapiro, Zinner, and Berkowitz (1977) regard combined family and individual therapy as essential in order to undo the disordered communication and projective identification that, in their view, pervade the families of adolescent borderline patients. They believe that the presence of the individual therapist in the concurrent family treatment helps with clarification of reality and can serve to bolster the alliance with the adolescent patient. They recognize the difficulties in this arrangement and acknowledge that some adolescents will refuse concurrent meetings with parents and that dropouts occur; nonetheless, they consider this model to be preferable to one in which patient and family are treated separately.

Friedman (1975) points out, correctly, that therapeutic technique with borderlines is often a function of theory; those who use an object-relations approach tend to advocate lengthy hospital treatment and "therapeutic" regression, while those who see the disorder in ego-psychological terms tend to propose more structured limit-setting techniques. Rosenfeld and Sprince (1965), for instance, strongly urge the use of supportive ego-building techniques that favor repression rather than uncovering approaches in the treatment of borderline children. Sugar (1979) proposes a multimodal program using virtually every available method—chemotherapy, individual group and family therapy, and what he calls "office network therapy," that is, the use of the patient's natural peer group as a therapeutic instrument.

I would go further than Friedman and suggest that in some cases, at least, both therapeutic technique and theory may derive from the particular personality styles of their authors, who, working in ways congenial to themselves, find that they have a therapeutic effect that they first consolidate and codify into a technical mode and then buttress with an explanatory theoretical system that is, no doubt, consistent with prevailing scientific constructs but that also serves to legitimize what they "naturally" do.

The value of biological treatment of the borderline adolescent is unclear. To my knowledge, no controlled studies of such treatment appear in the literature, although anecdotal reports of the use of medication in individual cases abound. Systematic research in drug treatment in borderline disorders in adults has yielded highly equivocal results, in the case of both neuroleptics and antidepressants. Certainly, it has failed to resolve controversies as to the diagnostic "location" of the borderline syndrome within the schizophrenic versus the affective spectrum. Gunderson (1986), in reviewing recent work in this area, concludes that, although neuroleptics may be of value in controlling acute psychotic symptoms, they do not appear to be effective in countering the specific and defining features of the borderline disorder and that a fair number of patients actually do worse with antidepressants. Clearly, further controlled studies of carefully selected populations of adolescent borderline patients will be required before any specific recommendations can be made for drug therapy in such cases.

Discussion

Areas of agreement, disagreement, and continuing ignorance emerge from this survey. There appears to be a fair consensus as to the clinical descriptive features of the borderline disorder in adolescents—impulsivity and self-destructive behaviors, affective instability, irritability and proneness to rage, substance abuse, and shallowness and fragility of object relations being prime characteristics, along with such "structural" (metapsychological) features as the predominance of the defenses of splitting and projection and the preservation of the capacity to test reality. There is also widespread agreement on certain of the developmental aspects of the syndrome; most students concur on the major importance of preoedipal determinants, though there is considerable caution regarding the specificity of particular phase or subphase issues.

With respect to treatment, however, a consensus is harder to come by. Although there is general assent to the view that psychotherapy of some sort is, at least in the present state of our knowledge, the treatment of choice, there is considerable dispute as to the precise mode or modes of therapy best suited to this group of patients. Recommendations range from classical psychoanalysis to the gamut of derivative psychotherapies, with no reliable data to suggest that any one or combination of these is more effective than any other. Indeed, although there are data that suggest long-term stability in this syndrome both with adolescents (Masterson, Lulow, and Costello 1982) and with adults (Barasch, Frances, Hunt, Clarkin, and Cohen 1985), there appears to be enough range of variation within the syndrome to support the applicability of a variety of treatment approaches. Further study would seem necessary to develop a subtypology that might promote the better specification of therapeutic modalities.

And what of the outcome of the available treatments? At present, little is available to clarify this. In fact, only Masterson et al. (1982) have reported such data with respect to adolescent borderlines (retrospectively diagnosed); they found that 58 percent of the patients treated in their long-term hospital-based program showed minimal to only mild impairment four years after treatment, while 42 percent were more seriously impaired. This, in their view, validates the effectiveness of their therapeutic method and, they concluded, "go[es] far toward laying to rest . . . the notion that borderline patients cannot benefit from psychoanalytic psychotherapy" (p. 519). On the other hand, McGlashan's (1986) long-term follow-up study on adult borderlines (also retrospectively diagnosed by DSM-III criteria) could not validate the benefit of similar therapy but did show that patients so treated functioned substantially better than schizophrenics after discharge and were comparable in most dimensions with unipolar depressives. At the least, the hospital experience did not prove deleterious; nor did it seem, as Friedman feared, to promote regression or further institutionalization. Pope, Jonas, Hudson, Cohen, and Gunderson (1983) found, on the contrary, that the outcome of their cases was considerably less favorable and that their borderline patients did only slightly better than a comparable group of schizophrenics and less well than patients with affective disorders.

Conclusions

It appears certain that a group of adolescent patients can be identified who essentially conform to the descriptive characteristics defined in DSM-III and other classifications (Gunderson; O. Kernberg) as those of the "borderline syndrome" or "borderline personality" in adults. Most clinical researchers in this field agree that the psychology of these patients is characterized by certain dominant defense mechanisms— particularly "splitting," projection, and (to Kernberg especially) "projective identification." Similarly, most agree that the crucial developmental issues are preoedipal and represent developmental defects rather than the compromise formations characteristic of neurotic symptoms.

Much, however, remains to be learned. It seems likely that most adolescent borderlines become adult borderlines, but their long-term fate remains uncertain with or without treatment. The relation of borderline disorders to schizophrenia on the one hand and to affective disorders on the other remains unclear. Treatment prescriptions are urgently needed; in their absence, it is difficult indeed to evaluate claims for efficacy or specificity. Further investigations of possible biological markers, predisposing neurochemical factors, and pharmacological therapies are surely in order, as are more systematic and less tendentious investigations of the developmental history of these patients, in order to tease out specific experiential elements. Indeed, refinement of diagnostic criteria for the entire range of personality disorders seems to be necessary in view of evidence of overlap and multiple diagnoses (Frances 1987). What is needed, thus, are fewer individual case studies and more systematic investigations of the biological substrate, specific diagnostic features, and the efficacy of therapeutic programs for these patients. After thirty years, we remain on the frontiers of understanding; it is likely that collaborative explorations across national and linguistic boundaries will further promote the scientific study and treatment of borderline disturbances in adolescents.

NOTE

1. In this respect, the studies of Cohen, Shaywitz, Young, and Shapiro (1983) on biological predisposition are of relevance.

REFERENCES

Akiskal, H. 1981. Subaffective disorders: dysthymic, cyclothymic and bipolar II disorders in the "borderline" realm. *Borderline Disorders* (Psychiatric Clinics of North America) 4:25–46.
American Psychiatric Association. 1987. *Diagnostic and Statistical Manual of Mental Disorder* (DSM-III-R). Washington, D.C.: APA.
Anderson, R. 1978. Thoughts on fathering: its relation to the borderline condition in adolescence and to transitional phenomena. *Adolescent Psychiatry* 6:377–395.
Andrulonis, P.; Glueck, B.; Stroebel, C.; and Vogel, N. 1982. Borderline personality subcategories. *Journal of Nervous and Mental Diseases* 170:670–679.

Barasch, A.; Frances, A.; Hunt, S.; Clarkin, J.; and Cohen, S. 1985. Stability and distinctness of borderline personality disorder. *American Journal of Psychiatry* 142:1484–1486.

Bird, J. 1980. The borderline patient and military life. *British Journal of Medical Psychology* 53:85–90.

Cahn, R. 1988. Discussion of Moses and M. Egle Laufer's Chapter. *International Annals of Adolescent Psychiatry* 1:75–78.

Cohen, D.; Shaywitz, S.; Young, J.; and Shapiro, B. 1983. Borderline syndromes and attention deficit disorder of childhood. In K. Robson, ed. *The Borderline Child: Approaches to Etiology, Diagnosis and Treatment.* New York: McGraw-Hill.

Ekstein, R., and Wallerstein, R. 1954. Observations on the psychology of borderline and psychotic children. *Psychoanalytic Study of the Child* 9:344–369.

Esman, A. 1980. Adolescent psychopathology and the rapprochement phenomenon. *Adolescent Psychiatry* 8:320–331.

Esman, A. 1988. Discussion of Moses and M. Egle Laufer's Chapter. *International Annals of Adolescent Psychiatry* 1:79–82.

Fard, K.; Hudgens, R.; and Welner, A. 1978. Undiagnosed psychiatric illness in adolescence. *Archives of General Psychiatry* 35:279–382.

Frances, A. 1987. Introduction to personality disorders. In R. Michels, ed. *Psychiatry,* vol. 1. Philadelphia: Lippincott.

Friedman, H. 1975. Psychotherapy of borderline patients: the influence of theory on technique. *American Journal of Psychiatry* 132:1048–1052.

Geleerd, E. 1958. Borderline states in children and adolescents. *Psychoanalytic Study of the Child* 13:279–295.

Giovacchini, P. 1979. The sins of the parents: the borderline adolescent and primal confusion. *Adolescent Psychiatry* 7:213–233.

Giovacchini, P. 1985. The borderline adolescent as a transitional object: a common variation. *Adolescent Psychiatry* 12:233–250.

Greenberg, L.; Haiman, S.; and Esman, A. 1987. Countertransference during acute hospitalization of the adolescent. *Adolescent Psychiatry* 14:316–331.

Grinker, R., Sr. 1978. The borderline syndrome. *Adolescent Psychiatry* 6:339–343.

Grinker, R., Sr.; Werble, B.; and Drye, R. 1968. *The Borderline Syndrome.* New York: Basic.

Gunderson, J. 1986. Pharmacotherapy of patients with borderline personality disorder. *Archives of General Psychiatry* 43:698–700.

Gunderson, J., and Kolb, J. 1978. Discriminating features of borderline patients. *American Journal of Psychiatry* 135:792–796.

Holm, K., and Hundevatt, E. 1981. Borderline states: prognosis and psychotherapy. *British Journal of Medical Psychology* 54:335–340.

Kernberg, O. 1967. Borderline personality organization. *Journal of the American Psychoanalytic Association* 18:800–822.

Kernberg, O. 1978. The diagnosis of borderline conditions in adolescence. *Adolescent Psychiatry* 6:298–319.

Kernberg, O. 1979. Psychoanalytic psychotherapy with borderline adolescents. *Adolescent Psychiatry* 7:294–321.

Kernberg, P. 1979. Psychoanalytic profile of the borderline adolescent. *Adolescent Psychiatry* 7:234–256.

Kernberg, P. 1983. Borderline conditions: childhood and adolescent aspects. In K. Robson, ed. *The Borderline Child: Approaches to Etiology, Diagnosis and Treatment*. New York: McGraw-Hill.

Laufer, M., and Laufer, M. E. 1984. *Adolescence and Developmental Breakdown*. New Haven, Conn.: Yale University Press.

Macaskill, N. 1982. The theory of transitional phenomena and its application to the psychotherapy of the borderline patient. *British Journal of Medical Psychology* 55:349–360.

Macaskill, N., and Macaskill, A. 1981. The use of the term "borderline patient" by Scottish psychiatrists: a preliminary survey. *British Journal of Psychiatry* 139:397–399.

McGlashan, T. 1986. The Chestnut Lodge followup study. III. long-term outcome of borderline personalities. *Archives of General Psychiatry* 43:20–30.

Mahler, M., and Kaplan, L. 1977. Developmental aspects in the assessment of narcissistic and so-called borderline personalities. In P. Hartocollis, ed. *Borderline Personality Disorders*. New York: International Universities Press.

Masterson, J. 1967. *The Psychiatric Dilemma of Adolescence*. Boston: Little, Brown.

Masterson, J. 1972. *Treatment of the Borderline Adolescent: A Developmental Approach*. New York: Wiley.

Masterson, J. 1973. The borderline adolescent. *Adolescent Psychiatry* 2:240–268.

Masterson, J. 1975. The splitting defense mechanism of the borderline adolescent: developmental and clinical aspects. In J. Mack, ed. *Borderline States in Psychiatry*. New York: Grune & Stratton.

Masterson, J.; Lulow, W.; and Costello, J. 1982. The test of time: borderline adolescent to functioning adult. *Adolescent Psychiatry* 10:492–522.

Masterson, J., and Rinsley, D. 1975. The borderline syndrome: the role of the mother in the genesis of psychic structure of the borderline personality. *International Journal of Psycho-Analysis* 56:163–177.

Michels, R. 1986. Borderline personality disorder: research issues and new empirical findings. *Journal of the American Psychoanalytic Association* 34:179–192.

Pine, F. 1974. On the concept of "borderline" in children. *Psychoanalytic Study of the Child* 29:341–368.

Pope, H.; Jonas, J.; Hudson, H.; Cohen, B.; and Gunderson, J. 1983. The validity of DSM-III borderline personality disorder. *Archives of General Psychiatry* 40:23–36.

Rinsley, D. 1968. Theory and practice of intensive residential treatment of adolescents. In A. Esman, ed. *The Psychiatric Treatment of Adolescents*. New York: International Universities Press.

Rinsley, D. 1978. Borderline psychopathology: a review of etiology, dynamics and treatment. *International Review of Psychoanalysis* 5:45–54.

Rosenfeld, S., and Sprince, M. 1963. An attempt to formulate the meaning of the concept "borderline." *Psychoanalytic Study of the Child* 18:628–635.

Rosenfeld, S., and Sprince, M. 1965. Some thoughts on the technical handling of borderline children. *Psychoanalytic Study of the Child* 20:505–512.

Shapiro, E.; Shapiro, R.; Zinner, J.; and Berkowitz, D. 1977. The borderline ego and the working alliance: indications for family and individual therapy in adolescence. *International Journal of Psycho-Analysis* 58:77–86.

Shapiro, T. 1983. The borderline syndrome in children: a critique. In K. Robson, ed. *The Borderline Child*. New York: McGraw-Hill.

Simon, H. 1984. The borderline syndrome in adolescence. *Adolescence* 19:505–520.

Slavin, M., and Slavin, J. 1976. Two patterns of adaptation in late adolescent borderline personalities. *Psychiatry* 39:41–50.

Stone, M. 1980. *The Borderline Syndromes*. New York: McGraw-Hill.

Sugar, M. 1979. Therapeutic approaches to the borderline adolescent. *Adolescent Psychiatry* 7:343–361.

Tarnopolsky, A., and Berelowitz, M. 1984. "Borderline personality": diagnostic attitudes at the Maudsley Hospital. *British Journal of Psychiatry* 144:364–369.

Zinner, J. 1978. Combined individual and family treatment of borderline adolescents: rationale and management of the early phase. *Adolescent Psychiatry* 6:420–433.

Zinner, J., and Shapiro, E. 1975. Splitting in families of borderline adolescents. In J. Mack, ed. *Borderline States in Psychiatry*. New York: Grune & Stratton.

LEWIS A. KIRSHNER

During adolescence, acting out may function in the service of developmental process. Through action, the adolescent may express in dramatic form the particular developmental issue with which he or she is struggling and, in doing so, attempt to evoke from the object the responses that are necessary for progression to a higher or more integrated developmental level. Describing the function of acting out in this way follows the important contributions of Blos (1966), who differentiated between the predisposition, the mechanism, and the function of acting-out behavior in adolescence and contributed a major developmental concept in noting the importance of enactments in reestablishing "temporal continuity" with unintegrated early memories and experiences within the developing ego. Blos's conception shares common features with the views of Erikson (1962) and Winnicott (1973), who noted a kind of claim on the objects of the adolescent for confirmation of his or her experience of reality and a phase-appropriate response. In this chapter, using case examples, I elaborate the developmental function of acting out addressed by these authors, utilizing the ego developmental model of Loevinger (1976) to demonstrate how the behavior of the adolescent reflects specific developmental stage issues.

Winnicott's (1973) views on this function of acting out were expressed in a talk about delinquency delivered to prison officials in Britain. In his talk, he observed that delinquents seemed to be youngsters who had initially experienced good-enough mothering but for whom some deprivation had then occurred that disrupted the developmental process in the integration of love and hate. Winnicott's view appears to be that without the connection with the caring object the child dares not risk expression of its hateful feelings and so fails to internalize a good object relation that can contain such feelings. With the subsequent expression of the delinquency, however, the adolescent makes a bid to reopen this rather early developmental issue, in a sense looking for the object to acknowledge the existence of hateful feelings and provide a structure in which it is safe to experience them.

In his well-known analysis of the Dora case, Erikson (1962) attempts to place this object-seeking aspect of acting out in a developmental context. What appears as "acting out," he observes, may contain "an adaptive, if immature reaching out for the mutual verification by which the ego lives" (p. 457). For adolescents, he proposes, such mutuality involves the capacity to pledge and receive "fidelity," an affirmation of genuineness and reliability. In Dora's case, her obstreperousness may, therefore, derive in part from her sense of betrayal by adults around her. Those members of Dora's family (and Freud himself, to the extent that he fails to support her) seem willing to disconfirm her sense of historical truth for their own purposes. In this framework, Dora is struggling to uphold a sense of norms for trustworthy behavior or of social reality, which are clearly tied to her attempts to achieve ego integration and identity.

If adolescent acting out can express a developmental need of the ego, making a demand on others to reestablish continuity with re-pressed or disavowed aspects of experience, as Blos argues, the phase of ego development must be of central importance. Winnicott's em-phasis on the need of the self to integrate loving and hateful feelings suggests an adolescent at an early phase of development, with a rather fragile sense of self, while Erikson's views on Dora correspond to his conception of the normative tasks of this stage of the life cycle, when a more secure self seeks a broader psychosocial "identity." Such dif-fering constructions of the self can be conceptualized as stages within Loevinger's model of ego development.

Loevinger's Theory of Ego Development

Loevinger's (1976) comprehensive view of what she terms "ego de-velopment" has now acquired a strong empirical base (Hauser 1976). Her work defines the ego as an organizing, meaning-making structure, more like an "experiencing self" than the ego in classic psychoanalytic theory. This "ego" represents a continuous attempt by the subject to construct a cohesive sense of self at different developmental stages that reflect progressive structuralization of the personality and differentiation from objects. While the early stages coincide with normal age landmarks of child development, any stage may also be retained into adulthood. This heterogeneity of stage of ego development is particularly characteristic of adolescence.

Briefly, Loevinger's stages may be grouped into three phases with intervening transition points. In the "preconformist" stages, the individual gains a sense of self from feelings and immediate perceptions. Needs are pressing and overwhelming, and the object is regarded largely in terms of gratification, frustration, or punishment rather than as an individual in his or her own right. Rejection or delays may be experienced as abandonment or attack by the powerful other, who must be fought, manipulated, or cajoled. Delinquents are most likely to operate at this level (Noam, Hauser, Santostefano, Garrison, Jacobson, Powers, and Mean 1984).

The mid-range conformist stage is characterized by an emphasis on similarity or difference from a reference group, membership in which defines the sense of self. The individual strives to be in harmony with the group and to hold appropriate attitudes and values, with self-reflection revolving around conventional feelings or beliefs acceptable to group norms. When an individual takes this step toward redefining a sense of self, in terms of a more abstract sense of similarity to others, he or she is making a momentous leap from the vulnerable self of the preconformist period, whose weak identity depends on the mirror held up by powerful others, to a more stable self who has entered the symbolic social order. Correspondingly, the individual now needs reciprocal relationships with others to sustain this sense of selfhood.

As the individual enters the postconformist phase, he or she becomes more sensitive to individual differences, and more self-evaluation becomes possible with this awareness of variability in realization of norms. The self is now experienced as partaking to a greater or lesser extent of different traits, thereby permitting awareness of a complex inner world and a greater sense of autonomy and separateness. The subject's growing acceptance of responsibility for his or her desires fosters an internalized morality, and others are evaluated more stringently. At this point, recognition of an autonomous self is sought from others rather than nurturing, mirroring, or approval.

The following cases illustrate differences in the developmental functions of acting out for adolescents at these three major phases. While the kinds of issues enacted in behavior are similar, involving early traumatic memories, separation conflicts, and intense affective states, specific developmental needs of adolescents vary and may require different responses from the therapist to support a therapeutic solution.

Fred: Establishment of the Preconformist Self

Fred, a troubled fifteen-year-old who had suffered traumatic separations as a child, already had a lengthy psychiatric history, including hospitalization as a "borderline" child. He had graduated from a day-treatment program the previous year and was attending a program for special needs children within a public high school when the incident to be discussed occurred. One day an urgent call came to the therapist from the school authorities demanding immediate hospitalization. Fred had been found in an empty office cutting his arm with a hunting knife, which he had brought into the school. He was described as angry and uncooperative, and the school psychologist considered him dangerous and unsafe. This was a serious setback to the months of apparently successful work with the boy and school administrators over the past year. With some negotiation, arrangements were made to have Fred brought for an emergency meeting rather than directly to a hospital as requested.

At the meeting, Fred was upset but in control as he poured out his story. He had recently formed an attachment to another special needs student about whom he had romantic thoughts. When he saw her befriending another boy, he became jealous and angry, insisting she meet him after school and telephoning her in the evening. She, in turn, had resisted his demands. Finally, Fred decided to bring the knife to school with a vague plan of somehow gaining her attention. When she seemed "mean" to him, he had gone to the room and scratched her initials on his upper arm. He conveyed that he had done this because he was angry and he loved the girl. He wanted to show her this by letting her see what she was doing to him, hoping she would respond. At no time did he intend to injure himself or others seriously, he insisted.

Fred's parents confirmed Fred's "crush" on the girl and noted his recent improvements in behavior. With their support, the school was approached to treat the incident as a behavioral problem displaying poor judgment on Fred's part and violation of rules rather than as an expression of illness. After considerable discussion, they agreed to allow Fred to return to class after a two-day suspension.

Among many possible meanings, Fred's behavior appeared to express his difficulty dealing with anger toward the girl and the narcissistic threat that her rejection posed for him. In this sense, he recalls Winnicott's (1973) delinquent, making a bid to reopen issues of aggression toward others who presumably might be expected to pay some attention to his hurts. By cutting himself, Fred announced that he was in pain over a kind of deprivation of response that he could not really express in words and that his selfhood was thereby threatened. The cut itself could then be viewed as an expression of the infantile experience of loss and abandonment that underlay his conscious sense of deprivation, thereby providing a continuity within the therapeutic discourse for memories previously unavailable to his ego, as Blos (1966) suggested. Fred could now speak of being hurt by one he loved, an important therapeutic advance, albeit the psychic boundary between this other one and him seemed still blurred—at the cutting point, as it were, of the initials carved on his skin. What Fred now sought, clearly, was a nurturant response to his wish to be loved and a recognition that his anger was not so much to harm the other as to express his plight. This intense need for immediate response, the unrealistic nature of his demands on the object, and the stress on the importance of his present feelings characterize the adolescent still struggling with the imperatives of a preconformist sense of self. In Fred's case, therapeutic consolidation of a stable self in relation to caring others had been a developmental achievement, which now entered a new chapter in attempting to integrate ambivalent feelings.

William: The Conformist Self Desiring to Belong

William was a boy who wanted very badly to be normal, "like other teenagers," despite a long history of traumatic events, beginning with the death of his mother at age four and culminating with the final breakup of his father's stormy and violent second marriage. As the target of scathing attacks by a jealous stepmother, he had demanded that his father do something, only to be admonished to be considerate of her rigid expectations. Struggling with his own problems, the father had arranged for William to be seen; but, apart from expressing a wish to return to the status quo ante with his dad, the boy had been politely adamant that he did not need psychiatric help. However, a few months later, his worried father recontacted the therapist to say that William had been caught by police breaking into his school gymnasium and damaging property.

At the ensuing meeting, William gave his account of events, which involved removing, fooling around with, and ultimately breaking the new school flag, recently hung by their principal on the gym wall. A bright, earnest fifteen-year-old without any prior history of serious misbehavior, William seemed regretful but realistic about the nature of this action and his own responsibility. It was "the wrong thing to do," definitely against the law (as the irate police officer had forcefully impressed on him), and he was sorry that he and his friend had gone so far. However, when queried why he believed such an incident might have happened, William was brought up short. Clearly, he had not so reflected, but, after a pause, he offered the opinion that it was not very important. "It was a prank, a joke. I thought it would be funny. It was a stupid idea. I'm sorry we thought of it." The gist appeared to be that no significant meaning was to be attached to the incident, and, no doubt, the affair did seem rather trivial. On the other hand, the timing of his "symptomatic act" raised some questions, as William was experiencing another year of failing grades at school, and his father was extremely concerned for other reasons about possible delinquent tendencies. After some fairly fruitless discussion, the therapist wondered what it was, after all, that William thought might be "funny." The young man now provided a fantasy. He imagined the look on the principal's face seeing his precious flag turned upside down in its mount (he had not intended to break it). What would that look be like? Of course, dismay, anger, feeling a bit of a fool. With this new scenario, William reluctantly admitted that he enjoyed the notion of upsetting the man, whom no one liked anyway. However, the point for him was irrelevant. He was not that angry at the school or the principal, he claimed, and that was not why they did it. More details could be provided, but their substance would be quite similar: minimizing the episode, resisting any introspection about it, and justifying his behavior within an acceptable framework of peer standards.

At a subsequent session, William returned to his topic in a new way. "Don't you think," he asked, "that the policeman overreacted by threatening me like he did and that my father is taking this whole thing way too seriously?'' To the therapist, the query held a certain urgency and demand for confirmation. If he chose to push ahead with his inquiry, no doubt the result would be further denial or, perhaps, more guilt in the form of feeling "stupid" for upsetting his dad. William wanted to be normal, after all, not a patient like his parents, and to have a regular teenage life, for which his father, despite some major failures in the past, was his only guarantor. Still, the therapist had reason to be concerned about the effect of the separation and the climate of violence preceding it on William's development, precisely because of his anger and disappointment in his father.

Like many adolescents, William appears to be struggling with issues of the conformist stage of ego development. He seeks to ground his identity in a field of relationships and group norms, minimizing his individual agency in favor of being "just one of the guys." What seems to threaten this developmental step is not simply the aggression expressed in his attack on the symbol of authority, aggression that he can scarcely acknowledge except in this symbolic action, with its metaphor of castration, but the deficiency in the enabling conditions of his interpersonal world, what the developmentalist Kegan (1982) has called the "embeddedness culture." In this respect, he is reminiscent of Dora, whose demand was for integrity from her father and a recognition of the corrupt conditions that had compromised her. Erikson insists precisely on the need for adults to ensure a structure in which ego ideals can be retained amid differentiation from parents. Here the central desire is not for mirror-like confirmation of the imperative needs that define the self at the preconformist phase, as with Fred. Rather, William's actions, like Dora's, call into question the arrangements of adult institutions in which he needs to place his trust.

In the ensuing therapy, William and his father were seen conjointly, freeing the boy from the unwelcome patient role and putting the focus on the problematic relationship. In fact, father quickly confessed some recent inappropriate behavior of his own, which William had witnessed (indeed, evoking dismay and anger, as in his fantasy of the principal). The therapeutic task now turned to finding ways to demonstrate to the father that he had not been living up to his responsibilities and to William that his anger about these failures was justified and normal and could be expressed. Pursuit of these unspoken aspects of life in the household brought relief. The boy was glad to "get things off his chest," including his accusation that, after all, it was his dad who had broken the important rules and not he. Vague memories of his father's drinking habits and unreliable behavior around his mother's illness, repeated during the recent separation, enabled him to explain some of his mixed feelings toward his father and to verbalize, to the extent he was able, his painful sense of betrayal and disappointment. The breaking of the school flag might be viewed, then, as a symbolic statement referring to the current unhappy state of his family as well as echoing the rage from the much earlier childhood loss, which had been repressed. Soon, William began to improve in his studies and decided to try out for a school team. Naturally, he was interested in concluding therapy, if the therapist agreed.

Lena: The Threat to the Autonomous Self

Since psychopathology and diagnosis do not necessarily coincide with level of ego development (Noam et al. 1984), it is possible to find fairly disturbed adolescents who manifest many of the markers of post-conformist stages such as a capacity for self-observation, an elaborated inner world of personalized values and perceptions, and a capacity to make individualized commitments to others. Lena, aged sixteen, represents this constellation. She was brought to a hospital emergency room by her mother and the police in a state of rage and defiance after attempting to force her way into the home of a girlfriend with whom she had been carrying on an increasingly stormy homosexual relationship. Ann's parents, intending to put an end to this situation, had forbidden Lena to visit, but, following several days quiescence, Lena presented herself once again on their threshhold, raging against her friend, and, ultimately, shattering a glass pane with a fist so that she received a severe laceration. The family called the police, who, failing to elicit cooperation, decided to pass the problem on to other authorities.

Lena proved to be astute and vocal, eager to relate her story, and, despite initial anger at being "railroaded" into the hospital, an unusually cooperative inpatient. She and Ann had been best friends, sharing musical and literary interests, until the past summer, when their friendship had become an infatuation. Both had other friends of both sexes, but, with their new romantic involvement, episodes of jealousy toward these others had begun to appear, first as mild and humorous jibes, later as deeper and more painful attacks. Confused by these intense emotions, the two decided to go separate ways, only to be drawn together by ever more painful feelings of rejection and rage with each perceived transgression of their formerly shared values and principles. Lena felt that Ann had unquestionably violated a pledge of personal honesty and loyalty by agreeing to date a classmate they had disliked and then fabricating an explanation about it. When pressed to justify this behavior, Ann had refused, culminating in the scene at her home.

Lena was curious about this relationship and her powerful feelings. She described a sense of isolation from her mother, who, she felt, had never understood her. The parents had divorced when she was five, partly a result of her mother's severe depressions, and both had subsequently remarried. An older brother had left for college, and Lena shared an apartment with mother and her working-class Italian husband. In therapy, she reported that issues of integrity and keeping one's word were very important to her and that her major disappointment with Ann lay precisely in that area. It failed to surprise her that her mother refused to support her actions and had agreed to the hospital admission. Her mother, after all, could not tolerate this kind of moral issue, having compromised herself by remarrying a rigid, uneducated dullard. Meanwhile, her father, despite high intelligence and cultivation, was painfully cold and distant.

When queried about her behavior, Lena insisted that Ann deserved to be embarrassed and punished for violating their understanding but did wonder about the intensity of her feelings and whether these could really all be caused by the breakup of the relationship. She was troubled by her tendency to make Ann "bigger than life" and was concerned that she felt so alienated from her family and school. She had planned to attend a top-level college, but now her plans were in jeopardy.

Lena was apparently very grateful for the attention she received from her therapist. She seemed to treat the hospital experience as a kind of field trip and joined staff in analyzing problems on the ward. With everyone supporting discharge and her enthusiasm for continuing therapy, she fairly quickly returned home. The initial week was stormy, with shouting incidents in school and arguments at home, both minimized by her, but brought to the therapist's attention by school authorities and her mother. The patient felt that seeing Ann was very painful and that her mother was a profound disappointment. She had a keen eye for hypocrisy at school and was provocative with teachers and the principal. Somehow, she felt that talking with her therapist, who seemed so perceptive and aware, would help her distance herself from these trivia of daily life so that she could focus energy on her artistic work, which would free her from the hurtful feelings. Unfortunately, this failed to occur, and she found herself unable to ignore Ann's behavior or to forgo being the recipient of her exclusive affection. Despite her conscious awareness of Ann's limitations and of her own responsibility for absorbing the loss, Lena remained consumed with moral indignation and, once again, decided to take her case to Ann's family, where she was arrested by the police and immediately returned to the hospital. There, she declared herself ready to be readmitted, as she was not capable of functioning in the world as she found it. The therapist decided to defer this decision, but her therapy now took a different course.

Lena was seen four to six times per week over the next year. She was told initially that she needed a reliable caretaker to turn to because she felt so abandoned and betrayed, and the therapist attempted to maintain an empathic, accepting stance. At first, she appeared to respond with a form of idealizing transference, which might be viewed as expressing her wish for a perfect father who could support her narcissistic aspirations. As time went on, however, she began to put herself into the posture of a helpless victim, and the therapeutic alliance assumed a passive quality of seeking magical fulfillment of immense expectations. At first, perplexed by the therapist's failure to cure her of her bad feelings, Lena grew increasingly bitter and enraged. Fits of sobbing and accusations of dereliction by various people, delivered in an angry, provocative manner, characterized the sessions. Therapy seemed to be useless and another disappointment in her life, and she sought another treatment solution. She brought in brochures about long-term hospitals that friends and teachers had told her about, demanded that the therapist admit her, and considered making a dramatic gesture to prove her distress. During some sessions, she slumped to the floor in a fetal posture and cried for the entire time. She was given permission to return after school to sit in the waiting room, which she considered soothing, and she occasionally did so. Meanwhile, the therapist experienced conflicting emotions of having to take care of a helpless and ill patient who might require residential treatment while often listening to the observations of a reflective and self-willed young woman who wanted to solve her own problems. The picture was confusing, and inpatient care, treatment with medication along a medical model of affective disorder, or some kind of day treatment were plausible alternatives. Fortunately, the father, for reasons of his own, took a strong stand against hospitalization and agreed to support outpatient therapy.

Within the regressive transference, the therapist attempted to explore Lena's intense rage that he, too, was not helping. The "too" referred, of course, to the mother, the one with whom Lena had been left when deserted by her father and who had been unable to respond because of her own depression. While remaining empathic in attempting to explore these early experiences, however, the therapist upheld a "developmental gradient" by not protecting Lena from the consequences of her actions and respecting her sometimes dubious decision making, refusing to cover for her when she stayed home or did not complete work, and encouraging her to put her feelings into words when this seemed a dubious undertaking. In the end, enough progress has been made for Lena to graduate and leave for college, carrying a somewhat detoxified but still intense set of feelings about her friend.

At times, Lena seemed like Fred, struggling with rage at early losses and unable to define a self apart from her feelings. Like William, however, she expressed a powerful desire to separate from disappointing and unfaithful objects into the larger structure of the social community of peers. Unlike those two adolescents, she maintained (most of the time) a capacity for self-awareness of her own inner moral and emotional conflicts. Her violent acting out condensed these themes and enabled them eventually to be spoken about, at a point in her life when the exclusive relationship with her friend, with its infantile pulls, seemed to be carrying too much weight as a guardian of a tenuous sense of self. Yet, in her therapy, it was finally this sense of self, capable of accepting the limits of entitlement and desire in a painful autonomy, which permitted her to withstand the enormous pressures of her infantile longings and disappointments.

Discussion

When Freud (1914) wrote his paper "Repeating, Remembering, and Working Through," he lacked the concept of an ego that could direct action in the service of development. Later, when the ego as an active organ of adaptation emerged in the theory, the notion of developmental stages was absent (Rapaport 1959). With Erikson's (1956) model of the life cycle, the conception of a developing self, which actively structures experience and interprets the inner and outer worlds, was added to psychoanalytic theory. The nature of the relation between life phase and developmental stage, however, is quite complex (Kirshner 1987; Noam 1985). The topic of acting out in adolescence provides an excellent illustration of this complexity, in part because the wide variation in level of ego development creates unusual problems and opportunities for meeting external and internal pressures.

A review of three major approaches to the understanding of adolescent behavior suggests that acting out can be placed on a continuum of levels of ego development (Loevinger 1976). Winnicott's (1973) notions about delinquency describe the adolescent at the early preconformist phase, whose sense of self derives from impulses and immediate needs. The inability of adults to hear the expression of rage, hypothesized by Winnicott, has fostered a mistrustful and wary personality, whose acting out may represent another try for connection with an object. Fred, in the present study, illustrates this issue. For Fred, the therapeutic task was to provide a holding environment in which his feelings could be acknowledged, confirming the integration of self at the preconformist level. The environment of choice at this phase is, of course, the family, and family therapy was the main modality of treatment.

Erikson's (1962) views on Dora were offered as a model for the adolescent struggling to achieve the organization of self at the conformist phase through fidelity to a normative order rather than by subjective experience. In the example of William, his acting-out vandalism drew attention to the failure of significant others to uphold this step. The lack of psychological mindedness characteristic of the conformist phase and the resulting need for an alternative treatment approach justified a conjoint therapy in which the enabling function of the parent could be restored.

Finally, postconformist differentiation in the direction of a more autonomous sense of self was portrayed in the case of Lena. While demanding recognition as a responsible subject, Lena demonstrated a marked regression to infantile conflicts. However, her developmental level permitted a psychoanalytic psychotherapy.

Conclusions

In all three cases, an episode of acting out drew attention to a break in the subject's sense of continuity of self. Unintegrated affects, painful losses, and historical realities spoke through the behavior, as past experiences of disruption were revived by current developmental challenges. The level of ego development dictated the form and structure of this revival and the kind of object needs associated with it. Choice of therapeutic intervention was related to this conceptualization.

REFERENCES

Blos, P. 1966. The concept of acting-out in relation to the adolescent process. In E. N. Rexford, ed: *A Developmental Approach to Problems of Acting Out*. New York: International Universities Press.

Erikson, E. H. 1956. The problem of ego identity. *Journal of the American Psychoanalytic Association* 4:56–121.

Erikson, E. H. 1962. Reality and actuality. *Journal of the American Psychoanalytic Association* 10:451–474.

Freud, S. 1914. Remembering, repeating, and working through. *Standard Edition* 12:145–156. London: Hogarth, 1961.

Hauser, S. T. 1976. Loevinger's model and measure of ego development: a critical review. *Psychology Bulletin* 33:928–988.

Kegan, R. 1982. *The Evolving Self*. Cambridge, Mass.: Harvard University Press.

Kirshner, L. A. 1987. Implications of Loevinger's theory of ego development for time-limited psychotherapy. *Psychotherapy* 25:220–227.

Loevinger, J. 1976. *Ego Development*. San Francisco: Jossey-Bass.

Noam, G. G. 1985. Stage, phase, and style: the developmental dynamics of the self. In M. Berkowitz and F. Oser, eds. *Moral Education*. Hillsdale, N.J.: Erlbaum.

Noam, G.; Hauser, S.; Santostefano, S.; Garrison, W.; Jacobson, A.; Powers, S.; and Mean, M. 1984. Ego development and psychopathology. *Child Development* 55:184–194.

Rapaport, D. 1959. An historic review of psychoanalytic ego psychology. *Psychological Issues* 1:5–18.

Winnicott, D. W. 1973. Delinquency as a sign of hope. *Adolescent Psychiatry* 2:369–371.

23 ADOLESCENT PSYCHOPATHOLOGY AND ATTACHMENT RESEARCH: MUTUAL CONTRIBUTIONS TO UNDERSTANDING

CHARLES JAFFE AND PETER BARGLOW

This chapter attempts to view the continuity of infant experience with adolescent psychopathology from multiple perspectives and to apply such insight to infant observation research. The emphasis in psychoanalysis on object relations, the development and transformations of the self (Kohut 1971, 1977), and the idea that the "richness of experience . . . can be defined both by the experiencing of age-appropriate conflict and by the sequences of syntheses, integrations, organizations, and reorganizations" (Lichtenberg 1983, p. 39) over time has opened the way to vigorous examination of psychoanalytic theories by infant observation researchers (Emde 1981, 1985; Lichtenberg 1983; Stern 1985). By contrast, this chapter reverses the direction of this emphasis through an attempt to apply insights obtained from adult analytic reconstructions and adolescent psychotherapy to enrich the process and yield of an area of infant research.

This collaboration between two therapists, one (C. J.) of an adolescent boy and the other (P. B.) of his mother, was stimulated by the effort to address questions left unanswered by an infant study (Barglow, Vaughn, and Molitor, in press).[1] The concurrent unfolding of the treatments, one a psychotherapy and the other a psychoanalysis, of two members of the same family by different therapists provided a special opportunity to make use of multiple perspectives to understand the infant-mother interaction of this now adolescent-mother pair and to shed new light on the research findings.

First, we will briefly describe the infant observation study that stimulated this collaboration. Next, we will report the presentation of an adolescent boy who as an infant displayed behavior that corresponded to that found in a study of infants of working mothers. Relevant reconstructions obtained from the mother's psychoanalysis will then be summarized, and we will show how the findings from both treatments were useful in beginning to answer a puzzling question raised by the infant research. Finally, we will consider some issues involved with efforts to combine the perspectives of psychoanalysis and developmental research.

The Study of Infants of Working Mothers

Ainsworth, Blehar, Waters, and Wall (1978), following Bowlby's (1969) work on attachment, studied the quality of infant-mother relationships in a laboratory setting by exposing twelve- to eighteen-month-old infants to a series of increasingly stressful separations. Today, this procedure is called the Strange Situation. The procedure involves a series of separation and reunion experiences involving the infant, the mother, and a stranger. The episode is rated and coded for proximity seeking, contact maintenance, avoidance, resistance, and crying. On this basis, infants are classified as secure, insecure/resistant, or insecure/avoidant. So-called insecurely attached avoidant infants ignore the mother's leaving and on her return actively avoid and turn away from her, refusing to communicate affectively with her. Considerable evidence indicates that insecure (particularly insecure avoidant) attachment constitutes a risk factor for subsequent social, educational, and psychological difficulty (Farber and Egeland 1982; Sroufe 1983; Vaughn, Deane, and Waters 1985).

The project of our interest (Barglow et al., in press) studied 110 low-risk, middle-class, infant-mother pairs with the Strange Situation.[2] It was demonstrated that avoidance scores of the group of infants of full-time working mothers who returned to work in the first three months postpartum were significantly greater than those for the group of infants whose mothers remained at home as primary caretakers. Specifically, 71 percent of the infants in the at-home group were securely attached, compared to 54 percent of the infants in the at-work group. Since these babies had care in their homes provided by a person outside the immediate family, this variation cannot be due to the effects of group day care.

The mothers from this sample had completed an extensive battery of pencil and paper measures prior to the infant's birth and had also submitted numerous reports concerning their own attitudes and the behavior of their infants during the first year of life (Joffe, Vaughn, Barglow, and Benveniste 1985). Several of these measures were selected on the a priori basis that they should index demographic (age, education, parity, and child's gender), attitudinal (mother's encouragement of independence and concern over control of infant's behavior), and personality characteristics (dominance, capacity for status, achievement via conformity or independence, intellectual efficiency, and femininity) that might distinguish mothers who went to work during the first year of the infant's life from those who did not. In addition to direct reports of their own attitudes and personality characteristics, the mothers provided their perceptions of infant behavioral style traits and developmental milestone achievements to permit evaluations of possible differences in maternal perceptions of the infant as correlates of work status. Statistical analysis contrasted and compared the two work-status groups on the demographic, attitudinal, and psychological variables selected a priori on the ten scores derived from the maternal perception measures of temperament (Carey and McDevitt 1978) and on overall developmental status (Ireton and Thwing 1972).

Of the thirty-seven tests using these variables, only one, parity, reached statistical significance to distinguish mothers who returned to work within the first three months from those who did not. The interpretation of the results was that many infants of mothers who return to full-time employment during the first year experience the repeated, daily separations from the mother as a rejection, leading to avoidance of her in the Strange Situation.

Main (Main and Weston 1982) proposed that the infant's avoidance of the mother in the context of the Strange Situation is a consequence of physical or psychological rejection of the infant by the mother. She suggested that rejected infants are particularly susceptible to behavioral disorganization in circumstances that lead to activation of the biologically based attachment behavioral system (see Bowlby 1969) such as the separation episodes of the Strange Situation. A conflict arises because the infant is simultaneously motivated to seek and to withdraw from contact with the attachment figure. In her view, avoidance (e.g., ignoring the mother's return, actively turning away from her, refusing to communicate with her) is a behavioral adjustment or adaptation of the infant that permits him or her to maintain control over a potentially disorganizing experience (see Main and Weston 1982, p. 54).

Despite this and other plausible interpretations of the infant's experience, important questions went unanswered in the study. What psychological factors could explain the finding that a little more than half (54 percent) the infants in the at-work group were securely attached to their mothers despite the repeated daily separations they experienced? Why did contrasts between personality factors in working and nonworking mothers not show any major statistical differences?

The following clinical material provided the impetus for concluding that maternal psychological traits promoted secure or insecure attachment in the infants and that the psychological test instruments used originally must not have been sensitive enough to detect this. Following the case presentation, we will return to the result of the application of new instruments to test the hypotheses drawn from the clinical material.

Psychotherapy of the Adolescent

Gregory, age eleven, was in the sixth grade of a suburban school.[3] He was referred for treatment after he had become "totally out of control," banging his head against a wall and threatening suicide. His mother said that Gregory had always insisted on having his own way and when frustrated would become verbally abusive and scream, even in public and in front of his friends. The mother indicated that Gregory would not allow her any privacy, to the extent of trying to force himself into the toilet with her. When the father was away on business trips, Gregory became terrified at being left alone and insisted on his mother's presence until he fell asleep.[4] The mother conceded to his demands rather than tolerate hours of bitter arguments. The mother had failed in her attempts at consistent rules and sanctions and reacted to Gregory's challenges with excessive compliance or harsh punishment. At times, she would lose control of herself and kick Gregory or throw a book at him.

The father was described as even more explosive than the mother. He yelled loudly at the child, scolded him for being slovenly, and often threatened physical violence. He blamed the mother for Gregory's behavior and to buy a few moments of peace frequently gave in to even the most outrageous demands. Both parents felt guilty that their quiet, six-year-old girl was overlooked in the excitement and turmoil.

The mother was also concerned about her son's behavior with friends and in school. Gregory fought with his boyfriends and displayed the same aggressive, bullying behavior with them that he manifested at home. After such an incident, Gregory would become consumed with worry about how long it would be before the rift was repaired. He tried to enlist his mother to speak to the friend's parents to be sure that he would not lose the friend. Gregory's relationships tended not to last because he was so pushy and selfish. Gregory's teachers repeatedly complained that he was a disobedient troublemaker, did not pay attention in class, talked continuously instead of listening, and often demanded special and extra attention.

Gregory's own report corroborated most of his mother's stories but differed from her conclusions in several ways. His chief complaint was that his mother did not spend enough time with him because she was always working or entertaining. He said that he had mentioned suicide only to get mother's attention. He also reported that his mother and father often fought bitterly and yelled and screamed at each other. He said that his father depreciated and insulted both him and his mother. When the father felt upset about his own behavior, he would try to win Gregory over by special favors such as making reservations to go to a football game, but then he often canceled at the last moment for business reasons. If Gregory protested, father sent him to his room while accusing him of being an intolerable burden. Mother also kept breaking promises that they would do things together. Gregory worried that his mother did not love him; sometimes, he said, mother hit him when they had arguments. Other than loud arguments, Gregory recalled little about his early relationships with either of his parents. He had always believed that his sister got better treatment.

Regarding his personal problems, Gregory reported that a year earlier he had had trouble with friends because he bragged too much about material possessions, such as the cars his father drove. He thought that perhaps he had not felt good about himself at that time. Since then, he had learned that what people own does not matter that much. He had recently found some new friends and now felt generally happy. He enjoyed sports, rock concerts, and summer camp. He professed no interest in girls. He said he liked school but often felt bored and had difficulty paying attention.

354

Gregory presented as a slightly built, compliant, young adolescent. He mumbled his words and was often difficult to understand. After being somewhat subdued in the first sessions, he became quite fidgety, moving about in his chair, chewing gum, or complaining about feeling tired. Gregory had little capacity for self-observation and little tolerance for delay or frustration. He acknowledged his mother's complaints and after some defensive self-justification revealed that, while he tried not to antagonize his mother "by bothering her all the time," he feared that, if he did not, she would forget about him. Later, he could see that his behavior did not live up to his own ideals for treating others but that he could not behave as he wanted when his fears were stimulated.

Gregory's mother had become pregnant as planned after six years of marriage. Pregnancy and delivery had been unremarkable, but there already had been considerable marital friction. Early motherhood did not go easily: "I was never a nature earth-mother type." The mother missed her job and resented the loss of privacy and the disruptions of her routines that the baby entailed. She reported that she did not like the tactile, messy aspects of infant care: "I'm not a touchy-feely type person. . . . I could hardly wait for the baby to become a child." The obstetrician overheard her talking to Gregory with the words, "How dare you continue crying," and commented that it sounded as if she were talking to another adult. Yet in other ways she was a very intelligent, well-informed, and competent mother who felt much love, loyalty, and devotion to her baby. The father also experienced deep affection for Gregory, though he shunned physical caretaking altogether, never changing diapers and rarely feeding the infant.

When Gregory was one month old, the mother returned to a demanding full-time job. She did not recall that she felt any distress at separation associated with leaving her son to go to work or that she had felt any significant longing for the baby while she was away. In retrospect, she believed she did miss him sometimes while on the job but mainly emphasized that she felt great comfort and pleasure with her own freedom rather than anxiety when she left the baby with the child's caretaker. Also, she vividly recalled Gregory's surprising response when she or her husband would leave him: "He didn't mind our going; he wouldn't notice at all or show me any reaction." "When I came back, he would usually ignore me, but he didn't cry or cling to me, and I was real proud of him."

Gregory ate well, gained weight on schedule, and seemed to be a happy, cuddly infant. Near the end of his first year of life, his parents considered him demanding and difficult. In response to frustration, "he would get his back up," assume a rigid posture, and scream. In his second year, he would sometimes hold his breath if he were not picked up. The mother tended not to yield to such behavior, thinking, "Just wait long enough and it will go away." Her husband, on the other hand, "couldn't stand up" to the baby and would usually give in, "taking the easy route," as she put it. The mother consciously wanted to keep some distance between herself and the baby since her own mother had been hovering and intrusive.

Gregory's motor milestones, speech development, and toilet training were not unusual, but in his second year of life there had been considerable problems with sleeping by himself in his own room. He could go to sleep only while touching one of his parents, and, when they tried to put him into his own bed, he would cry for prolonged periods. Often, the parents gave in, letting him stay all night.

In psychotherapy, Gregory would present some problem, then be unable to elaborate. He insisted that his therapist identify as "bad" any person who angered him and that he directly answer such questions as, "When will so and so talk to me again?" or, "Will you call mother and tell her to change her mind?" It was very difficult for him to experience the treatment as useful unless the therapist could answer his questions. Efforts to clarify the situation or his feelings were usually felt as accusations. At times of such disruption, Gregory would erupt with violent fantasies and would feel disconnected. At other times, he would lapse into apathetic silence, rearrange his schedule, or lie to his mother so that he would miss appointments. At one point, he announced that he would not continue to come regularly and felt that the therapist had to accept his decision without question. He was astounded to be told that treatment was a mutual decision, that the therapist did not have to do whatever he proposed, and that treatment was important enough that it merited regular attendance.

In addition to individual psychotherapy, Gregory was seen weekly with his parents. The interactions followed a consistent, inflexible pattern. Gregory would have little to say, not wanting to talk about things that would start an argument. The mother would launch into a string of complaints to which Gregory would respond defensively. Each would accuse the other of distorting or lying. Mother would then point to

Gregory's defensiveness as a manifestation of his problems and as a justification for not wanting to be involved with him. Father would sit impassively while the argument ensued, then either attempt to placate Gregory with the promise of rewards for good behavior, lecture him on proper conduct, or berate his wife for creating the problems with Gregory in the first place. Mother would then complain about father's lack of support. All would eventually turn to the therapist for support in viewing the others as the culprits. None could see their own contribution to the disruption.

Reconstruction of aspects of Gregory's early experiences was not a focus of his psychotherapy. However, some statements about transference configurations and their meaning were possible. If Gregory perceived the therapist as irritated with him, this quickly recalled father's anger and touched his own fears of destructiveness. His image of father was of a potentially harmful, destructive man who must be placated or avoided so he would not become enraged and retaliate with abandonment, punishment, or lectures on moral conduct. The relationship with a distracted, disappointing, and inconsistent mother who could not tolerate strong expression of emotion or support Gregory's achievements was intensely reawakened when he experienced some need for the therapist. More generally, the quality of interaction with Gregory suggested that his manifest pleadings for concrete solutions, his provocative behavior, and even the transference configurations overlaid a sense of lack of connection associated with a conviction that any involvement was fruitless. When he made any move to reconsider this stance, the slightest perception that the therapist was unavailable to help alleviate fears and tensions was seen as an emergency and required active reassurance to quell the ensuing panic. Gregory seemed desperate for a calming relationship but was so mistrustful and expectant of disappointment that he could not contain his anxiety. In treatment, as he had been as a child, he was pseudo independent, attempting to hide his feelings and maintain self-control by minimizing the importance of his parents' or therapist's unavailability.

The Psychoanalytic Treatment of Mother

The patient, a thirty-five-year-old married woman of Greek ancestry, was a management consultant. At the time she began treatment, she felt she had not been promoted as rapidly as she should have been, as predicted by her earlier academic success, her charm, and her proven creative and intellectual capability. She thought she might be unwittingly "self-defeating." Even more troubling were daily fights with her husband, what she described as an "awful sex life," and increasingly distressful battles with her eleven-year-old son, Gregory. The patient felt "hopelessly trapped," in conflict between commitments to her demanding job and to her two children. She also had a six-year-old daughter and was obsessed with guilty worry because she preferred this cheerful, easy-going girl to the difficult Gregory. It quickly became clear that her favoritism toward her daughter duplicated her own mother's preference for her brother, who was three years younger than she. The patient felt that her own mother envied her since, during all her childhood, she had been criticized and scolded by mother for being vain, selfish, self-indulgent, and sinful in a Greek Orthodox religious sense. This situation "cast a black shadow over my growing up."

In the first year of analysis, the patient's appearance was that of an innocent, compliant flower child ground under the heel of a brutal husband. In her analytic hours, she usually appeared perplexed, flustered, or scatterbrained, an appearance that belied her tough competence in an important job. For instance, when entering the office from the waiting room, she would often stagger in with such an overflowing array of objects that several things would drop to the floor.

The patient had been her father's favorite, and he responded to such "sweet helplessness" with vigorous efforts to assist her. She was obviously healthier and brighter than her brother, and, because of this, her father admired and spoiled her while neglecting her sibling. The patient reported that her father teamed up with her against her mother in almost every family dispute. Typical of their relationship was an incident in which he had once provided her in advance with the answers to questions on a major school exam that he had obtained through a teacher friend. She recalled that she could have done well without his help but that she accepted such unusual assistance from him because of her insecurity about her mother's love, which caused her intense self-doubts about almost every area of performance.

In the second year of analysis, a transference incident manifested by fantasies that her analyst was corrupt and licentious led to the reproduction of the pregenital relationship to her mother. Unconsciously, she was sure she deserved a corrupt, sadistic analyst because she herself was a greedy, deformed, dishonest person, just as her mother had claimed. At this time, she also dreamed of herself as the Greek statue *Winged Victory,* but a version that had a large vertical black crack through it that threatened to demolish the whole torso. (As a child, she had been given a toy copy of this statue by her father.) While this image was related to sexual mutilation anxiety, it also represented the "damaged goods" self-view that early in treatment had been defended against by the presentation of the naive, squeaky-clean, little-girl image.

The patient remembered how often during her childhood her mother had considered her to be devious, evil, or devil possessed, a concern that reached its height in an accusation of incest during her early adolescence. Her mother's condemnatory attitudes toward both the patient's alliance with her father and her unsought superiority over her "fat, asexual" brother established or reinforced unconscious beliefs, first, that genital sensations and, later, heterosexual wishes were bad and destructive. Such concerns extended to other body parts and sensations. For example, mother would express her distress at the patient's touching her lip or the skin around her fingernails with the admonition, "You look just like an ugly, greedy monkey."

The patient had originally managed such maternal (and self-) negative views of bodily functions, sensations, and activities by open defiance, as was illustrated by a memory of masturbation in front of her mother to embarrass her. During latency, she had attempted a conscious disidentification with her mother: "I wouldn't let her get to me, or reveal I felt anything. . . . She would scream, cry, and threaten. I would get tough and stony faced."

Later, the analysis produced insights related to the patient's problems in caring for her son in the first years of his life. The patient was dominated by relentless self-criticism and self-debasement that indicated the extent to which she had internalized her mother's early life portrait of herself as a "bad seed." She compensated for feelings of inferiority by heavy investment in her work performance. At this time of the treatment, she found analytic silences almost intolerably painful. She often felt criticized during silences and would have an upsurge of hostility toward the analyst or toward her children. Her defensive posture was to attempt desperately to control the analyst's responses through the creation of arguments about appointment times, vacation schedules, and fee-payment procedures. Similarly, she had managed feelings of helplessness stimulated by her baby's needs by becoming ritualistic, demanding, and controlling. If the analyst did not respond quickly with verbal interventions other than an interpretation, she would speed up her associations and her verbalizations so that she would become slightly breathless, as if her inhalation were impeded. The symptom's origins were found to be related to an obsessive hyper-awareness of breathing and related to struggles over control during her second year of life, when, as her parents recalled, she often had tantrums and had transitorily become a breath holder. Gregory's mid-childhood and adolescent clinging and his forceful intrusion into all aspects of her life made her feel suffocated and helplessly "held down," making her want to escape.

These observations led to further analysis of the patient's defenses against her mother's intrusiveness and eventually to a better understanding of her contributions to the symptoms of her adolescent son. Her son's clinging and invasion of the patient's social activities, his ceaseless efforts to control all her actions, duplicated the reconstructed intrusive relationship that the analytic patient had had as a child with her own mother. Often, she felt forced to escape the child with the use of sweet helplessness, excessive compulsivity, emotional withdrawal, and denial of the pain of separation from emotionally important objects such as those represented by her analyst. The patient and the analyst could agree retrospectively that something similar had occurred during Gregory's first years. For prolonged time periods, she had retreated into her shell or escaped with eagerness to work-related activities in which her competence had nullified sharp feelings of guilt and inadequacy about her child-care functioning.

The Application of the Reconstructions from the Mother's Analysis to the Understanding of Pathogenesis in Gregory

The mother's experience of Gregory's infancy as reported in her analysis enriched the understanding of Gregory's early relationship with his mother. The final reconstruction of the childhood situation suggested that the birth of Gregory presented his mother with overwhelming burdens and demands that reawakened self-images of badness and threatened to recapitulate her own mother's invasions. The consequent psychic regression, potentiated by the normative regression of pregnancy, remobilized the wide array of Gregory's mother's psychic escape mechanisms that were explored and analyzed during psychoanalysis.

The mother had felt very ambivalent toward Gregory as a newborn, her hostility further intensified by a displacement to the baby of hostile feelings toward her withdrawn husband. Her anger had also been mobilized by concurrent feelings toward her own mother, who had visited her during the early weeks of the baby's life. The grandmother rejected her daughter's career aspirations and reinforced her shame over distressing feelings of inferiority by demonstrating how much better she was at infant rearing. As a result of all these converging factors, the patient shrank from tactile contact with Gregory, utilized rigid feeding and sleeping schedules, "refused to be manipulated by the baby," and followed the "tough care" methods of her own parents while wishing that the baby would rapidly grow into an independent child. By moving away affectively when her infant sought contact, the patient illustrated what empirical researchers have termed "anticontingent behaviors . . . contradictory to the intended goal of the infant's behaviors and signals as interpreted by the observer" (Greenspan and Lieberman 1980, p. 280).

At other times, the adult patient, identifying with the parenting devotion of her own father, would compensate for her times of inadequate provision of baby care by exaggerated expressions of love, slavish devotion, and unrealistic permissiveness, which was, however, a stance difficult to maintain. It was this emotional alternation that contributed later to Gregory's personality deficits and accounted for the habitual "avoidant" behavior of his early infancy. Later, however, this avoidance proved inadequate, and intense separation anxiety was prominent in his relationship with peers and teachers. Still later, in early adolescence and during psychotherapy, Gregory manifested a good deal of clinging behavior, fear of loss of love by his peers, hypersensitivity to rejection by his mother, and intense efforts to regain equilibrium through forcing reunions. These events of specific early maternal deprivation, based on both the developmental history and the mother's style of parenting as reconstructed during psychoanalysis, enabled us to reach a deeper understanding of Gregory's adolescent psychopathology and psychotherapy.

Evaluating the Findings of Infant Observation from the Perspective of Gregory's Infantile Experience

Data from Gregory's psychotherapy and developmental history and reconstructions derived from his mother's analysis all suggest that he had an "anxious avoidant attachment" relationship with his mother. The mother's description of the child's earliest reactions to separation is typical of infants in this category: "He didn't seem to mind at all, or show us any feelings." "There was no crying and he didn't notice I was going or gone." "When we came back he ignored me and didn't seem to hold a grudge."[5] Gregory's later school behavior is also characteristic of once-avoidant infants. In the classroom, these children have been described as being highly dependent, seeking attention in negative ways, showing poor peer relations, and having little sensitivity to other children. Sroufe (1983) wrote, "Whenever a child so infuriated a teacher that he or she wanted to isolate the child . . . it was inevitable that this child had a history of chronic parental unavailability or rejection and had been a Group A (anxious avoidant) infant" (p. 76).

Gregory's mother had worked full time at an outside job since the second month of her son's life, a social variable associated statistically with this kind of avoidant infant response to separation. However, review of the clinical material obtained from the treatments of Gregory and his mother suggested that the mother's response to separation from her infant might be a crucial contributing factor that would explain the increase of avoidant attachment in infants of working mothers. This hypothesis based on the reported treatments led the research team to administer a psychological test that had been designed specifically to measure the mother's separation anxiety on leaving her infant, defined as "an unpleasant emotional state reflecting a mother's apprehension about leaving her child" (Hock 1984, p. 40). This scale targets anxiety consciously related to leaving the baby to go to an outside job or transferring the infant to another caregiver. When administered to a population of about fifty women, working mothers of insecurely attached infants scored lower, $p < .05$ (i.e., experienced less conscious separation anxiety), than did working mothers of securely attached infants (Barglow et al., in press). In addition, the working mothers of babies that scored high on avoidance had demonstrated a higher incidence of depression and other dysphoric symptoms when they were interviewed for the first time during pregnancy. These two findings were consistent with the hypotheses originating in the study of Gregory and his mother. The mother's avoidance of Gregory was causally related to Gregory's avoidance of her. The infant Gregory's avoidance was related not only to the repeated daily fact of separation from the mother because of her work but also to the psychopathology of the mother, manifested by her need to flee the baby and the demands of the infant-mother relationship that she experienced as intrusive.

The insights from these dual clinical experiences made more comprehensible and meaningful the empirical generalizations derived from infant observation. The research finding that many infants of working mothers were securely attached, although significantly fewer than those of nonworking mothers, was more clearly appreciated. The psychoanalytic perspective had provided a direction for a fruitful search for factors aside from maternal work status that affected the quality of infant attachment.

Issues in the Use of Multiple Perspectives

In both the clinical and research settings, much is currently made of the relationship between caretakers' empathic availability, adjustment in infancy, and the presence of pathology in adolescence (see, e.g., Lichtenberg 1982; Wolf 1982). Our work examines this continuity from a number of perspectives and, in so doing, makes many assumptions, all of which are subject to scrutiny. The first is basic to psychoanalytic theory, namely, that one can reconstruct early problems with mother-infant relations through the psychoanalytic process and that these problems influence current behavior, that is, that there is continuity between early relationships and those formed later, not so much in manifest behavior as in the meaning of the new relationship or situation. We also make the assumption that reconstructions from the mother's analysis tell us something important about her son's early experiences, even in the absence of his confirmation. In addition, we assume that there is a relationship between events in the research setting and those in the consulting room that allows data from one area of observation to generate hypotheses and to validate data from the other. Clearly, we can only summarize some of the issues at hand.

As to the validity of psychoanalytic propositions, is it justified to apply knowledge gained through reconstructive efforts when that very knowledge is in question? Of course, much has been said on the topic of proof in psychoanalysis, while little has been resolved. In that regard, however, among many questions one could ask are, Did Gregory really display insecure avoidant behavior as a child? Can the mother's recollections be trusted on this point, or did she, by virtue of the very defenses reported, not attend to Gregory's actual behavior? Since Gregory's treatment did not involve the kind of helical process of deepening mutual conviction that results in even those reconstructions that might be accepted as valid by some (Basch 1983; Peterfreund 1983), can the speculations based on transference enactments and his current presentation be valued as useful in understanding his infantile experiences and their relation to his current behavior? Can we say that the mother's experience of Gregory's childhood experience is at all useful in this regard?

In essence, what one considers proof of psychoanalytic propositions depends on whether one requires going beyond psychoanalytic method to supply such proof. One is not likely to look beyond the consulting room if one's position is that the only truth analysts can seek is the development of a cohesive narrative (Ricoeur 1977). From this vantage point, the hypotheses about Gregory's infancy may not be particularly convincing. There was really no process wherein analyst and patient convincingly achieved a coherent story of the patient's psychic reality. Since the evidence for such a conviction is something only the patient could achieve (Peterfreund 1983), the mother's analysis and any research from other fields would be irrelevant. Also, if one believes that theories are not and should not be translatable (Goldberg 1986), efforts to find bridges to enrich knowledge are of little merit.

On the other hand, if one believes that it is the thematic affinity of data originating from clearly different spheres of observation that may constitute the best proof of the validity of psychoanalytic reconstruction (Edelson 1986) or that proof in psychoanalysis consists of "substantiations" from many related areas (Peterfreund 1983), then the fact that this work includes evidence from multiple perspectives that converge in similar findings supports the validity of the reconstruction of Gregory's early experience and the continuity of meaning between his current relationships and those he developed in the past.

Regarding the validity of the hypothesis that Gregory was an insecure infant, Barglow's research team found in the current study a high concordance between parental recollections of infants' home responses to separation and researchers' categorization in the laboratory test situation. While the maternal research sample was selected for "normality," many subjects who had insecurely attached offspring manifested psychopathology as severe as that of Gregory's mother. In a follow-up study, Barglow et al. (in press) found that a group of working mothers with insecurely attached infants had lower levels of separation anxiety when leaving their infants and more psychopathology than did mothers of securely attached infants. Gregory's mother experienced no discernible distress when she was away from the child. Descriptions of the typical psychological traits of mothers of avoidant infants by several empirical investigators again point strikingly to the personality of Gregory's mother. Main and Goldwyn (in press) found that an infant's avoidance in the reunion episodes of the Ainsworth Strange Situation correlates statistically with the mother's perceived rejection by her own mother. Avoidance by infants is also predictable from the mother's explicit dislike of physical contact as well as from maternal insensitivity to infant signals during the first three months of life (Ainsworth et al. 1978). Further, Main (Main and Stadtman 1981; Main, Tomasini, and Tolan 1979) found the mothers of avoidant infants to be generally low in emotional expressiveness.

Regarding the issue of continuity, adolescence has always been considered a time of major transformation, the vicissitudes of which are based on current challenges, earlier developmental mastery, and unresolved conflict. The factors in adolescent transformation have been of interest to classical theorists (Blos 1962), self psychologists, (Wolf, Gedo, and Terman 1972), and infant observers (Lichtenberg 1982) alike. However, although the tapestry of development becomes richer as new information is gathered regarding temperament, cognitive development, or the capacity for the use of new objects to modify the self developed in the first years of life, the threads of the fabric seem to remain discernible. For example, Sroufe (1983) demonstrated in preschool follow-up studies that early avoidant behavior by the infant is superseded by typical patterns of defiance, manipulation, rage episodes, and dependent clinging behavior, and Main, Kaplan, and Cassidy (1985) reported continuity of attachment relations done at twelve months and six years. From another perspective, Main et al. note that parents had enduring conceptualizations of their own early attachments that were correlated with their child's attachment classification. It would certainly be of interest in understanding adolescent behavior disorders and transference enactments such as we observed in Gregory if studies were done that demonstrated the continuity of attachment patterns from infancy to adolescence. Detailed reports such as ours can contribute useful information about the type of relationships and patterns of expectation seen in these adolescents that may lead to useful methods for studying attachment in this population.

Another issue deals with the confluence of theories of psychoanalysis and those of other fields. Kohut (1959) defined psychological data as those that are gathered through introspection and empathy. In contrast, data in research are usually thought of as obtained through the senses, as objective or empirical. This would suggest that the events under study are observed with very different instruments and, therefore, lead to theories that are hard to relate. On the other hand, if one's position is that all knowledge is gained through introspection and that the distinction between data derived from sensory and introspective input is spurious, then theories from research and from the psychoanalytic process are potentially integratable. This is related to the concept that all information is derived from a combination of observation and integration with prior expectation. A corollary concern is who is doing the observing. Grunbaum (Holzman 1985) would consider the fact that the analyst in this instance was also the principal researcher to be a fatal flaw because therapeutic intent contaminates observations and successful outcome of treatment cannot be used to validate psychoanalytic theory.

A further issue in integrating theories is the compatibility of the underlying assumptions. The assumptions underlying work with the Strange Situation are that attachment behavior relates to an enduring affective bond, that attachment behavior, promoted by the infant's capacity for signaling, is related to the function of inborn biological-motivational control systems and serves a primary function as opposed to operating as an avenue for drive reduction, and that individuals construct internal working models of self and attachment figures that guide interpretation and production of behavior (Joffe and Vaughn, in press; Main et al. 1985). In addition, the concept of internal working models takes into account the presence and consequences of unconscious motives that may be incompatible with conscious ones, that awareness of both models may be experienced as painful or disorganizing, that these models are affective/cognitive and are formed by action schema as well as symbolic representation, and that there may be multiple actively maintained models that are operant in different circumstances (Bretherton 1985; Main et al. 1985). In contrast to social learning theories that take the position that attachment is solely the interactions between infants and caregivers or that it can be defined as a series of discrete behaviors (Joffe and Vaughn, in press), the assumptions underlying developmental research with the Strange Situation are clearly related to such psychoanalytic principles as unconscious motivation, defense, and repetition and seem compatible with newer psychoanalytic theories of self and self-organization.[6]

Conclusions

Such epistemological and methodological questions certainly are often posed and continue to demand effort to resolve. As early as 1905, Freud wrote, "The direct observation of children has the disadvantage of working upon data which are easily misunderstandable; psychoanalysis is made difficult by the fact that it can only reach its data, as well as its conclusions, after long detours. But by cooperation, the two methods can attain a satisfactory degree of certainty in their findings" (p. 201). The preceding has presented an effort to attain such collaboration, an endeavor that seems useful both in the service of furthering psychoanalytic knowledge of the continuities and transformations in development and in the service of informing the study of issues that have broad social policy and clinical implications.

NOTES

1. This material presented here is part of a larger study led by Peter Barglow that examines in detail the reciprocal contributions of psychoanalysis and research to the validity of psychoanalytic reconstruction.

2. The sample was chosen to eliminate errors due to unusual sampling populations (middle-class, intact, physically healthy family), the possibility of poor infant care (care was by nonfamily member in home), and coding inconsistencies.

3. Gregory was in psychotherapy with C. J. at the same time as his mother was in analysis with P. B. Both analysts independently obtained and evaluated clinical data about Gregory, his mother, and their interaction before any discussion between analysts took place.

4. This sleep disturbance had precursors during the second year of Gregory's life. At both times, night distress seemed to be related to daytime absence of father, an association perhaps related to the phenomenon of father "hunger" described by Herzog (1980). Absence of the father to buffer aggressive impulses toward the mother during the regressive influence of sleep could have produced a traumatic hostile attack of the child's self, which was particularly vulnerable because of the developmental changes of early adolescence.

5. It is always possible, of course, that the mother's recollections of her son during her analysis were not entirely accurate. Did Gregory really not protest at all his parents' leaving, or did they simply refuse to recognize it or now not remember it?

6. Stern (1985, p. 25) notes that "attachment is a set of infant behaviors, a motivational system, a relationship between mother and infant, and a life-span subjective experience for the infant in the form of 'working models.' " This last he considers close to the selfobject concept and to his ideas about the infant's subjective experience. However, he differentiates the working model concept from representations of interactions that have been generalized (RIGs) in a number of ways (pp. 114–115). (1) An RIG relates to a specific type of interaction, while a working model represents a repertoire of interactions that changes as new RIGs are included or deleted. (2) Working models have emphasized expectations concerning felt security, while RIGs include expectations of a variety of interactions, among which are arousal, affect, mastery, and curiosity. (3) Working models have been conceived mainly in cognitive terms and remain experientially remote, while RIGs relate more closely to affective experience that does not undergo cognitive transformation to act to appraise or guide change from average expectation.

REFERENCES

Ainsworth, M.; Blehar, M.; Waters, E.; and Wall, S. 1978. *Patterns of Attachment: A Psychological Study of the Strange Situation*. Hillsdale, N.J.: Erlbaum.

Barglow, P.; Vaughn, B.; and Molitor, N. In press. Effects of maternal absence due to employment on the quality of infant-mother attachment in a low-risk sample. *Child Development*.

Basch, M. F. 1983. Empathic understanding: a review of the concept and some theoretical considerations. *Journal of the American Psychoanalytic Association* 31(1): 101–126.

Blos, P. 1962. *On Adolescence*. Glencoe, Ill.: Free Press.

Bowlby, J. 1969. *Attachment*. Vol. 1 of *Attachment and Loss*. New York: Basic.

Bretherton, I. 1985. Attachment theory: retrospect and prospect. In I. Bretherton and E. Waters, eds. *Growing Points of Attachment Theory and Research*. Monographs of the Society for Research in Child Development, vol. 50, serial no. 209. Chicago: University of Chicago Press.

Carey, W., and McDevitt, S. 1978. Revision of infant temperament questionnaire. *Pediatrics* 61:735–739.

Edelson, M. 1986. Psychoanalytic dialogue: Freud as scientist in the Rat-man and Wolf-man cases: a controversy about the scientific value of clinical data and the case study method of psychoanalysis. Paper presented at the fall meeting of the American Psychoanalytic Association, New York, December 20, 1986.

Emde, R. 1981. Changing models of infancy and the nature of early development: remodeling the foundation. *Journal of the American Psychoanalytic Association* 291:178–220.

Emde, R. 1985. From adolescence to midlife: remodeling the structure of adult development. *Journal of the American Psychoanalytic Association* 33(suppl.): 59–112.

Farber, E., and Egeland, B. 1982. Developmental consequences of out-of-home care for infants in a low income population. In E. Zigler and E. Gordon, eds. *Day Care*. Boston: Aurburn.

Freud, S. 1905. Three essays on the theory of sexuality. *Standard Edition* 7:135–245. London: Hogarth, 1975.

Goldberg, A. 1986. Translation between psychoanalytic theories. *Annual of Psychoanalysis* 12/13:121–135.

Greenspan, S., and Leiberman, H. 1980. Infants, mothers, and their interaction: a quantitative clinical approach to developmental assessment. In S. Greenspan and G. Pollock, eds. *The Course of Life: Contributions toward Understanding Personality Development*, vol. 1, *Infancy and Early Childhood*. Department of Health and Human

Services publication no. ADM. Palo Alto, Calif.: Consulting Psychologists Press.

Herzog, J. 1980. Sleep disturbance and father hunger in 18–20 month old boys: the Erlkonig syndrome. *Psychoanalytic Study of the Child* 35:219–236.

Hock, E. 1984. Working and non-working mothers with infants: perceptions of their careers, their infants' needs and satisfaction with mothering. *Developmental Psychology* 14:37–43.

Holzman, P. 1985. Psychoanalysis: is the therapy destroying the science? *Journal of the American Psychoanalytic Association* 33:725–770.

Ireton, H., and Thwing, E. 1972. The MCDI in the psychiatric-developmental evaluation of the preschool child. *Child Psychiatry and Human Development* 3:102–114.

Joffe, L., and Vaughn, B. In press. Infant-mother attachment: theory, assessment, and implications for development. In Wolman, ed. *Handbook of Developmental Psychology*. New York: Prentice-Hall.

Joffe, L.; Vaughn, B.; Barglow, P.; and Benveniste, R. 1985. Biobehavioral antecedents in the development of infant-mother attachment. In M. Reite and T. Field, eds. *Psychobiology of Infant Attachment*. Orlando, Fla.: Academic.

Kohut, H. 1959. Introspection, empathy, and psychoanalysis. *Journal of the American Psychoanalytic Association* 7:459–483.

Kohut, H. 1971. *The Analysis of the Self*. New York: International Universities Press.

Kohut, H. 1977. *The Restoration of the Self*. New York: International Universities Press.

Lichtenberg, J. 1982. Continuities and transformations between infancy and adolescence. *Adolescent Psychiatry* 10:182–198.

Lichtenberg, J. 1983. *Psychoanalysis and Infant Research*. Hillsdale, N.J.: Analytic.

Main, M., and Goldwyn, R. In press. Predicting rejection of her infant from mother's representation of her own experience. *International Journal of Child Abuse and Neglect*.

Main, M.; Kaplan, N.; and Cassidy, J. 1985. Security in infancy, childhood, and adulthood: a move to the level of representation. In I. Bretherton and E. Waters, eds. *Growing Points of Attachment Theory and Research*. Monographs of the Society for Research in Child

Development, vol. 50, serial no. 209. Chicago: University of Chicago Press.

Main, M., and Stadtman, J. 1981. Infant response to rejection of physical contact by the mother. *Journal of the American Academy of Child Psychiatry* 20:292–307.

Main, M.; Tomasini, L.; and Tolan, W. 1979. Differences among mothers of infants judged to differ in security. *Developmental Psychology* 15:472–473.

Main, M., and Weston, D. 1982. Avoidance of the attachment figure in infancy: descriptions and interpretations. In C. Parkes and J. Stevenson-Hinde, eds. *The Place of Attachment in Human Behavior.* New York: Basic.

Peterfreund, E. 1983. *The Process of Psychoanalytic Psychotherapy: Models and Strategies.* Hillsdale, N.J.: Analytic.

Ricoeur, P. 1977. The question of proof in Freud's psychoanalytic writings. *Journal of the American Psychoanalytic Association* 25:835–871.

Sroufe, L. 1983. Infant-caregiver attachment and patterns of adaptation in preschool: the roots of maladaptation and competence. In M. Perlmutter, ed. *Minnesota Symposium on Child Psychology,* vol. 16. Hillsdale, N.J.: Erlbaum.

Stern, D. 1985. *The Interpersonal World of the Infant.* New York: Basic.

Vaughn, B.; Deane, K.; and Waters, E. 1985. The impact of out-of-home care on child-mother attachment quality: another look at some enduring questions. In I. Bretherton and E. Waters, eds. *Growing Points of Attachment Theory and Research.* Monographs of the Society for Research in Child Development, vol. 50, serial no. 209. Chicago: University of Chicago Press.

Wolf, E. 1982. Adolescence: psychology of the self and self-objects. *Adolescent Psychiatry* 10:171–181.

Wolf, E.; Gedo, J.; and Terman, D. 1972. On the adolescent process as a transformation of the self. *Journal of Youth and Adolescence* 13:257–272.

24 THE EMERGENCE OF
THE ADOLESCENT PATIENT

VIVIAN M. RAKOFF

My grandmother—and probably your great-grandmothers—was married at sixteen. She was not delinquent or promiscuous (although the
retroactive virginalization of the old and deceased seems to be an
atavistic and normative mechanism of idealization). She was in fact my
grandfather's second wife, and she took her place after the death of
his first wife, her older sister, during childbirth, an ancient and accepted
arrangement about which I never heard a single word of complaint,
either directly or indirectly. She assumed the responsibility for her
sister's surviving daughter and immediately started to bear her own
family. She had her own son before my grandfather left for South Africa.
He worked there for ten years before sending for her to join him—and,
when she finally did, she immediately became pregnant and had, as
fast as is humanly possible, another three sons. My grandfather was
probably eighteen when he first got married. Altogether he fathered
six children.

All this happened at the turn of the century. It is not a particularly
remarkable story; it can be reduplicated thousands of times. Nor was
it true only of poor Eastern European Jews. Young lords and ladies
were locked into marriage and childbearing at about the same age, and
also peasants and workers in Europe were fixed in their niches—economic, geographic, and marital—very early in life. Where, one asks,
were their opportunities for "authenticity," the temptations into "identity diffusion," the experimental role playing, and explorations of the
adolescent "moratorium"?

Compared with many of her contemporaries, my timid grandmother
was a great adventurer. She left her hometown village and voyaged

with two children to the end of the earth. Although context clung to her like the clods of earth adhering to the roots of a fallen tree, and although she may not have known anything about the revolutionary process responsible for her voyaging, she was, in her modest way, one of the makers of a new way of realizing life's possibilities. But did she or thousands like her have, in our terms, an "adolescence"?

To ask the question—let me say right off—is not to invalidate the concepts. After all, the playfulness of a relatively unencumbered "good enough" childhood and the normative dependence and modestly expressed sexuality are real, even though for much of mankind child labor, begging, sheepherding, gooseherding, mine working, chimney sweeping, silk cocoon unraveling, lace making, domestic labor, newspaper vending, and so on might have seemed so appallingly common— so almost universal—that the whole notion of a psychology of a dependent, nurtured childhood could be questioned, radically questioned and discussed either as a bourgeois luxury or as an interesting but isolated anthropological curiosity. Even babyhood and infancy are not inescapably given; the psychological, sociological, and biological components are variously expressed (Aries 1962).

But we know, sociology, anthropology, and economics aside, that the epigenetic unfolding of infancy, childhood, puberty-adolescence, and adulthood as purely biological phenomena is universal. Babies are small and vulnerable, their survival predicated on an ethological choreography of signals sent back and forth between parent (mother) and babe, a hard-wired near reflex pattern of interchange that allows a noisy, dirty, almost parasitic stranger, a consumer of time, energy, sleep, and economic resources, to be perceived as valuable, delightful, cute, and a source of joy. That is a baby! The child is obviously malleable and growing, not yet wise enough or strong enough for true independence, capable of being helpful or exploitable, but not full grown mentally, physically, or sexually. And it is clear that childhood comes to an end with puberty. The endocrine storm works its well-known transformational magic, and out of a process that metaphorically recapitulates labor, or from another point of view adumbrates the legend of a phoenix, the child gives birth to a new changed but continuing self—the adolescent, the hairy, sexually fired, intellectually adept adolescent, the focus of our preoccupations.

Something, however, sets the adolescent phase, stage, or condition apart from the preceding stages: infancy manifestly comes to an end with weaning, walking, and speech; childhood ends with puberty; adolescence begins with puberty; but where does it end? The other stages have an inescapable biological framework, a strong physical cage that contains all the varieties of anthropological and economic circumstance, which will affect both somatic and psychological characteristics. Poor nutrition, lack of opportunity, and disaster may all affect the potential capacities of infant and child, but they will remain, however distorted, recognizably as being within a particular life state.

The adolescent phase is curiously indeterminate in its later boundary. Indeed, the entity itself has been recognized or labeled as a discrete life stage only very recently. Aries places its specific recognition at the end of the nineteenth century, and, while Freud's collected works have more than 150 references to puberty in the cumulative index, there are only six—perhaps seven—to adolescence. Certainly, in his consideration of puberty in the "Three Essays on the Theory of Sexuality" (Freud 1905), he addresses the specific task of achieving a mature sexual identity—something most of us would consider an essential characteristic of what we call adolescence. But he does so in the context of biological puberty, and he does not label it adolescence. He was writing, if I may remind you, not far from the place where my grandmother had waited to be sent for from South Africa and only two years after she had rejoined her husband (after a wait about as long as Ulysses' odyssey). He also wrote in a Vienna where the crown prince had had his fatal love affair with Marie Vestsera, a seventeen-year-old aristocrat. She was barely older than the often-cited fourteen-year-old Juliet, but she was "in society," ready for a relationship full of secrecy and disastrous potential. And she did not sneak out of a top window on a ladder; she was jeweled and gowned and pushed into the matchmaking whirl of balls and parties where sexual intrigue and courtship were an accepted and, in fact, central purpose. She was—this tragic kid caught in a tragedy—young, youthful, a *"suesses maedel"* (Salvendy 1988), but not in her society's terms what we call adolescent.

Thus, when Anna Freud (1958) suggests that the interest and discovery of adolescence is attributable to psychoanalysis, she is only partially correct. It is associated with the development of psychoanalysis, and both psychoanalysis and, I suggest, adolescence are products of a particular phase of historical development—a theme to which I will return. The first major work specifically devoted to the "adolescent" is Hall's (1904) two-volume *Adolescence*. Freud's three essays were published in 1905, and it was not until the 1920s that Jones (1922) produced his single essay, "Some Problems of Adolescence," and Bernfeld (1923) published his important work on troubled young people. From then on, there was an accumulating body of papers that have become the classical milestones of psychodynamic theory in this area: Anna Freud's (1936) postulation of turmoil; Blos's (1967) elaborate exegesis of the attainment of sexual and social adulthood; and Erikson's (1964) magisterial formulation of the tasks of adolescence. Together these and many others defined an entity that we now all recognize—the adolescent of the twentieth century. Not that it is true only of the twentieth century. There are earlier adumbrations in the almost clichéd notions of youth with its associations of love, adventure, recklessness, energy, beauty, lack of foresight, and excess of emotion. But none of this approaches the definition of adolescence as a discrete life phase that has emerged during the past fifty or sixty years (Rakoff 1980).

While psychoanalysis and psychiatry were becoming aware of youth and adolescence, other nonpsychological (if there are such things) currents in society were giving increasing support to the idea that human beings at various life stages required support and recognition. Babies, as I have said, are obviously babies, but, as Aries (1962) has documented, children were not always obviously children. They required free public schooling, child labor laws, and public free hospitals to emerge from their role as miniadults, often rachitic, undersized, doomed to forced labor and an early death. Adulthood, if adulthood means responsibility and a fixed point of social status, earnings, and an end to experimentation and mobility, started frighteningly early—by our standards—for most of mankind. If little children—again by our standards—were dressed and treated like adults with the full expectation of assuming moral responsibility for their actions and a more or less major degree of responsibility for their economic lives, how much more so were the postpubescent youths who would now be called adolescent.

There is a poignant picture in Richard Hoggart's (1957) "The Use of Literacy" in which a group of working-class British teenagers are dressed much as their fathers were. They were doing as workers what they expected to be doing for the rest of their lives, and their income would hardly increase. Barely beyond their first growth of body hair, they were fixed in their adult identity for life. I have referred to this picture in the past, but I failed to make the observation that, if they were made old before their time, their fathers, by the same historical

375

token, were stultified in their mature years. Deprived of what we would consider a full adolescence, they were also deprived of their full range of adult capacities: locked into dead-end unfulfilling jobs, without many options, barely literate or illiterate, their life situation was not something to which youngsters could ambitiously aspire—because in most significant ways the young men had, only too quickly, become their fathers. There was very little intermediate phase between childhood and adulthood—one fell into adulthood.

It is very difficult for those of us brought up in even modestly prosperous circumstances in cities to appreciate the full degree of constriction of working-class lives as recently as fifty or sixty years ago here in North America. (I am fully aware that there are groups even today who probably suffer in similar ways.) On a personal note, it became vividly clear to me when I once had the privilege of appearing on a panel with Buckminster Fuller. After the meeting, we found ourselves housed side by side in guest apartments in the university. As many of you know, he was a marvelously talkative man, endlessly anecdotal and reflective. He had the interesting characteristic that as he told one a story he also speculated about the general implications of what he was talking about. He eventually told me about his troubles as a late adolescent. He had got into trouble at Harvard, had a bad emotional experience, and squandered a lot of money. He ran away from Boston and worked for a while in a factory in Sherbrooke, Quebec. I will quote what he had to say: "I never swear, and I made a decision with myself never to swear because when I was working in the factory with grown men, big men with beards and wives and children, I realized that they knew nothing. They could not read, they could not write, and their talk was nothing but swear words. They were not stupid men; I think a lot of them were a lot smarter than I was. But their lives were as small as a walnut. Anybody who thinks that it was so grand back then should know that for most people, life was horrible and without any kind of vision, except, I suppose, they went to church on Sundays."

I am perhaps overstating matters: boys did run away from home to go to sea, to join the army, to become horribly vagrant, or they were contracted into apprenticeship. But the greater number stayed where they were and did what their fathers before them did. Their period of transition was marked in many societies by initiation rites: the circumcision rituals of Africa and other simple societies and the similar rituals for young girls were more or less associated with the menarche. Even these brief rites de passage were often lost in the great move from countryside to city that accompanied the Industrial Revolution and the alteration of social structure and social expectation, which was heralded by the American and French revolutions.

Of course, there was always a small group of young people who did have some leisure, some years of relative freedom from intense economic pressure, some time for experimentation. These were the cadets referred to by Aries or students or young aristocrats allowed a year or two for travel and "sowing wild oats." Yet, for all the appearance of freedom, they too had to settle for a relatively restricted range of adult responsibilities determined by hereditary class and fortune. However, compared with the great majority of mankind and indeed the women of their own class, they had many degrees of choice. They could mould their destinies through talent and character.

The literature of any society is a fair reflection of both "what is" and what society thinks "should be." Until the nineteenth century, there are few serious characters in the drama who were not gentry of one degree or the other. Dr. Johnson remarked that tragedies happen to a "very fine fellow." Let us consider tragedy: in its most classical sense, a tragedy happened to a fundamentally virtuous man betrayed by a characterological flaw in a crisis. The essence of the tragedy is the play of character in action, not economic opportunity or mere circumstance. It implied the choice—as I have just previously noted—available to the socially privileged, notions of personality as an attribute fundamentally affecting the outcome of one's life. The sufferings of the humble by contrast were not tragic but "comic," which is to say "not real." In classical times, the comedy at the end of the tragic trilogy was a "satyr play" acted in grotesque masks and huge swollen phalli. The characters were often ordinary people caught in the silly plots of mistaken identity, twins substituted for one another, the stuff of farce through Roman times until today. Ordinary people, although obviously human, did not have the density of personality or effectiveness in the world of the aristocrats. In that sense, they were deprived of "the right to tragedy" (Rakoff 1970).

In the nineteenth-century novel, the literary form of capitalism reflected a different social perception. Merchants, small landowners, orphans, and laborers were given the right to character previously granted to "my lord." While the church had always believed in the democratic distribution of souls and physicians plied their craft in the democracy

377

of anatomy, the nineteenth century saw the democratization of choice and the right of character to influence major life events.

The forces that brought about these changes were fundamentally political, and they represented a transfer of concerns for every individual from the domain of theology—the church—to the social and political. Being true to oneself, as Polonius sententiously instructed Hamlet, became a democratic virtue. Obedience to the law, to the ethical commands of the church, to the king, duke, landowner, or—wait for it—one's parents or fashion were no longer as pressing or good as they had been up to the end of the eighteenth century. "Sincerity" became a new kind of virtue (Trilling 1972).

Am I being excessive if I suggest that the central task of the Eriksonian adolescent—the establishment of a secure identity—is first sketched out—as Trilling suggests—in Diderot's *Rameau's Nephew,* in which the demands of the court are placed against the inner needs and feelings of a young man? By the end of the nineteenth century, the vocabulary of Erikson's description of the adolescent had been developed along both its positive and its negative axes: "alienation" and "anomie," the economic and social components of disconnectedness and meaninglessness underlying identity diffusion, were the negative pole, while "authenticity" and adventurousness, choices made in good faith, were at the positive pole.

But before Erikson, Anna Freud, and Blos, Freud had constructed his model of psychological man. While Freud's particular understanding of the psyche was a unique achievement, he was very much a product of his time and the inheritor of intellectual structures that had been developed—one could almost say matured—during the preceding century. As a rough starting point, the dialectic "invented" by Hegel suffused subsequent European thought in one form or the other. The dialectic was itself a product and reflection of the sociopolitical forces that had erupted in the French and American revolutions. Stable, eternal, secure fixity had been lost, and in its place was constant struggle between opposing forces that were, however, contrasting aspects of a containing unity: thesis, antithesis, synthesis. The map of history and economics, throughout the nineteenth century, became the map of psychological man, transformed by Freud into the knot of id, ego, and superego. It was as though the challenge to fixed and eternal verities, the sociopolitical emphasis on individual rights and individual struggles, the bourgeois assertion of the single person's entrepreneurial right and capacity, were all reflected in a shift of the locus of psychological concerns from the "objectively moral" to the subjective. Subjectivity became something of a philosophical cause. I have already alluded to Marx's "alienation," Kierkegaard's "authenticity," Nietzche's call to move beyond "good and evil" to a self-defined life's journey, and, as a warning bell, Durkheim's "anomie."

The rights and dangers were becoming clearer, and knowing oneself was translated from the cool, rational Socratic task to the complex arational exploration of the subjective. It will by now be apparent to you where this too quick and simple argument is leading: let me try to make it explicit. A vision of human life and opportunity had been hammered out by a wide range of thinkers of whom Freud was the conduit to the medicopsychological. As Rieff (1959) suggested, Freud transformed questions of moral-ethical struggle into medical problems to be examined dispassionately and correctly in a context of the therapeutic with the hope of cure at the end. The process also defined the patient in terms of a cultural hero of our time—a subjectively guided explorer of life's opportunities, intent on discovering the true self, rejecting of history.

If not a new human type, then a new emphasis on some perennial human capacities had been fashioned. And the notion of self-determination, allied with economic opportunity and a distrust of received historical forms, accompanied the emergence and definition of adolescence as an epoch of development. The striking thing is that the adolescent, as we have come to describe him, is not simply a young adult or an older child but perhaps more than any other patient group conforms to the model of the culture hero of our time: idealistic, authentic, adventurous, choosing among many alternatives, a model for all the adult life stages.

Within the larger category of the adolescent patient, it may be useful to make some distinctions between three categories of concern: the ailments and adjustments surrounding the pubertal phase, the disorders of young adulthood, and the problems of historically fostered adolescence. The distinctions may be arbitrary or inconclusive, but the immediate self-discovery of physical and intellectual powers and the realization of sexual and emotional characteristics following the transitions of puberty are perennial and historic, affecting all humankind and all social classes. These things did not happen because of the rise of entrepreneurial capitalism, the American and French revolutions, the migration from country to city, the growth of prosperity, and the extension of middle-class options and choices in the twentieth century. They were, are, and will be normative components of development.

The disorders of young adulthood for psychiatry are the onset of the major psychoses during the teen years and the early twenties. Schizophrenia, alas, has appalling uniformity in its time of onset and its epidemiology across cultures (with minor arguable variations). It appears to be true that characterological disorders or turbulence postulated by Anna Freud as stage specific in adolescence are, according to the studies of Offer (1975) and Masterson (1967), not phase specific. They are—it seems—the warnings of life-long problems or at least long-lasting problems. The turbulence of the adolescent years appears to be in many instances simply the entry to adult turbulence. However, there do appear to be syndromes generated by the epoch-dependent or historically determined adolescence about which we have been speaking: most notably the increase in suicide and depression during the years fifteen to twenty-five, anorexia nervosa, substance and drug abuse, and subtle forms of religious malaise and anomic rootlessness. The list is not exhaustive but will serve to focus discussion. I am not here proposing to replace the useful and well-established categories of early adolescence, mid-adolescence, and late adolescence. Nor am I discounting the flowering of talents, intellectual capacities, and sometimes pathology in the adolescent period. Rather, I am proposing that there is a particular aspect of the entire period that is characterized by dilemmas and opportunities of choice and the expression of individual personality. It is this era-dependent or historically permitted adolescence that may indeed, as I am about to suggest, extend far beyond the period we normally designate as adolescence.

Adolescent suicide as a major public health problem is not a perennial phenomenon. There are, however, anecdotal reports of waves of suicide, but these are unconfirmed and expressed romantic yearning and weltschmerz carried to an extreme. However, Klerman (1988) writes, "For each successive birth cohort in the 20th century there are increasing cumulative rates of illness and particular earlier age of onset rates for females higher than males. . . . Cohorts born after 1936 who reached adulthood after World War II have early age of onset (of melancholy) and higher rates of depression than the cohort born earlier in the century" (pp. 8–9).

In every birth cohort the rates are higher in women than in men. Klerman is concerned with the influence of a given "period" on the epidemiology of melancholy and its expression in suicide and depression. He is in this study particularly involved with the baby boom generation and afterward—the group who generated the chilling statistic: suicide as the second highest cause of death in the "later adolescent period." He asks a question that he does not attempt to answer. What is the mysterious pathogenic factor—the agent blue—in this period that generates increased melancholia?

The suicide rate among young Canadian Indians and Innuit has become a topic of national concern. Malcolmson (personal communication, 1988) reports that at least one-third of the teenagers in a particular settlement had attempted or completed suicide during the past four years. When asked if they knew the cause of these suicides, the other youngsters invariably used the same words: those who killed themselves were "bored."

The populations considered by Klerman and those described by Malcolmson are very different. Klerman's youths (like those in most studies of adolescent suicide) were principally urban, from the most developed and prosperous countries in the world, whereas the Innuit youths are little different from the inhabitants of the oasis described by Haliburton (1933). Is there indeed a common pathognomic factor?

Perhaps Durkheim (1950, p. 252) still holds the key to the pathogenic "factor blue." As he considered the apparent increase in suicide in Europe toward the end of the nineteenth century, he wrote,

When society is disturbed by some painful crisis or by beneficient but abrupt transitions, it is momentarily incapable of exercising this influence; thence come the sudden rises in the curve of suicides. But the man who has always pinned all his hopes on the future and lived with his eyes fixed upon it has nothing in the past as a comfort against the present affliction. For the past was nothing to him but a series of hastily experienced states. What blinded him to himself was his expectation always to find further on the happiness he had so far missed. Now he is stopped in his tracks; from now on nothing remains behind or ahead of him to fix his gaze upon. Weariness alone, moreover, is enough to bring disillusionment, for he cannot in the end escape the futility of an endless pursuit.

Adolescent suicide, however, is not simply a stage-specific phenomenon. It reflects as do other characteristics of adolescence the almost prototypical reflection of general social phenomena. The rate of adolescent suicide has increased as suicide in general has increased. Although adolescent suicide rates have increased more than the rate for the general population has (Sakinofsky and Roberts 1987), there are other significant variations; for example, while male suicide rates have increased steadily from 1944, female suicide has remained fairly steady for the past fifteen years. But, in most of the statistics-keeping world, the suicide rate has shown a steady increase—except in Japan, where rates are declining (Kato 1969).

Like suicide, anorexia nervosa/bulimia has shown a similar rate of increase in the Western world. Jones, Fox, Babigan, and Hutton (1980) reported that the incidence of anorexia doubled in the period 1970– 1976 compared with the period 1960–1969, and the condition has always been associated with economic prosperity (although the class showing tends not to affect male patients). For the purposes of our discussion, it is important to note Garfinkel and Garner's (1982) observation that the condition appears to be spreading to lower economic levels. Anorexia nervosa is not a new disorder. Its classical description as a clinical entity goes back to Gull and Laseque in the 1870s, and there are obscure earlier reports, but it too has become democratized in the past few decades.

Does the "agent blue" responsible for the increase in suicides also generate the increase in cases of anorexia/bulimia? Garner, Garfinkel, Schwartz, and Thompson (1980) have charted the profound effect of fashion on the growth of anorexia nervosa/bulimia. But fashion as "agent blue" begs the question. What does fashion reflect? From where does a fashion derive that women should look like men or that "thinness" is almost a moral condition? Fat is not only ugly and nonsexy; it is a moral lapse. Yet it is intensely demonstrative and is not secret and intimate. It is a signal to the field that, in addition to any other messages, also conveys, See how I can control myself (and you). In short, it is contextual and manifests a considerable degree of field dependency, a conformity to some ideal perceived by the patient as necessary for self-acceptance and acceptance (Rakoff 1983).

An audience of adolescent psychiatrists does not need a reminder of the peculiarly adolescent phenomena of cult seeking and religious preoccupation, the various fluctuations but the persistence of substance abuse, or the horrifying fact that automobile accidents are the major cause of death in the age group. Taking the family car on a seemingly empty highway and guiding it like a rocket in an ecstasy of self-determination—the goal is not a place but a state, a state of being powerful, and in some celebratory way anomic.

Bernfeld (1923) commented on the "protracted adolescence for males going on for longer than even we allow for adolescence" and emphasized the positive components of the phenomenon: "tendency toward productivity whether artistic, literary, or scientific and by a strong bent toward idealistic aims and spiritual values." The argument I have been developing takes this notion several stages further; adolescence, in addition to being a life stage bracketed between puberty and adulthood, is also a set of characteristic social expectations and opportunities that may extend throughout much of the life cycle. When the circumstances permit, adolescent behavior reappears not so much as a regression but as the mobilization of a constant potentiality. The openness of choice and self-determination may present in mature individuals with the same or similar enthusiasm or difficulty as it does for youths or young adults. In its positive aspects, it promotes the capacity for adventure, risk taking, creative change, enthusiasm, idealism, and healthy skepticism. The negative is the fostering of anomie, alienation, and despair with the accompanying phenomena so frequently noted of suicide, alcoholism, increased accident rate, divorce increase, and so on and at a less serious level the so-called mid-life crisis, which rarely affects the unsuccessful or those people whose jobs are closely tied to the simple business of earning a living.

The adolescent, while being a young adult, is also the essential embodiment of the social opportunities and dilemmas developed during the past two centuries, reaching an accelerated crescendo during the past fifty years—opportunities in the ideal—available to people of every age. The increase in suicide in adolescence accompanies a general increase in suicide rates that probably reflects the anomic forces in society to which the adolescent like the older lonely male is especially vulnerable. The components of anomie—detachment, mobility (paradoxically), the drive to the future, and the discontent with the present—which affect the whole of Western society, particularly affect the adolescent. Marriage is delayed; career choice is fostered; mobility is an ever present possibility. The question can be asked, How does this describe the Innuit, the native Indian youth, the young ghetto blacks who also kill themselves more frequently than previously? Opportunity for them is severely limited. But they are embedded in a societal context that pours in on them, invalidating their actuality with television and movie visions of tormenting and sometimes spurious models of possibility. As Durkheim (1950) wrote, "With increased prosperity desires increased. At the very moment when traditional rules have lost their authority, the richer prize offered these appetites stimulates them and makes them more exigent and impatient of control. The state of deregulation or anomie is thus further heightened by passions being less disciplined precisely when they need more disciplining" (p. 253). He emphasized the danger of expectation without fulfillment. There are some expectations that cannot be fulfilled: perfect authenticity, total satisfaction with one's place in the world, being virtuous enough, for some being rich enough, beautiful enough, or tragically—frivolous though it may sound—thin enough. When these tormenting expectations are experienced without a sustaining set of guiding values, the groundwork of many different kinds of trouble is laid down.

Conclusions

Perhaps a blanket term can cover—to some degree—these problems: disorders of aspiration. The label cannot capture all the nuances or psychodynamics of identity diffusion, adolescent suicide, drug and substance abuse, anorexia nervosa, traffic accidents involving young people, or devotion to cults; but it relates to a crucial component of all these. Durkheim described the dissatisfaction with the given, the daily, as a factor in anomic suicide. It affects, I suggest, all those who yearn painfully for "the orgiastic future" or whose actual circumstances have been depleted of local myth and history to be replaced by a cargo cult of distant riches. It is also clearly a component of anorexia nervosa: young women with enough money but little power exert their will on what is closest to them, and they sculpt their bodies into existential art. They rarely know what motivates their "relentless pursuit of thinness," but the percolated-down fashion with its signals of lightness, fleetness, control, and peculiar asexual sexuality gets through to them. At its most subtle, the disorder of aspiration affects many lives with a sense of inadequate achievement. It shows itself in constant self-doubt, erratic behavior, restless yearning, and searching.

The great currents of history and social change do express themselves in individual opportunity and individual pain. Opportunity as we all know is both a privilege and a threat. When the opportunity is coupled with the ethos of achievement, an intense concern with individuality, and what Durkheim called "the morbid desire for the infinite," fragile, self-doubting, deprived, or in other ways vulnerable individuals, left to their own resources, feel themselves unequal to the opportunity and unable to cope. That inability may be reflected in a variety of clinical syndromes, only a few of which have been addressed in this chapter.

REFERENCES

Aries, P. 1962. *Centuries of Childhood.* London: Cape.
Bernfeld, S. S. 1923. Über eine typische Form der männlichen Puber-tät. *Imago* 9:169–188.
Blos, P. 1967. The second individuation process of adolescence. *Psychoanalytic Study of the Child* 22:162–186.
Durkheim, E. 1950. *Suicide: A Study in Sociology.* New York: Free Press.
Erikson, E. 1964. *Childhood and Society.* New York: Norton.
Freud, A. 1936. *The Ego and Mechanisms of Defense.* New York: International Universities Press, 1966.
Freud, A. 1958. Adolescence. *Psychoanalytic Study of the Child* 13:255–278.
Freud, S. 1905. Three essays on the theory of sexuality. *Standard Edition* 7:125–230. London: Hogarth, 1953.
Garfinkel, P. E., and Garner, D. M. 1982. *Anorexia Nervosa: A Multidimensional Perspective.* New York: Brunner/Mazel.
Garner, D. M.; Garfinkel, P. E.; Schwartz, D.; and Thompson, M. 1980. Cultural expectations of thinness in women. *Psychology Reports* 47:483–491.
Haliburton, R. 1933. *The Flying Carpet.* London: Blis.
Hall, G. S. 1904. *Adolescence.* New York: Appleton.
Hoggart, R. 1957. *The Uses of Literacy.* London: Chatto & Windus.
Jones, D. J.; Fox, M. M.; Babigan, H. M.; and Hutton, H. E. 1980. Epidemiology of anorexia nervosa in Monroe County, New York: 1960–1976. *Psychosomatic Medicine* 42:551–558.

385

Jones, E. 1922. Some problems of adolescence. In *Papers on Psychoanalysis*. London: Bailliere, Tindall & Cox.

Kato, M. 1969. Self-destruction in Japan: a cross-cultural epidemiological analysis of suicide. *Folio of Psychiatry and Neurology* 23:291–307.

Klerman, G. 1988. Youthful melancholia. *British Journal of Psychiatry* 152:4–14.

Masterson, J. J. 1967. The symptomatic adolescent five years later: he didn't grow out of it. *American Journal of Psychiatry* 123:1338–1345.

Offer, D. 1975. Adolescent turmoil. In A. Esman, ed. *The Psychology of Adolescence*. New York: International Universities Press.

Rakoff, V. 1970. *The Longing for Significance*. Toronto: C.B.C.

Rakoff, V. 1980. History in adolescent disorders. *Adolescent Psychiatry* 8:85–99.

Rakoff, V. 1983. Multiple determinants of family dynamics in anorexia nervosa. In P. L. Darby, P. E. Garfinkel, D. Garner, and D. V. Coscina, eds. *Anorexia Nervosa: Recent Developments in Research*. New York: Liss.

Rieff, P. 1959. *Freud: The Mind of a Moralist*. Chicago: University of Chicago Press.

Sakinofsky, I., and Roberts, R. 1987. The ecology of suicide in the provinces of Canada. In B. Cooper, ed. *Psychiatric Epidemiology*. Baltimore: Johns Hopkins University Press.

Salvendy, J. 1988. *Royal Rebel: A Psychological Portrait of Crown Prince Rudolf of Austria-Hungary*. London: University Press of America.

Trilling, L. 1972. *Sincerity and Authenticity*. Cambridge, Mass.: Harvard University Press.

25 DISCUSSION OF VIVIAN M. RAKOFF'S CHAPTER

ROBERT W. BUCHANAN

In his presentation, Professor Rakoff proposes that adolescence is both a life stage and a particular configuration of social opportunities and dangers and that, because the emergence of adolescence accompanies many social forces, what we label "adolescent" may in fact be a condition found throughout life. He illustrates this first by presenting a rationale for the emergence of a person whom we call an adolescent from a historical perspective. He then develops his theme of the emergence of the adolescent patient with current, well-known clinical entities and connects them with that very historical development.

Rakoff begins with a warm description of his grandparents as an example of life during an era when lives were fixed and marriage, child rearing, and responsibility occurred early. The idea of the existence of an extended, nurtured childhood, which later would be called adolescence, could be questioned or considered a bourgeois luxury or an isolated curiosity.

He moves to the established biological viewpoint with its accepted landmarks. Infancy is reasonably clear cut when it comes to defining boundaries. "Rakoff's baby" is a hard-wired parasite who can be perceived as a valuable source of joy. Childhood is also clearly defined as existing between infancy and puberty. Adolescence seems to begin at puberty, but where or does it end? Or does it?

Rakoff then discusses the emergence of adolescence as a life stage within both psychoanalysis and psychiatry and what he calls "nonpsychological currents." In the field, he names Aries, Sigmund Freud, and Anna Freud. To Miss Freud he gives only partial correctness to her view that adolescence is attributable to psychoanalysis. Rakoff says that adolescence is associated with the development of psychoanalysis and that both are products of a particular phase of historical development. This is the beginning of the development of his theme, that is, a shift from stable eternal fixity to an emphasis on the subjective and on individual rights and struggles. He then mentions other prominent contributors to the idea of adolescence, including Hall, Jones, Bernfeld, Aichorn, Blos, and Erikson.

To the other nonpsychological currents he gives credit for recognizing that various life stages do require certain types of support and recognition. I believe, moving back to the psychological realm, that this recognition has been greatly enhanced by the researchers and writers in the field of self psychology, which I will comment on later.

Rakoff returns to the theme of the restriction imposed on working-class lives when children are viewed as miniature adults with the assumption they will quickly assume the identity of their fathers. He postulates that being deprived of an adolescence leads to lives that are deprived and unfulfilling. Rakoff demonstrates how one can use the literature of a society to reflect what is and what the society thinks should be. Before the nineteenth century, the serious characters in drama were the gentry. The essence of tragedy is a character flaw in an otherwise virtuous man of high social standing. His life outcome was not determined by economic opportunity or circumstance but by choices he was able to make because of his socially privileged status; that is, he had options. Rakoff states that the suffering of the common man was not regarded as tragic but as comedic or "not real." I am not sure if this means that the common man was regarded as a mere caricature of a real, whole man. Is the man of high social standing then the forerunner of the "cultural hero" who is to come?

There was a shift in nineteenth-century literature in that novelists began to give character to the regular man. Rakoff describes a democratization of choice and the right of character to influence major life events. Obedience to authority—the law, church, king, and parents—was giving way to individual consideration. The American and French revolutions were external reflections of these changes in the social view of man.

This shift from stable fixity to struggle between opposing forces characterized the atmosphere surrounding Freud and, therefore, according to Rakoff, set the stage for Freud's view of psychological man. Increasing emphasis on the individual, subjectivity, authenticity, and alienation—all what I would call inner experiences—leads to notions of opportunity, hope, and expectations. It also leads to the defining of what Rakoff calls a "cultural hero." This "hero" is an explorer of life's opportunities, one who distrusts history, one who is idealistic and adventurous. But Rakoff points out that this "adolescent" is not merely a young adult but more a model for all the adult life stages.

The chapter shifts at this point to a more familiar, to me, clinical perspective. However, just as I was about to get comfortable, I was introduced to a new way of viewing adolescent psychopathology. Rakoff would like us to consider three categories. The first he calls ailments and adjustments surrounding the pubertal phase. This relates to the usual problems related to sexual awareness and increased physical and intellectual power. The second category he calls the disorders of young adulthood, a category that comprises the major psychoses. As he is trying to describe those illnesses of adolescence, which are phase specific, he has intentionally left out the adolescent character disorders that appear to be associated more with life-long problems. The third category is called the problems of historically fostered adolescence and consists of those clinical entities on which the rest of the paper focuses.

The word "adolescence" in this case does not seem to be referring to that period between ages thirteen and twenty but more to the human qualities we have heard before—idealism, authenticity, adventurousness, facing choices and opportunities. Rakoff believes that many clinical problems are generated by the historically determined adolescence he has developed thus far. These clinical syndromes are adolescent suicide and depression, anorexia nervosa, substance abuse, religious malaise, and anomic rootlessness.

Rakoff cites several statistical studies that show increases in the incidence of these syndromes and asks if there is a common factor, or "agent blue," if you will. Durkheim, commenting on the apparent increase in suicide in Europe at the end of the nineteenth century, wrote, "when society is disturbed by some painful crisis or by beneficent but abrupt transitions, it is momentarily incapable of exercising this influence; thence come the sudden rises in the curve of suicides" (1950). Is the influence Durkheim refers to the opportunity for choices that Rakoff is asserting? The beneficent transitions in the syndromes

Rakoff has included appear to be the increased opportunities and the individual expression available to the adolescent—the very factors that led to the development of adolescence in the first place.

I would like at this point to present a quote from Rakoff that captures the essence of the argument (p. 383):

Adolescence, in addition to being a life stage bracketed between puberty and adulthood, is also a set of characteristic social expectations and opportunities that may extend throughout much of the life cycle. When the circumstances permit, adolescent behavior reappears not so much as a regression but as the mobilization of a constant potentiality. The openness of choice and self-determination may present in mature individuals with the same or similar enthusiasm or difficulty as it does for youths or young adults. In its positive aspects, it promotes the capacity for adventure, risk taking, creative change, enthusiasm, idealism, and healthy skepticism. The negative is the fostering of anomie, alienation, and despair.

It is a compelling idea that Rakoff has advanced—the view that adolescence is a set of characteristic social roles, expectations, and opportunities that may present in mature individuals at any adult stage. I believe that it is true that these attitudes characterize healthy adulthood but that they have changed since adolescence by the process of growing up. Reality and life experience of the adult shape and change these "adolescent" points of view. I do not see how the choices one makes at age fifty can be done with the same enthusiasm or difficulty that occurs with the adolescent.

Why do opportunities lead to such devastating negatives? Rakoff believes that increased opportunities lead to increased expectations—expectations that all too often are unrealistic and that cannot be fulfilled. He states that we could refer to these as "disorders of aspiration." He adds that he does not intend to disregard the importance of individual psychodynamics or specific nuances related to each of the clinical entities mentioned but that he is rather trying to find an underlying common component.

I believe that this opens the door for more critical work in understanding adolescence. The idea that adolescence ends at a certain age to be followed by adulthood is simplistic and basically not true. One can see from clinical work with our patients as well as by examining our own selves that issues related to adolescence are present through-out life. I think that the experience one has as an adolescent with parents, teachers, and friends will provide lifelong models for living and making reasonable choices. But these models are constantly being transformed throughout life.

Self psychology has given us a way to understand important if not critical emotional requirements that must accompany the opportunities and choices we have been referring to here. The old psychoanalytic theory of adolescence as a recapitulation of the oedipal conflict has been joined and enhanced by newer thinking. Palombo (1987) states, "Adolescents arrive at this phase with specific developmental needs for particular responses from their caretakers. The nature of the self-object functions required at this stage is different from those of prior stages. The ability to be responsive to the adolescent's needs are de-termined not only by the relationship they have had to their child prior to that phase, but also to the issues that are activated within them by the adolescent".

I believe that these crucial selfobject needs and functions underlie the success or failure of the opportunities the adolescent or adult is given. Understanding this has important implications for helping our patients, raising our children, and understanding ourselves. We cannot provide opportunities alone. They must be provided in the context of a human relationship. It is this combination—an opportunity in the context of a supportive relationship—that will allow the adolescent to turn the opportunity into a vital part of his life experience. Without this crucial selfobject function, the experience feels meaningless.

I see a man who is thirty-five and recently divorced after ten tu-multuous years. He grew up in a wealthy, educated family and had more opportunities than most. As he was complaining to a longtime family acquaintance about his current status of no job, no meaningful relationships, and not much prospect in the future for either, the other said to him, "I don't understand, Bill. You've had every opportunity." Bill had the opportunities alright, but his life lacked the selfobject involvement necessary to incorporate the opportunities.

Conclusions

Rakoff has given us a creative and new way of conceptualizing ad-olescence. Far from the standard view of adolescence as a period of time in human development, Rakoff sees adolescence as a set of characteristic social expectations and opportunities that may extend throughout much of the life cycle. This is a presentation about human potential and how opportunities can lead either to a fulfilling, productive life or to a life of emptiness and despair. Opportunities alone are not sufficient. Opportunities must occur in a psychological environment that will allow them to be integrated into a whole adult being. The enthusiasm of adolescence needs to be nurtured for it to become a vital, functioning part of adulthood.

NOTE

Presented at the American Society for Adolescent Psychiatry Training Institute V, Seattle, Washington, February 28, 1988.

REFERENCES

Durkheim, E. 1950. *Suicide: A Study in Sociology.* New York: Free Press.
Palombo, J. 1987. An outline of adolescent development. Paper presented at the tenth annual Self Psychology Conference, Chicago, October.

PART IV

PSYCHOTHERAPEUTIC APPROACHES IN ADOLESCENT PSYCHIATRY

EDITORS' INTRODUCTION

Despite the proliferation of biological treatment methods in recent years, psychotherapy in various forms remains the heart of clinical work with adolescents. New developments—the AIDS epidemic, the explosive spread of various intoxicants, the emerging concern about adolescent suicide—keep hospital services for adolescents filled and test the ingenuity and dedication of the therapists who seek to deal with the psychological aspects of these problems.

Alexander Gralnick, a pioneer and proponent of adolescent psychiatry, presents an overview of adolescence, adolescent development, and hospital treatment of the adolescent. He discusses the definition of adolescence, stages of development, social influences on adolescents, the hospital, and the hospital of the future. Gralnick is deeply concerned about social, cultural, political, and economic forces over which we have little control. He is adamant about deinstitutionalization and its effect on chronic illness. He believes that the hospital is guided by a simple thesis, that the patient becomes ill in an unhealthy environment but can become well only by being immersed in a sound one. The goal, then, is not merely to remove symptoms but to eradicate basic psychopathology. Gralnick outlines the dimensions of the "future hospital," one whose social nature can successfully nurture the sickest of patients back to mental health.

Myron Stocking describes the treatment of an adolescent girl who had survived a catastrophic family event. He discusses the nature of the catastrophe, the patient's initial adaptation, the internal experience of the patient as she dealt with the trauma of past events, and the technical problems of the therapy that included working with an oppositional extended family as well as finding a balance in the individual therapy between intrapsychic focus and family work. Stocking postulates that the processes of trauma and mastery are often mirror images of one another; both are responses to the interplay within the patient between unconscious fantasy and external reality.

Debra Schnall and Joseph Youngerman discuss treatment in impoverished communities of families encumbered by severe social and economic factors. They recount their experiences when severely dysfunctional families and their antipodal problems are encountered in hospital treatment of disturbed adolescents. The authors conclude that deeply rooted transference and countertransference issues of institutional dependency must be directly confronted. They present a case example in which either the entire family should be hospitalized or the fundamental premise of hospital treatment had to be radically altered. They illustrate the use of paradoxical therapy techniques to prevent overly dependent merging by needy, symbiotic families.

James M. Jones, Glen T. Pearson, and Rhonda Dimpero examine the vicissitudes of hospitalizing an adolescent by a family. They describe the process involved in developing an alliance in which trust and mutual respect provide a context for examining conflicts and working together for change. The authors propose a conceptual model for integrating the psychodynamic inpatient treatment of the adolescent with the systems-oriented approach to the family. Jones, Pearson, and Dimpero conclude that the classical phases of treatment should be conceptualized as overlapping periods each of which contains all the elements of resistance, regression, alliance, working through, separation, and emergence from the hospital.

Helen A. Widen, as a college psychotherapist, sees increasing health- and life-threatening behavior in the young adult population. Widen believes that therapeutic parameters must be introduced by the clinician in order to modify concepts and theoretical techniques. She sees disavowal as a defense against accepting the need for change and introduces the option of discussing questionable behavior when it reaches life-threatening proportions.

26 ADOLESCENCE, THE ADOLESCENT, AND HOSPITAL TREATMENT

ALEXANDER GRALNICK

Offer (1987) writes that adolescence did not start with the Industrial Revolution but was known as such by the Romans, Greeks, and Egyptians, only "to have almost disappeared during the Dark Ages." It was stated in 1556, he reports, that "the third age, which is called adolescence . . . ends in the twenty-first year . . . and it can go on till thirty or thirty-five. This age is called adolescence because the person is big enough to beget children" (pp. 8–9). Further, Offer believes that in our country the stage of adolescence has been prolonged, particularly in the middle classes, in which the young continue economically dependent.

In our culture, we think of childhood and adolescence as periods that should be rather carefree and happy. The emphasis is on pleasure, and there is something of a deemphasis on values, as though they are for a later, more serious stage. Certain basic virtues, of course, are taught, but with hardly the necessary urgency.

We judge the adolescent's age range differently. Some think of it as from twelve to eighteen and others as from fourteen to eighteen or twenty-one. Some date it from the onset of the physical and physiological changes that begin usually at age twelve. Often, one's occupation and level of responsibility is taken into account, with the age extended for the student or otherwise economically dependent person. The marital status may be considered as well as whether the individual in question is living singly or with a mate. The eighteen-year-old working to support a family or taking care of a household is less likely to be considered an adolescent than is the high school, single, dependent student or even the older college student.

Legal considerations also determine our judgment. The adolescent teenager may do or be permitted to do many adult things. He may work, she may bear children, and both may refuse to be hospitalized or may sign themselves out once in. They may enlist in the army, be engaged in military action, and actually kill other human beings or be killed. In the same culture, at different times, the concept of the adolescent will change. Before the child labor laws, it was common for children to work and contribute to the family's support in a very adult manner. My father often told the following story with both pleasure and pride. He came to the United States from Russia at the age of eleven. The very next day he went to work carrying a brown paper bag filled with a roll and a banana. He knew what a roll was, and he knew how to work, but he had to be told what a banana was and how to eat it. He grew to adulthood before he was eighteen.

Other cultural considerations enter into one's concept of the adolescent as well as of what the adolescent years are. Our typical native adolescent is quite different from one in Iran or in Ethiopia, who is starving or witnessing family members starve to death, or, for that matter, in Rio de Janeiro, where hundreds of thousands of young people roam the streets as orphans fending for themselves. They, too, grow and become wily adults very quickly. At least, the age range of the adolescent and his other characteristics and problems are closely related to his culture. Our judgment, our expectations, and our goals for him are also related to our values as they are learned from our culture.

Society tends to protect the adolescent, if only by extending this period of life it regards as needing supervision. However, the question is whether we, as psychiatrists, have been protecting the sick adolescent as well as we might. I think we may have emphasized understanding his psychodynamics and protecting his civil rights at the expense of his right to treatment. In so doing, we have acquiesced together with too many others to his deinstitutionalization.

I tend to fault American psychiatry as a profession for having readily accepted deinstitutionalization (Gralnick 1983, 1985). This iniquitous practice has denied hospitalization to too many people who, in the community, have been exposed to the drug scene and other abuses that have worsened their lot. Now there are mounting numbers of adolescents chronically to hopelessly sick. At the least, their outlook is grave.

In the heyday of the state hospital, the cry was that long-term hospitalization caused chronicity and deterioration, particularly for the majority of patients who then were diagnosed schizophrenic. In the community, exposed as they now are to alcohol and hard drugs, neglect, and homelessness, these youths seem to present a new breed of illness, variously alluded to as borderline, dysthymic, or character disordered. Some now think of this cohort as "dysfunctional" rather than psychotic.

What we are really seeing is the schizophrenic patient with an overlay that is due to the different situations to which he has been exposed. Otherwise, the paranoia and other delusions, the poor judgment, bizarre life-style, and the like indicate the underlying diagnosis. As with the previously long-hospitalized patient, the disease process marches on, with the resulting deterioration, perhaps somewhat different from the way it appeared in the hospital but a deterioration nevertheless. The psychotic process becomes fixed, and ordinary efforts at resuscitation are uniformly unsuccessful. The only difference is that now the patient is in the community, not in the hospital. Those who diagnose these patients differently seem content because they are now not as terrified as they were of the diagnosis of chronic schizophrenia. In reality, however, these patients, regardless of diagnosis, are no less terrifying, and we may be equally pessimistic about their future.

The consideration of adolescence cannot be separated from that of adulthood. Maturity is also hard to define, yet we use the term to separate off the adolescent from the adult. It may mark the very end of adolescence and the start of adulthood. Yet we know many a teenager who is quite mature, just as we know adults who never mature and are veritable adolescents all their lives. These are common observations that must prompt us to think carefully.

The matter of "adolescent turmoil" also requires attention. Many hold this phenomenon to describe an aspect of the disturbed adolescent but also think of it as typical of the developmental process of the normal adolescent. It is supposed to describe the psychological and emotional disequilibrium, rebellion against authority, and changeable and unpredictable behavior as natural to the youngster. Many actually think that, if the adolescent does not live through this turmoil, he will remain overdependent on his parents, have trouble establishing his identity, and have difficulty in relating to peers. In other words, the adolescent cannot mature without turmoil and a struggle with his parents.

I think this view of matters is based on the theory that somehow there is a grand design that inevitably determines the course and stages of our lives. The instinctual and libidinal forces are such that their resolution can be only by fire—Sturm und Drang. It is as though these developments are unrelated to other conditions, including the nature of the parents, their philosophy and values, and the social conditions under which the person is raised. I cannot accept that view of things, and I urge its reconsideration.

Offer (1987) tells us that normal and usual adolescents do not necessarily experience adolescent turmoil. He believes that most psychiatrists have been misled by their experience with the disturbed adolescent and have misapplied knowledge of him to all adolescents. He says that the usual young person enjoys life, is happy with himself, and enjoys work and a job well done; he is work oriented and hopeful about the future, he accepts his body changes, and he is not apprehensive about sex; further, he gets along with his parents. Offer concludes that adolescent turmoil is not part of the normal process of growing up. According to him, only about 20 percent of adolescents have real problems and need the psychiatric help that, unfortunately, only a small percentage receive.

The youngster, influenced by his culture to believe that he is only an adult when he is on his own, independent, and self-sufficient, will have trouble as he grows from his teens. The one raised to appreciate the importance of others, especially those who have reared him, who accepts his indebtedness to them and is, therefore, concerned for them, will accept that human beings are interdependent rather than independent. He will individuate in a mature and rational manner, for his is a different value system.

In the hospital, we find adolescent patients confused about their true role in relation to others. They suffer from too much self-involvement, too much self-centeredness, and too little concern for others. They have no concept of interdependence and its importance and feel too little responsibility toward and for others. We consider it a major part of our work with them to challenge this value system and to change it so that it comes closer to that of our own. Values thus play a vital role in our therapeutic work.

Stages of Adolescent Development

There is a logic to the way psychiatry divides the human being's life into stages, each somewhat distinct and separate from its previous one and the ones to follow. The theories on which we base our approach and techniques would anticipate that action. Freud described the earliest stages of development—the oral and anal—as well as the id, the ego, and the superego. Belief in the theories of the instinct and libido almost foretold what was to be thought and described as fact. The Oedipus and castration complex formulations were also natural to this belief system. In our hierarchical culture, it is also natural to think in stages of development, each an advance over the other.

I think that there are particular advantages for those who think this way. There is a certain comfort to be gained from such rather simple constructs of an otherwise complex being. Further, it fits nicely with our basic theories, seems to support them, and, thereby, gives us additional confidence in our formulations. It affords us ready explanations of what we see, and that also makes life a lot easier. Not only can we describe the individual patient, but we can also describe and diagnose whole groups as though they were one, and that, too, is quite an accomplishment. Further, we can afford understanding and prescribe remedies for many more than one at a time. What could be more gratifying than that? Individuality need not concern us, particularly.

At any rate, what we have offers us a feeling of stability or, perhaps, the appearance of such, for, in truth, the results we get are not that good. However, I am not so sure that we will be content for long with the look of things so much as better accomplishment for our efforts.

There are two sides to a coin, and, where one finds advantages, there will he discover disadvantages. First, our conceptualization of stages of development supports a formulation that is increasingly open to question. In that respect, then, it may be hindering progress in our theorization and hampering our technical creativity. We may be in something of a trap with one construct feeding on another and be prevented from seeing a truer continuity in human development. We could miss seeing the seeds of later stages in the earlier times and lose the opportunity of developing and affecting their course. At any rate, we are, in fact, frustrated in our efforts to understand and treat the adolescent more successfully.

I guess I am suggesting that we question how we think about the adolescent, let alone that we question our concepts and techniques. I do not think that what we see in the youngsters of middle-class America is universal or, as Offer (1987) says, even true across the board in the United States. I would prefer thinking in terms of life as more of a continuum with less sharply demarcated stages. This would permit more flexibility in our thinking and allow us to see each youngster individually. There is no reason for each human unit to fit into a group because of his age anymore than because of his color. It tends to stereotype. Is there any reason why a particular eighteen-year-old should not be considered an adult rather than an adolescent even though he is a student? I sometimes think that seeing the adolescent as a "stage" disconnects him from his life, both past and future. There may be some validity to the belief some hold that adolescence is a luxury our society can no longer afford.

Social Influences

It is undeniable that early life experiences play a part in the development of one's personality. Very much has been made of early experiences, especially with mother and father. It is thought that these leave indelible imprints in the brain that, in turn, unconsciously influence one's functioning, if not predetermine it. I am beginning to believe, however, that this is hardly as true as believed and that continuing later experiences are at least as effective in determining our behavior, including matters of a social, political, and economic nature over which we have little control.

I think I can believe that unconscious forces are not necessarily at play—that we have reason to question the whole theory of the unconscious—and that pressures of a very conscious nature are at play. I do not think in terms of memories buried in an "unconscious" and exerting forces beyond our control. I now believe that there are conscious conflicts created by our contradictory value systems and that these wreak havoc in the human being. I think that value systems are adopted by children much earlier than we believe and play a more important role than we realize. The exercise of values is not more common to the adult than it is to the adolescent.

I would like to question Offer's (1987) belief that things have not changed any too much when he states, "Indeed, it is a mystery how the more things change, the more they remain the same" (p. 7). He believes that ethics and religions are much the same and that the family is still the anchor of the socialization process. I would suggest, instead, that, in the past three generations, society, globally and within our borders, has been changing quite radically. Large sections of the world have turned away from capitalist democracy and have embarked on social and economic paths that, by their very nature, will change the quality of man's values and thinking and the nature of human relationships. The fact of their existence has an effect on the thinking and standards of people throughout the world and particularly on the thinking and emotions of many in our country. This has been true to such an extent that the most powerful proponent of the socialist world has been established as the "evil empire." Nothing positive dare be said about it. Its people are but robots who must be saved. Its leaders are taking the people down the path of world conquest, and we must be prepared to prevent this no matter what the cost. This has an effect on the psychology of our adolescents and is a change of which we must be quite aware. The threat of nuclear annihilation has affected another tremendous change in the psychology of the people of the world.

Revolutionary changes and struggles are going on within nations. Religions and ethical standards are radically different, very much so in recent years within the United States. There is a heightening concern people have for themselves and an ever lessening one for the welfare of others. Witness the equanimity with which we accept the great numbers of homeless, that one of five children lives under the poverty level, that we have such numbers of homeless mentally ill. Witness these and the Iran/Contra affair and its effect on the psychology of people. I am sure that the pessimism and cynicism, if not hopelessness, of people is up many-fold. Innumerable other examples could confirm the lowering of ethical standards in our country.

I think, further, that we may question that the family is the anchor of the socialization process, at least the family as we once knew it. There are too many one-parent families, either the result of death, divorce, or desertion; too many parentless families, families with unwed mothers; and far too many reconstituted families, the result of combined part-families following divorce. We can no longer linger with past ideas of the family and its effect on the socialization process. I think we must be prepared now to see a different psychology and set of standards among our young and to see them continue to change. The effect on their mental stability has yet to be fully understood.

I am not saying that childhood is not different from adulthood or that these so-called stages should or need not be studied. If described, however, they might be seen from another perspective. I am saying that these stages do not come solely as a result of some grand design— as a result of biological and/or instinctual forces—but are determined as largely, or more so, by continuing social, cultural, economic, and political forces of a global nature that determine the stage of one's development, perhaps unrelated to age.

I think there is reason to question the thinking that all youngsters of a certain age act more or less the same and experience the same emotions and developmental problems. What a person thinks and feels and how he behaves is more a matter of his social experience and the strata of society from which he arises. The sixteen-year-old black or Hispanic dropout raised in the ghetto is hardly similar to the sixteen-year-old raised in the suburbs and attending private school. Their systems of values are radically different, as are their sexual appetites and habits, their aspirations, and their hopes. These rather obvious matters tend to be overlooked when one thinks in terms of instincts and an order of events predetermined, in the main, by physiological changes and sexual drives. If there is similarity in the lives of any group of youngsters, it would be because they are of the same class and social experience.

When adolescence starts is not so much a matter of difference as is when it ends. We hear eighteen, twenty-one, and as distant a number as thirty-five. The physical markers thought to usher in its onset are easy to see, though its psychological and emotional ones are not. Physical changes do not mark its end. What then does? What emotional and psychological changes mark the earlier evidence of adolescence? We generally point to attraction to the opposite sex. But is that enough, let alone valid? What about attitudes toward one's self and others? What should be their quality? What about love and concern for others? What about values and their nature? These could be psychological markers that we should define and relate to adolescence as a stage. What would they have to be to mark the end of adolescence or the beginning of adulthood? What must be one's real life situation to at least be an adult? I ask these many questions without having answers. Nor do I believe anyone else has given them satisfactory responses.

If adolescence covers years fourteen to eighteen, what are satisfactory developments at the annual markers of fourteen, fifteen, sixteen, seventeen, and eighteen? Do we or can we satisfactorily define them? What do we mean when we say one is a "mature" sixteen-year-old? Is he developed beyond the usual sixteen-year-old? Is he then no longer an adolescent but an early adult?

We speak of the demands parents and society make on adolescents as contributing to their problems, causing their turmoil, and accounting for their unhealthy reactions. But is it not true that we are making demands of the growing person from birth? Think of the many things we expect of the newborn—to notice us, to smile, to laugh, to respond to our touch, to toilet train, and so on. Should we not then deal with the common factors in all stages of life that affect and perturb the growing person?

The Hospital

Deinstitutionalization has resulted in the discharge into the community of a host of young people exposed to an entirely different life experience from that of the state hospital. It has also resulted in the denial of hospital care to untold numbers until they are chronically sick. Pepper, Ryglewicz, and Kirshner (1982) have called these the "uninstitutionalized generation." In both instances, they have been treated inadequately and heartlessly, if not cruelly. They have been exposed to the drug scene, seedy single-room hotels, homelessness, flop houses, soup kitchens, starvation, exploitation, rape, and prostitution.

We know that most current systems of care do not attract or hold them and that they do not comply with recommended treatment (Caton 1981; Pepper, Kirshner, and Ryglewicz 1981; Sheets, Provost, and Reilman 1982). Lamb (1982) and Schwartz and Goldfinger (1981) point out that psychiatrists and hospitals tend to reject these patients and actually find ways to terminate their treatment prematurely. Thus, the nature of their psychopathology really counts against them. There is a tendency to avoid seeing them as the psychotic people they are and to see them instead as a new generation of dysfunctional young adults. I am distressed by the trend to call them "clients," and the sense I get is that they are given short shrift because they do not recognize that they need treatment. There is the suggestion that they should know better rather than the recognition that they are too sick to be reasonable.

With the foregoing as one's basic orientation, how then does one accomplish two essential things? First, how does one conceptualize an institution for the study, treatment, and reconstruction of the adolescent who enters its doors? Second, how does one organize it, determine and express its philosophy, administer it, study it and its results for the profession, and, finally, gain allegiance from staff so that they will implement the program as it develops?

As to the concept, our hospital is seen as a society of its own, with a past, a present, and a future. It is of such a stable nature and so soundly and rationally structured as to have a therapeutic effect on its patients. It is a substantially sane society to which the patient is brought for healing and, further, for reconstruction into a healthier individual. The intent is that he become sounder and, thereby, abler to withstand society's pressures. The hospital is guided by a simple thesis, namely, that the patient decompensates in an unhealthy environment and must then be immersed in a sound one in which he can become healthy, not just freed of leading symptoms. It is not a complex to which he is brought to receive some specific single treatment or set of treatments but a society that in itself has a health-producing effect. The concept is that there has already been something basically unhealthy about the patient for him to have developed the symptoms with which he comes.

The goal of the institution, then, is not merely to render the patient symptom free but to eradicate more basic psychopathology. It is not enough to allay anxiety, or eradicate a delusion, or erase a hallucination. The goal should be to correct the patient's misconceptions about himself and his distortions of the nature of his relationships. It should be to affect the patient's value system, so vital to his functioning: first, to make him aware that he has one, that it affects him and those about him, and that it does so in a positive or negative fashion; second, to examine his value system for its inconsistencies and how these frustrate his progress, produce crippling anxiety, and threaten his stability; and, third, in this manner, to challenge his value system as it contrasts with that of the society in which he is now living and with which he has to contend. The challenge, particularly, is to all that is egocentric for the purpose of helping him to be more concerned for those about him. This, of course, is in the face of most of what his culture has been emphasizing, namely, that he comes first.

The goals outlined are not ordinary, and accomplishing them is not easy. They are, nevertheless, achievable. However, before indicating how and in what setting this may be done, several items need discussion. In office practice with the neurotic patient, these goals may be sought and gained through the analytic process. The elements of transference and countertransference are present; the transference neurosis can be established, worked through, and resolved, and even the patient's values explored and affected, if the analyst believes that is his legitimate concern. However, when one is dealing with the psychotic patient, these elements are not available to us. The patient cannot develop a transference, and the transference neurosis cannot be established, let alone worked through. The office-practice relation is not at our disposal.

We have heard of, and some of us have known, exceptionally talented analysts who have been able to establish effective therapeutic relationships with selected schizophrenic patients. However, these are singular people. The stark reality is that those who mainly treat the hospitalized patient are well trained and good at their work but very often are residents in training and those who are not too far into their experience as psychiatrists. I would hazard the guess, nevertheless, that, even if an institution were populated completely with the most talented and skilled analysts, it would need the social structure I will attempt to describe.

The currently hospitalized psychiatric patient, regardless of diagnosis or age, is ordinarily very sick. In today's scene, he may be already chronically ill, although not previously hospitalized, or have had one to several short hospitalizations. In these brief encounters, little but symptom relief had been achieved. The patient may then have been seen irregularly, or not at all, for a shorter or longer period of time before the next decompensation brought him once more for hospital treatment. We know that the rule is to have brief rather than extended hospital care in most every case, regardless of the number of the episodes. The brief encounters have merely been temporary care, but the pathologic process, nevertheless, marches on insidiously. We finally have the chronic schizophrenic and the other patients who are now besetting us.

My own belief is that the first episode should be treated most seriously and for an extended time to get quickly at the root of things and to correct matters. As it is now, in most instances, it is after several short hospitalizations that extended care is sought. At such time the patient is already chronic, the pathology has solidified, and the prognosis is bad. Nevertheless, the hospital is expected to produce a good and lasting result. The opportunity to treat the patient thoroughly has been lost from the start. This custom prevails, though we know empirically that, the earlier we treat thoroughly, the better the result. Conversely, the later we treat, no matter how and with what, the worse the result.

Now, with that as a preamble, what more do we think and do to sometimes very effectively help the chronic patients who come to us for extended treatment? Note that I say "treatment," not "care," for we are a hospital, not an asylum.

To begin, we do not see the therapeutic result as issuing solely, or evenly mainly, from the dyadic therapeutic relationship, important as that may be. Similarly, we do not think of any one factor as the most important, unless it be the total hospital milieu and the effect of its system on the patient. I think of this total hospital system as a process that effects the patient, arrests his psychopathology, and, if given a chance, will allow a healthy human being to evolve from one who was quite basically sick, not just ridden with some symptoms.

We think of the psychiatric hospital not as an asylum but as a therapeutic environment. To us it is a social structure in which the staff live with, relate to, and contend with patients, and vice versa. It is a culture of its own, with staff and patients drawn from different cultures and of varying ages, sexes, colors, religions, sizes, habits, inclinations, and social and political persuasions. All are brought from their own milieu with its accustomed ways to this new culture to which they must adapt. The task of doing so is complicated by the fact that the patients, at least, may be confused, unstable, agitated, depressed, possibly suicidal, and suffering with delusions of one sort or another. They may be overcome with suspicion and distrust, antagonistic—sometimes to the point of being combative—and with their own ideas of what is going on, quite unrelated to what really is. They have their own ideas of what they hope to accomplish, very different from our knowledge of what we must achieve with them. Not the happiest or easiest set of circumstances but, nevertheless, the cold reality!

I have alluded to the fact that those who reside in a psychiatric hospital and treat patients and those who come to it for treatment essentially constitute a culture. Each comes to the institution with his own way of viewing things and ways of acting and interacting. Each has his own wants and will be intent on their fulfillment. Of course, what we have then is the makings of a conflictful situation—not different from that of life globally or within the family. If one sees this as the true situation within a hospital and faces it, one can put it to good use. If one cannot use the transference neurosis, he can consciously use this conflict-laden situation to gain awareness of the patient and help the patient grasp the unhealthy and healthy aspects of his personality and behavior. An essential part of the process, of course, is to help him learn and perform more healthily. This is worked out very consciously in a constant and minute study of the patient's performance as compared to how he might or should react and interrelate.

The aim of this tactic is to furnish the patient the insight into himself not otherwise available by the analytic process but, nevertheless, important if he is to progress. In this manner, insight is gained by an examination of the current life scene without recourse to a recollection of life's early happenings. We now look on the study of conflict within the hospital, that is, between groups as well as between individuals— be they between patients, or between staff, or between patients and staff—and the resolution of that conflict as the essence of the therapeutic process.

One's awareness and use of values is critically important to the proper resolution of conflict and the insight that can be gained thereby. At the hospital, we are keenly aware of its value system, study those of the individual patients and those of their groups, and constantly study the clash between them. In the seeking of their resolution, all of us gain a fuller awareness of ourselves. The patients, the staff, and the hospital as a society gain from such knowledge. I can tell you that, as the result of this process, the hospital is a constantly evolving institution. And that is as it should be. It is not only that we learn certain techniques better and better but that all of us who compose the hospital are that much more stable, more rational, and that much more capable of helping the very sick.

Conclusions

If an institution is to be worthy of itself, it is vitally important that it subject itself to self-study. We have been doing this rather exhaustively for many years. Since I am convinced that we must utilize the hospital as a main tool in our armamentarium, at least until we know a lot more about the origins of mental illness and considerably more about its effective treatment, I should say a bit about the future hospital.

If any future hospital is to be really effective with the psychiatric patient, it must have access to him at length very early in the course of the illness. It will have to be, and be seen, as a society of its own under the leadership of psychiatrists supported by sufficient multi-trained professionals, all dedicated to the following common goals: in a treatment atmosphere, to render fully adequate therapy to all on as individualized a basis as possible; in a caring atmosphere, to render as emotionally protective, supportive, and humane an environment as possible; in this milieu for there to be an ever-present and emphasized therapeutic attempt to have the patient know himself increasingly well and to learn the healthier ways of relating to others; in an educational atmosphere, to expand the knowledge of nonprofessional as well as professional staff for the better treatment of patients both in the hospital and in the community when they are discharged to it; in a research atmosphere, to discover the earliest signs of mental illness, particularly of schizophrenia, so that it may be more successfully treated in its infancy; and, finally, to search for the genetic, biologic, constitutional, and pathophysiological origins of mental illness and, with equal assiduousness, to study and discover the social nature of the psychiatric hospital so that it may even more successfully nurture the sickest of our patients back to mental health.

NOTE

Presented to the New York Society for Adolescent Psychiatry on April 20, 1988.

REFERENCES

Caton, C. L. M. 1981. The new chronic patient and the system of community care. *Hospital and Community Psychiatry* 32:475–478.
Gralnick, A. 1983. Deinstitutionalization: origins and signs of failure. *American Journal of Social Psychiatry* 3(4): 8–12.
Gralnick, A. 1985. The case against deinstitutionalization. *American Journal of Social Psychiatry* 5(3): 7–11.
Lamb, H. R. 1982. Young adult chronic patients: the new drifters. *Hospital and Community Psychiatry* 33:465–468.
Offer, D. 1987. The mystery of adolescence. *Adolescent Psychiatry* 14:7–27.

Pepper, B.; Kirshner, M. C.; and Ryglewicz, H. 1981. Young adult chronic patients: overview of a population. *Hospital and Community Psychiatry* 32:463–469.

Pepper, B.; Ryglewicz, H.; and Kirshner, M. C. 1982. The uninstitutionalized generation: a new breed of psychiatric patient. In B. Pepper and H. Ryglewicz, eds. *The Young Adult Chronic Patient*. New Directions for Mental Health Services, no. 14. San Francisco: Jossey-Bass.

Schwartz, S. R., and Goldfinger, S. M. 1981. The new chronic patient: clinical characteristics of an emerging subgroup. *Hospital and Community Psychiatry* 32:470–474.

Sheets, J. L.; Provost, J. A.; and Reilman, J. 1982. The young adult chronic patient: three-hypothesized subgroups. In B. Pepper and H. Ryglewicz, eds. *The Young Adult Chronic Patient*. New Directions for Mental Health Services, no. 14. San Francisco: Jossey-Bass.

27 CATASTROPHE AND THE CAPACITY TO WITHSTAND IT: AN ADOLESCENT RESPONDS TO PERSONAL TRAGEDY

MYRON STOCKING

Some years ago I treated an adolescent girl who had survived catastrophe. I saw her for nine months. This limited period of treatment proved helpful to her and enlightening for me. In this description of our work, I will address the following issues: (1) the nature of the catastrophe and the patient's initial adaptation; (2) the internal experience of the patient as she dealt with the trauma of past events; and (3) technical problems of the therapy, which included working with an oppositional extended family as well as finding a balance in the individual therapy between intrapsychic focus and family work. Both forms of treatment were necessary in order to sustain the continuity of the patient's treatment and to help her develop a sense of inner worthiness.

Preliminary Literature Review

The diagnosis of posttraumatic stress disorder was first established as a discrete diagnostic entity within the official diagnostic nomenclature of American psychiatry (American Psychiatric Association 1980). As described there, the disorder is characterized by a pattern of symptoms arising in response to the experience of a traumatic event, "an event that is outside the range of usual human experience and that would be markedly distressing to almost anyone" (p. 236), evoking intense fear, terror, and a sense of helplessness. Over time the survivor reexperiences important elements of the original trauma in dreams or intrusive thoughts that reevoke uncontrolled and powerful states of emotional distress. Periods in which feelings are dissociated alternate with affective arousal. The victim may experience emotional numbing and a general loss of emotional responsiveness. Victims may subsequently avoid stimuli associatively linked to the original trauma, with a resulting constriction in adaptation to life. The helplessness, anxiety, and affective disturbance must persist for at least one month to establish the diagnosis and may recur for life.

Sigmund Freud published the first psychodynamic formulation of posttraumatic stress. His developing ideas on the issue are interspersed throughout his entire published works (1886–1937). He was the first to demonstrate clearly the relation of subsequent symptom formation to a previous real life traumatic event. His initial formulations in collaboration with Josef Breuer were based on studies of patients with hysterical symptoms, including flashbacks, dissociative fantasies, anxiety dreams, and psychosomatic symptoms, in which the original trauma was reexperienced at an interval of time after its occurrence. They showed how unconscious symbolism disguised the relation of subsequent symptoms to the original traumatic event (Breuer and Freud 1895). In their view, hysterics suffered from memories of actual trauma unmastered when first experienced.

Freud evolved over time a theoretical model of the structure of the mind. Early, he hypothesized a "stimulus barrier" against the external stimulation arising from the perception and recall of life events. During this period, he believed, "the common traumatic neurosis is a consequence of an extensive breach being made in the protective shield against stimuli" (Freud 1920, p. 31). The mental apparatus is "flooded with large amounts of stimulus and another problem arises . . . the problem of mastering the amounts of stimuli which have broken in and of binding them" (Freud 1920, p. 29). Later, Freud (1926) delineated a scheme of psychological defensive operations triggered by signals of external danger or fears evoked by internal anxieties. He came to place such emphasis on the role of unconscious fantasy in triggering neurotic symptomatology that he minimized the importance of actual life events in hysterical and obsessional symptom formation. However, with subsequent experience with patients suffering traumatic neurosis in World War I, he reestablished a more balanced emphasis on the interplay between underlying fantasy and actual life events in producing traumatic states.

Horowitz (1986), who subsequently elaborated Freud's theoretical approach, has emphasized the cognitive dimension of Freud's formu-

lations. As summarized by Horowitz, Freud's theoretical model conceptualized a feedback loop: "Suppose that there is a continuous
perceptual sampling of an ongoing external stress event and that the
degree of processing of this information can be regulated. The degree
of this modulation, in turn, depends on the magnitude of aroused emotions such as fear or anxiety. Initially, as the information input increases, signal emotions, such as anxiety, also increase. The anxiety
encourages an increase in defensive inhibitions, and so there is a reduction in information processing" (p. 87).

Horowitz went on to integrate the work of contemporary cognitive
theorists with Freud's earlier formulations. He delineated a new theoretical construct, "the completion principle," that summarized the
human mind's intrinsic tendency "to continue to process new information to bring up to date the inner schemata of the self and the world"
(Horowitz 1986, p. 93).

Lenore Terr, Robert Pynoos, and Spencer Eth are representative of
those who have addressed the posttraumatic stress disorder from a
developmental perspective. Terr (1981) has contrasted the response
over time of children of varying ages who were kidnapped and left
buried in a school bus to the characteristic patterns of response of
adults to severe trauma. In the group she described, the children experienced no amnesia for their experience. There was no alternation
between intrusive reexperience of the trauma with periods in which
they were symptom free; nor did the children experience flashbacks.
Their play was a primary mode by which they attempted to master
their trauma. The use of play in childhood appears to overlap in its
psychological function with the dream experience of traumatized adults.
Children actively reenact their experience in contrast to the passive
reexperience of adults who feel no control over the repeated intrusion
of the traumatic event into their daily lives. While Terr found these
significant differences in the response of children and adults, she did
not detect significant variations in response of children at different
developmental stages within childhood.

In their studies of a sample of children who had witnessed the homicide of a parent, Pynoos and Eth (1985) described distinct differences
in the adaptive efforts of preoedipal, oedipal, and latency children and
of adolescents in responding to their traumatic experience.

In addition to the literature alluded to thus far, which has been focused on inner reactions of individuals who have faced extraordinary

stress, there is a body of literature that focuses on various external factors that affect the course of a posttraumatic stress response. Some studies have placed an emphasis on the specific nature of the traumatic event itself, for instance, Wilson, Smith, and Johnson (1985). Green, Wilson, and Lindy (1985) have emphasized the importance of the recovery environment in contributing to the response of the traumatized individual to his trauma. The last two works cited appear in *Trauma and Its Wake,* a series of volumes edited by Charles Figley that provide an excellent ongoing view of the continuing research and clinical work in the field of response to trauma (Figley 1985).

Statement of Purpose

I have given a brief overview of the extensive literature on psychic trauma and, more recently, on posttraumatic stress disorder. The literature has been more devoted to the elaboration of theory than to the description of actual clinical experience. Despite a plethora of clinical anecdotes and condensed case summaries, there remain remarkably few case presentations describing in detail the process of psychotherapy. There are still fewer detailed descriptions of the therapeutic process with individuals who have been able to use their treatment to master to a considerable degree the traumatic experience to which they were originally exposed. A significant exception to these generalizations about the literature is represented by *The Reconstruction of Trauma* (Rothstein 1986), which includes a number of admirable clinical accounts, some condensed, but others in moderate detail.

In the presentation that follows, I describe the therapy of an adolescent who appeared to adapt with great strength to potentially traumatizing experience. My primary goal in this account is to describe the treatment process in a way that permits the reader to differentiate clinical process and theoretical inference. I try to describe the therapeutic process with sufficient clarity, objectivity, and detail that the reader may use the account to enlarge on his or her own experience in a way that permits independent theoretical inference.

Clinical Case Study

In August of the year she was still fourteen, Patricia Moriarty's father shot and killed her mother, her grandfather, and then himself as Patricia and her boyfriend, Bill, fled the house. Pat's initial response to the murders included the shock, fear, and sense of loss one would expect. For the subsequent three months, she was plagued by nightmares and insomnia. However, her anxiety and sadness then subsided, and she appeared to resume the ordinary tasks of her life. Her schoolwork was as good as it had ever been. She appeared to make a smooth adaptation to a foster home, which her uncle and guardian, Jim Moriarty, had felt might pose problems. Her social adjustment appeared good. It seemed unlikely to those around her that anyone could integrate so serious a loss and trauma with so little outer evidence of distress and so little loss of confidence in herself and her world. Yet, by Christmas, she told her foster mother, Christie O'Donnel, that this was the "best Christmas of my life."

When new difficulties emerged ten months later, it was not immediately obvious that they were related to the losses of the summer before. Over time, after Pat and her sister had moved in, Christie and her husband, Wendell, confronted the daily tensions of living with two new daughters, one a teenager. As their frustration mounted, they became increasingly critical of Pat. Their concern and anger focused on her attachment to Bill, her boyfriend. They felt the relationship was too exclusive and too intense. They felt she was closing herself off to other relationships too early. Her foster parents' negative response to her boyfriend evoked the first obviously negative responses Pat had shown them. For the first time she became passively aggressive. Beneath a surface compliance she became increasingly provocative. In her house, Christie expected respectful acquiescence. As Pat resisted her opinions about Bill and other life issues, the difficulties and bitterness between them became increasingly serious.

Pat's uncle, Jim, tried to stay out of the arguments in the foster home. He understood Christie's point of view, although he did not share it. Bill struck him as a fine young man. While their relationship was intense, Bill and Pat cared for one another; neither was prepared for anything beyond that. Jim shared the foster parents' concern about a second issue that was generating increasingly bitter controversy. Wendell and Christie agreed that Pat was too involved emotionally in the affiliated groups of Alcoholics Anonymous (AA), to which she devoted much time. To them, it did not seem natural for a fifteen-year-old girl, who had never herself had any problem with drinking, to spend two, three, or even four nights a week at Al-Anon or Alateen meetings.

Wendell took it as an insult. He felt it reflected on Pat's happiness in their home and felt it was a "put down" of his own drinking habits. Long before he knew Pat, he had decided he was not an alcoholic, and it troubled him now that Pat's preoccupation again brought the issue of drinking to the forefront of his life.

Faced with what they experienced as new challenges from Pat, Christie and Wendell responded as they did with their own children. They provided Pat with a structured but increasingly rigid set of rules and expectations to govern her conduct. Pat was to limit herself to seeing Bill one night a week during one of the Alateen meetings they both attended. In addition, they could talk on the phone one time a week for fifteen minutes. Further contact between the two was prohibited. Further, Pat was to return home immediately after school in the afternoon. She was to help Christie prepare the evening meal and then do her schoolwork. Her limited freedom would be to pick her own television shows and to follow her own interests (such as sewing) while around home.

If we think a moment about what is expectable in a young adult whose hard life experience has taught precocious and brittle control of emotion, we will understand that real trouble lay just ahead.

The Assessment

It is arbitrary to separate assessment from treatment. Treatment begins when the therapist first makes direct contact that has potential effect for the one treated. The clinician's assessment of therapeutic possibilities begins immediately with his first knowledge of facts relevant to the treatment process and does not end as long as he continues to think actively or creatively about it. From the first time I heard Pat's situation, I was confident treatment would prove helpful. My primary question was whether I would be able to engage the critical people in her life adequately so that they would permit treatment to take place.

I began assessment of Pat by interviewing her guardian and uncle, Dr. Jim Moriarty. He was a reserved man who did not trust easily. I saw him three times before I ever met with Pat. This was more time than I usually allot for attaining background information when I work with an adolescent. My purpose was to solidify my relationship with Dr. Moriarty so that, if Pat decided to leave the O'Donnels, I would continue to have his support for my work with her.

417

After telling me of Pat's childhood in his first two interviews, Dr. Moriarty told me about his own life in the third session. He felt guilty that he had not reached out more to his brother in the months before his suicide. He felt badly that he did not have the temperament to take in his brother's children. As he recounted his own life, expressed his guilt, and met with acceptance from me, he began to feel some confidence and trust.

It was Dr. Moriarty who made the decision to obtain psychiatric assessment for Pat. His primary concerns were, first, that Pat's nightmares had returned recently. He was also worried about Pat's adjustment to living in Christie and Wendell's home. As Christie employed increasingly severe sanctions as punishment for impudence or argument, a new equilibrium was being established that placed a great deal of pressure on Pat. Uncle Jim suspected Pat would soon insist on leaving if Christie stuck by the new regime. He knew of no suitable alternative possibilities for placement. He feared Pat might be pushed to elope with her boyfriend Bill. Finally, Jim was concerned with Pat's participation in the affiliated groups of AA. She accepted the AA philosophy, immersed herself in AA social structure, and seemed to let it dominate her life. He worried that Pat's involvement would focus her concern on past difficulties rather than on present possibilities. He thought that it might draw her inextricably into a social network of deeply disturbed people and that, over time, she might come to define herself negatively. Dr. Moriarty was a good historian. While he was not Pat's parent, he was well informed on many events of her life. I will not focus on her early history except to note that, in Pat's infancy, her mother lived an isolated life. While she was pleased to have a child, her own life was difficult. She may have been drinking heavily during this period.

It is certain that Pat's father drank heavily, and, by the time Pat was five, his drinking was of alcoholic proportions. That year, he suffered a job reversal to which he never adapted. From then on, he drank away his paycheck. Mrs. Moriarty went to work days to keep the family afloat. By the time Pat was ten, she had assumed the responsibility of housekeeper, caretaker to her younger siblings, and companion to her father.

Initial Contact with Pat

Pat was plain in appearance. At first she was subdued. From the start, however, she talked in a straightforward way and had the ability to establish emotional contact. Contact with her flowed spontaneously and without artificial barriers. When we first met, I told Pat that I needed to learn of her experience from her own point of view. I said I knew she had been through some unusually painful experiences, but I was impressed by what others told me about how strong she was in facing things.

"I've had a whole lot of help." She began to tell me about the people she knew in AA and how much they had done for her. She described simply, and without self-pity, her life before her parents' death. She had been trapped in a situation she had found nearly unbearable for the six years before her parents had died. During this period, not only was her father critical and contemptuous of her, but for about three years he had been physically abusive as well. No part of their life together had been too trivial to elicit disagreement. If she cooked rice, he wanted potatoes; and if she prepared potatoes, he wanted rice.

Pat experienced her mother as a kind of naive person who did not know how to cope with her father and was unable to protect the children from him. Her mother never acknowledged the seriousness of her father's drinking problem until a few months prior to his death. Pat and her mother had joined Al-Anon despite Mr. Moriarty's objections. It was through their experience in the group that each stopped minimizing the difficulties in the family relationship.

Mother's life had been one of pressure and privation. While she and Pat had been close earlier, she became increasingly irritable and demanding of Pat over the period when Pat needed to be much more heavily dependent on her. With the help of Al-Anon, a group for family members of alcoholics, Pat learned to stand up to her father in a way that she felt was healthy and helped restore her pride.

While her view of herself became much more solid, her father felt the groups were "turning her against him." He responded with increased violence. He often hit Pat; on one occasion, he broke her wrist. He injured her mother in one fight, and Pat had to call the police three times. One time she and her sister and brother were locked in the bedroom, and he wanted her to unlock the door. She refused. He never got over his anger about that. Later, at a time when feeling sorry for himself, he threw the incident up to her as an example of her pride and lack of appropriate respect for her father.

Finally, mother, with Pat's support, realized that her husband had to leave if any of them were to survive psychologically. Without the exploration, understanding, and support of the AA groups, neither Pat

419

nor her mother would have been ready to take this stand. Even then, mother opted to tell father by means of a note she left him one morning explaining that he had to leave that day. When Pat returned from school that day, her father had been drinking. He was enraged. He told Pat he was being kicked out. Pat told him that his drinking was a sickness; she hoped he would get over it. For now, it would be better if he were out. On the other hand, she had come over the last months to separate some tender feelings for her father from the hatred and frustration she felt toward what she now defined as his "illness." She told him, "I love you, Dad, and I hope you will be okay."

He stalked out but returned later and began to attack her verbally once more. His feelings became increasingly intense. He told Pat he was going to kill her. She realized fully the danger. She called Bill on the phone. When he rushed over, her father was gone. They decided to leave, but the ignition on Bill's car had been disconnected.

At about this time, Pat's mother, grandfather, and stepgrandmother arrived. They had assembled to decide what to do. Soon her father returned. He ordered Bill to take Pat outside. She defied him, staying where she was. She went over and turned on the television. Events then blurred. The next she knew, her father was back and had a gun. He shot her grandfather in the stomach. She, Bill, and her mother ran out of the house. She heard a shot and saw her mother fall. There were two more shots, then silence. She knew it was all over.

When the police arrived, it was 8:55 P.M. No one acknowledged that Pat's parents were dead until midnight, but Pat knew. She felt furious that no one talked to her. She felt angry in particular that "everyone spoke to me like I was a small child." She was not permitted to watch television or read the newspapers. "The grown-ups decided all the questions for the grown-ups." Pat's anger did not subside. When she was addressed, it was as a "poor little girl." "I did not look at it that way. I felt lucky to be alive."

Pat recalls a period of anxiety and tenseness that lasted until the funeral, when for the first time she cried. The night after the deaths, she and Bill went for a ride to get some time away. In a filling station, there was a tire-changing machine that made a noise like a gun. It went off just as they were driving away, and Bill nearly drove off the road. Pat felt the depth of her loneliness and sorrow at the funeral. Again, the adults made decisions to meet their own needs. Her mother and father were not buried together. Out of respect for her stepgrandmother who had survived, it was decided that the grandfather and Pat's mother should be buried together; Pat's father was buried elsewhere. It hurt Pat to think of her father as now so alone. Her mother had always stayed with him until the end. Except for the alcoholism, Pat was convinced that they loved one another.

It was clear in the first two interviews that Pat was intelligent and thoughtful. She seemed able to use me constructively, despite my sex, and was ready to work on her own behalf. Nonetheless, I felt it was essential to talk with Pat's foster mother, Christie O'Donnel, during the assessment before I decided to move ahead with individual psychotherapy. After the tragedy, Pat had taken part in an individual therapy with a school counselor. Christie had disrupted that treatment abruptly when she felt the counselor's stance had implied a criticism of her foster home situation. It was important that I have an alliance with Christie if a traumatic disruption in Pat's therapy was not to be repeated.

When I first met Christie, she seemed uncomfortable but also a strong and determined person. She was working class and spoke crudely and directly. She had qualities I admire, and I believe my respect was obvious. It helped in my initial contact that I had no illusions about the strength of my position with Christie. Pat had cautioned me that, if Christie felt left out or in any way pushed, she would "get her back up."

I know most people respond poorly if they feel themselves to be coerced within a relationship. So I approached Christie with no idea of getting her immediately to change her approach but rather with the goal of befriending her and offering her any help I might in a situation that I knew was difficult for all. Perhaps the fact that Christie had interfered in Pat's treatment at school helped her align herself behind treatment now. While she had won that first battle, she had since come to feel she might lose the war.

In any case, during the course of our first interview, Christie appeared to relax and to accept me as a straightforward person that she could trust well enough. Her manner and her words made it clear she would call the shots on the rules in her home. I would be useful if I could help Pat adapt to them. Christie was surprised to think treatment might involve weekly meetings for Pat. However, as she thought it over, she felt sure that Pat had not fully worked through the sadness of the experience of her parents' death, and she hoped that perhaps Pat could learn to be more open with her and less hostile. Finally, she hoped Pat might get more distance from the involvement in AA. She told me I had her permission to move ahead with treatment if I thought I could help.

Psychotherapy

It is helpful in describing Pat's treatment to isolate four important lines along which it developed: (1) the development of our own relationship and a therapeutic alliance, processes that were at first fostered by our focus on Pat's current life relationships with the people around her and by the process of reexperiencing the events of the tragedy and the emotions appropriate to them; (2) our joint meetings with others significant to Pat; (3) our work with intrapsychic issues, specifically the acknowledgment and understanding of her own intense sense of guilt in relation to her parent's death; and (4) supportive work in helping her to accept her adult sexuality as she came to acknowledge it more openly and to address the issues of sexual intimacy and birth control.

The Development of Our Relationship:
Pat's Relatedness to Others:
Reexperiencing the Emotions of the Tragedy

From the start Pat talked openly. She seemed hungry for a relationship and the opportunity to share her feelings and her experience. In the first two sessions, but to some extent in almost every session during the first six weeks of treatment, Pat reexperienced the day of the shootings. At first she seemed to relive the experience in telling it, permitting herself to feel the sadness fully. She would check out my reaction to what she had been through, wondering if I saw things differently than she and reassuring herself about "mistakes" she had made that avoided might have prevented the tragedy.

Equally important to our early relationship was her need for me to understand and accept her experience in Al-Anon and Alateen. Before she took part in the meetings, Pat had shared very little of her thoughts or feelings with anyone. She was shy and ashamed and did not open herself to others. In the self-help groups, she had always received

respectful attentiveness. When she participated, she was always encouraged to stand up for herself assertively.

My own ignorance of AA and its methods, not unusual at that time
for therapists dynamically trained, may not have been a total disadvantage. Pat was able to take the active role in educating me. I believe my
attitude of acceptance in contrast to her foster parent's rejection of Al-
Anon was a factor that strengthened our alliance. By the end of our first
three months of work together, there was a strong trust between us.

Joint Work with Significant Others

From time to time throughout the treatment, it became important to
Pat for me to intercede for her in the relationship with others critical
to her life circumstances. At other times, she just wanted to be sure I
knew "who she was talking about." Usually, we arranged that I meet
the person currently important, most often in a joint interview with
Pat. These interviews were scheduled at Pat's request. In responding
to her cues, I respected her autonomy. For Pat, this was a new form
of response from an adult. She had grown up in an authoritarian environment. Her foster parents and her father attempted to dominate
her behavior, blind and deaf to her inner feelings. They openly belittled
her AA experience. Her own mother too had used Pat psychologically
to meet her own needs—for her personal and emotional survival as
well as for the sake of family peace. The adults in AA had responded
sensitively to Pat's need for support, but their message to her was
determined by their own philosophy as much as her internal state. It
is my impression that I succeeded in establishing a climate in which
her foster parents could experience a more accepting way of reacting
to Pat. They were accessible because it mirrored their own individual
experience with me. I had respected the feelings of each and never
directly confronted their need to be in control.

I will describe two interviews. One was between Pat, Christie, and
myself; another was with both foster parents. Both were critical to the
success of the overall treatment endeavor.

During the course of the joint session with Christie, Pat was able to
relate differently to her than she had before. Until this point, Pat had
observed Christie carefully when they were together but was usually
passive, saying little. In this interview, for the first time she actively

described her own feelings to Christie. She explained graphically, but not hostilely, how frightened she had felt at others' anger ever since the day of the "accident." She described to Christie the intensity of her father's eyes and the anger in his voice before he left the house on that last day. She told Christie that now when the two of them fought together Pat felt a stronger reaction inside than made sense. She said she could understand now that her own behavior made Christie angry because she was learning to see things from another's point of view.

Christie responded in a very human way. She told Pat of some of the violence she had experienced in her own household as a child. She explained how she felt now when Pat would not obey. She pointed out that, while she knew she yelled, she had never hit Pat. She would have hit her own children if they had ever made her feel as deeply hurt and angry as Pat had made her feel.

Following this session, there was a significant shift in their relating to one another. They did not find that their difficulties evaporated, but Pat always had a feeling thereafter that she did not really need to feel deeply afraid of Christie. Over the week that followed this interview, the communication remained more open, if not always less tempestuous. In talking with me, Pat began to refer a lot more to Wendell. "He's coming out of the woodwork. He made jokes with me about when are Bill and I getting married. He said he had decided on his engagement present—he was going to get Bill a ladder." Pat could see the hostility in this line of banter at a time when Bill and she were trying to resist the idea of running off together, but "at least you can deal with him" when he said what was on his mind.

Pat felt it would be useful if she could talk with both foster parents together with me. She noticed that, when she related to them alone, "they play each other off with me," and she thought that, if we could all three talk directly together, it would be a help. Also, she was feeling increasingly ambitious, and she thought maybe she could help them become less hostile to the idea of her role in AA.

So I agreed to contact Wendell and see if he would be willing to come in. There followed a number of communications between us (some transmitted via Pat or Christie), culminating in a couple of telephone calls. First, he established that if we were to have contact he would call the shots. Second, if we were to meet it would have to be on the basis of his schedule. No daytime hours would do, so we had to set it up in an evening meeting. I deferred to Wendell for at that stage, if there had been any power struggle I had insisted on winning, he would have refused to participate.

When Pat, Christie, Wendell, and I finally sat down in the office, I felt a pall in the air. Wendell was a heavyset man with all the hostility of an Archie Bunker but without Archie's wit and charm. I admired Pat's self-possession as she took over the proceedings during the lengthening pause that followed after I introduced myself to Wendell. In the heaviness of the silence, Pat turned to me and said, "I told you I wanted to share a poem last time we talked, so I brought it along." The poem, entitled "A Day without Prayer Is Like a Day without Sunshine," was written by a friend in school. It was written in adolescent argot. While the poem was long, the lines were spare and terse. It described the feelings of an adolescent who had experienced a number of disappointments. She sits down discouraged, jealous of others around her, and criticizes God for not helping. The poem concludes:

> Why didn't you help me today
> Was it too big of a task?
> God came down and said to me
> "Kid you didn't ask!"

I was touched by her reading of the poem and by Pat's attempt to reach out to the adults around her by sharing it. I commented, "Wendell, that does say something to me; what's your reaction?" He replied, "I'm not into poetry. Most poets are trapped in the big I." I replied spontaneously with blank misunderstanding, "What do you mean? . . . they are too selfish? . . . too tied up with their own point of view?"

Christie broke in, "What he means is, he doesn't understand it." The ice was broken. Wendell then rose to his own defense, elaborating his response rather than hiding it. He expressed his concern that, even though Pat had had big problems, "She sinks into them too much. With all the Al-Anon and Alateen, sometimes she doesn't have anything left over for her sister Peggy, her brother Joseph, or the rest of us." That was why he and Christie felt it was so important to limit her. For them, limiting the meetings was trying to limit what they experienced as self-involvement that was hard on the family.

Pat did not back down from her point of view. She managed powerfully and economically to convey the degree she still felt troubled by

425

a sense of guilt in her life. She made clear the importance of the AA experience in helping her deal with that sense of inner unworthiness. She responded somewhat concretely to Wendell's accusation that she did not care for her brother Joseph.

She said she could not stand to see Joseph at that time because she felt so badly about his being left to be raised by Aunt Priscilla. Aunt Priscilla, her mother's sister, represented the worst for Pat. She thought her a self-centered lady who had intruded into the lives of others to meet her own needs. Pat was convinced she remained, despite denial and deception, an alcoholic who was drinking daily before noon. Priscilla had her own need to establish a version of the tragedy, which Pat felt was not accurate. When she differed with Pat's assessment of the family difficulties, she accused Pat of distorting what had happened. Her hatred of Pat's father had led her to place all the family's difficulties on the father. Furthermore, at times when she felt irritated she told Pat that if the tragedy was not her father's fault it was Pat's. Priscilla said the parents would not have argued so much with one another if Pat had been less difficult.

Finally, Pat complained she could not stand Priscilla because she tried to control Pat's behavior. When Pat visited for a week at Thanksgiving, Priscilla had granted and withheld the privilege of going to Alateen meetings because she found that with these manipulations she could successfully control Pat's behavior. For the first time, Christie and Wendell were able to see their own attempts at controlling Pat in a new perspective. Negotiation around the group meeting attendance was still required after this session, but Pat felt the interaction changed its quality. Thereafter, Christie and Wendell listened more often to her reasons without blindly trying to control her actions.

I believe my presence with Wendell, Christie, and Pat played a role in shifting the equilibrium between them while we were together. Each felt a little less beleaguered, less under pressure, and more able to observe, listen, and reflect. Even a small shift in this dimension was significant for them because it helped them form a nucleus of experience with one another that was new and could subsequently grow. When they had responded more directly together, attending to the other's perception as well as their own, there were shifts in their perspective of one another. This experience carried over into their interaction when they were apart.

The Emergence of Intrapsychic Issues

Following this interview, the climate shifted significantly at home. There was much less fighting, and Pat did not feel so submerged in nameless anger. As she felt less bad, she was able to enter a period in therapy during which her focus shifted from the frustrations of her relations with others, and she had energy available to examine her own inner life.

In a subsequent interview, Pat came in looking frightened. She told me there was a large spiderweb on the stairs leading to my office. She remembered that once, when she was five years old, she had awakened one morning to find a spider sitting on her nose, "right between my eyes." She had been terrified. The image of the spider led her thoughts to Christie. Part of her problem with Christie was, she said, that "I feel she's trying to take my mother's place. I don't feel I can be open with her. If I let her take my mother's place then my mother will be really gone." She began to think of how much she missed her mother now. There had been a long period in her life when she had felt no gratitude to her mother. When her mother left to go to work, Pat had missed her terribly. She felt hurt and angry to be left alone with her father with no protection from him. Since that time when she met with other mothers from the Al-Anon group, she could look at her own situation more realistically. She felt bad when she thought back on how artificially high her expectations of her mother had been and the depth of the disappointment she had felt with her.

Further, she felt guilty recalling when, after her mother had been going to Al-Anon, she had turned to Pat asking if she should leave her husband. Pat had told her that she should. Even now when she thought how directly that particular decision had led to the tragedy that followed, she felt queasy. She continued to talk of her view of her parents. Her relation with her mother had troubles in it, but she could always evoke a clear image of her mother as someone who knew how to comfort her with a hug or a kiss.

With her father it was different. She could not evoke pleasant images of him when she recalled their experience. "Nice pictures like that would be unreal. Really he drank and beat me. That I will never miss. The only father I can miss is one that could have been, not one I really knew."

Nonetheless, as she permitted herself to recall some of her experiences with her father, we did uncover germinal events that had never fully flowered, that had provided fragmentary experiences of a better kind. Pat had never been able to integrate these as a consistently positive part of her life that she could reliably evoke by herself. It was true that her father had drunk heavily and had been largely unavailable as his problems became increasingly insurmountable. Earlier, though, Pat recalled that it had been father who taught her to drive. She had been eleven then. Her father had needed her to drive to the liquor store when he was too drunk to drive himself. He was dependent on her in that way and tried at times to stay on her good side so she would comply.

Pat recalled some other more pleasant times. Unhappily, the good experiences had themselves been interwoven with more painful ones. An example arose when she told me of a repetitive dream that bothered her. In the dream her father shot her. While its libidinal overtones were obvious, I responded to this dream at first as if it were only a relatively simple anxiety dream, a traumatic repetition of the death scene she had so narrowly avoided. The dream led her to memories of actual life experiences in which she had learned to shoot a gun with her father. One of his few friends during the years of hard drinking was a drinking companion, a black policeman. The three had enjoyed some good times together. Pat learned to shoot a gun under the guidance of her father and his friend.

In the appointment before her seventeenth birthday, Pat came in in a lightly ironic mood. She said, "Sweet sixteen and never been kissed. Isn't that a laugh? Nowadays most girls who are fourteen have had intercourse." She let her thoughts wander freely, and soon she was feeling sad as she shared with me how inhibited and frightened she felt with Bill at times when, enjoying their kissing and caressing, he had pushed for greater intimacy. The mixed feeling of excitement, discomfort, and something near disgust she felt when she thought of her genitals being stimulated may have helped her recover memories that followed.

Pat had known the O'Donnels for years before she lived with them. Their son, Willy, had been Pat's closest friend. She now recovered a series of memories in which Willy and she had been with her father together. The mood had not been hostile. Father showed the two of them his camera and let them use it. On one occasion, he persuaded

Willy to be photographed in the nude. He urged Pat to take part as well. She had refused to pose, but she still found the idea of her father's interest in exhibitionist sexuality exciting. It was when she recalled the nature of her feeling then that she began to understand her experience of guilt in her current life in a new way.

Underlying her conscious sense of guilt (if she and her mother had not taken part in Al-Anon and threatened father with the loss of their relatedness, if she had taken the bullets out of his gun before the accident, if she had called the police) there was a guilt that was even more powerful despite the fact that it had been unconscious. It was only as Pat got near her sense of unconscious longing for and repulsion by a forbidden infantile sexuality with her father that she could find relief from the powerful sense of self-criticism that stubbornly shaped her feelings about herself in her current life.

In the final phase of treatment, Pat's focus shifted back to current concerns. She became quite interested in learning about her body. She read *Our Bodies/Ourselves* (Mayhew 1971) at my suggestion. She found it helpful, and she and Bill read it together. Together, they confronted their sexual relationship in a new way. They shared their own feelings and responses with one another, talking together.

Despite the new energy and interest in their sexual education, they decided that they did not want to have intercourse for the present. While they educated themselves on birth control, they decided to defer intercourse for now. They decided that, while their relationship was a deeply serious one, they were not ready to make a final commitment to one another. While Bill bought her a ring that looked to my eye very like an engagement ring, they explained that they were not "engaged." The ring was just to be a real symbol of the seriousness of their intentions to one another. For the time being, they decided Bill should enter the service and get more advanced technical training. This plan would necessitate a year's separation. After that period, they would have the chance to be together again, and then they would reassess their long-range expectations and hopes for one another.

After nine months of therapy, Pat decided that she felt comfortable with the main issues inside herself and with her life. She wrote me about six months later. She said her life was going well. She had graduated from high school, had a job that pleased her, and was happy. Bill was in the service, still away, and both were looking forward to resuming their relationship when he returned.

Discussion

As we have seen, Pat underwent an extraordinary experience that threatened her life as well as her psychological equilibrium. She lost her grandmother. She lost her mother. She lost her father. Each loss was acute and unexpected. She narrowly escaped being murdered. The murderer was her own father. She witnessed a multiple murder–suicide. Despite the enormous potential of Pat's experience for causing trauma, she adjusted with a minimum of symptomatology and made a promising initial adaptation. Her psychological growth did not appear to be blocked. Her failure to be more grossly traumatized by such extreme life experiences poses issues for the psychoanalytic theory of trauma. For the purposes of this discussion, I will refer primarily to an earlier theoretical synthesis not alluded to in the earlier review of the literature, that of Rangell (1967). Rangell's articulation of the dynamic metapsychological framework has particular relevance for Pat's experience. Using a mixture of historic, descriptive, and metapsychological approaches, he arrived at a "composite description—still not rigorously a definition of trauma" (p. 80): "A traumatic occurrence is characterized by the intrusion into the psychic apparatus of a stimulus or series of stimuli (the traumatic event), varying in their qualitative manifest contents, in their quantitative characteristics, and their time relationships, which set up an unconscious train of intra-psychic events (the traumatic process) beyond the capacity of the ego to master at that particular time."

The central elements in Rangell's definition are traumatic event, traumatic process, and the resulting state of dysfunction resulting from the ego's unsuccessful attempts at adaptation and mastery. The core of his concern is the convergence of painful external reality and underlying unconscious vulnerability. This definition of trauma is broad enough to encompass a wide range of external stimuli; yet the formulation takes account of the delicate balance between external reality and internal psychological state, appropriately placing emphasis on the "unconscious train of intra-psychic events (the traumatic process)" that is set off by real life experiences.

Rangell (1967) differentiates the manifest (conscious) and the latent (unconscious) aspects of the traumatic process, stating, "It is the latent and unconscious meaning of the psychic event that is most crucial in determining the course and outcome" (p. 66). This distinction provides

430

us with a basis for understanding why Pat's initial adaptation to her loss was so much smoother and quicker than we might have expected.

Pat's unconscious experience as expressed in the quality of her self- and object representations and their differentiation from one another underwent a dramatic reorganization following the catastrophe. The balance between negative inner images derived from unresolved aggression and positive ones expressing loving energies shifted dramatically, with positive images becoming predominant.

Following her parents' death, for the first time in her life Pat had the possibility of consolidating positive parental images and the emotional associations they engendered. Her parents no longer intruded on her daily in hurtful ways. Their death provided her a moratorium for the reintegration of her prior experience.

I believe Pat had had solid early mothering, which met the predominance of her needs well during her infancy and toddlerhood. The negative maternal images arising from later life experiences when her mother was not available physically and psychologically were not all she had to draw on. Pat had always been able to evoke a comforting inner image of a mother who cared for her. At the time of the catastrophe, Pat's positive inner maternal images now converged with an actual life experience in which her mother died while trying to help her separate physically and psychologically from the father who tormented them. Her mother had taken a stand for her children, and her death was experienced as a loving and heroic act by Pat. Her image in death became a protective and caring one. She had given her life for Pat. Her actions taking a stand with Pat against the father evoked loving feelings in Pat and a view of herself as cared for and worthy of care.

Simultaneously, also at the latent level, positive images of the father, although tenuous and dissonant, from her actual life experience could consolidate once he was gone. Pat succeeded in segregating what was oppressive in him as part of an "illness," his alcoholism, from which he suffered as truly as did the other family members. Further, she integrated latent unconscious fantasies of a good father rarely experienced with isolated and inconsistent islands of positive experience remembered from real life. It was her father who taught her to drive. Her father had shared his policeman friend, and they had taught Pat to shoot. Even the repressed experience of her father's sexual interest in her had left her with the feeling that she had some potential effect

431

on his impulses and that, at some level, she was a positive object of his desire.

At the manifest level of her experience, Pat's participation with the Al-Anon groups had a particular effect on her because it was highly appropriate developmentally. At a time when she was actively struggling to establish her autonomy, her experience in the group offered her an enhanced understanding of her life situation, and the members of the group fostered her independence from her parents and provided her a caring network of people outside her home. Her relationship with her boyfriend, Bill, consolidated her sense of herself as a person who was taken seriously, admired, and loved. The psychotherapy experience with me gave her a conscious understanding of the reality and power of her sense of guilt about her relationship with her parents while they were living. The experience with Al-Anon, Bill, and me converged to support at both latent and manifest levels Pat's successful adaptation.

Rangell's (1967) differentiation between traumatic event and traumatic process addresses a significant confusion that permeates early psychoanalytic theorizing about psychic trauma. In the early literature on trauma, the single term "trauma" was used to allude to the internal state produced in a person who had undergone a difficult life experience as well as to allude to the difficult life experience itself. In theorizing on trauma, many early authors focused primarily on a population of patients distinguished by their severe and persistent states of disorganization following the difficult life experience. A conception of trauma resulted that emphasized the dysfunction of the traumatized individual. No adequate consideration was given to the experience of individuals who faced extraordinarily difficult life events and were subsequently able to adapt to or even to master them.

While it is not a central focus of his discussion, Rangell (1967) seems sensitive to this issue, noting at one point "a positive effect of trauma that stimulates efforts to confront and overcome it," as well as "a negative effect that aims toward repression and avoidance" (p. 77).

It is my impression, on the basis of my work with Pat, that she actually emerged stronger and freer, following the hard experience of loss, than she had been before. I believe that the processes of trauma and mastery are often mirror images of one another, two sides of a single coin. Both are responses to the interplay within the individual between unconscious fantasy and external reality.

Some vulnerable individuals find a confirmation of destructive fantasies in traumatic life experience. The trauma is experienced unconsciously as a justifiable event consonant with their bad inner state. Hence, the disaster cannot be dismissed as a fluke, meaningless psychologically, over and now in the past; but it lingers in the mind, shaping future expectation. A persistent sense of unworthiness becomes the matrix of future life experience. The individual with an unconscious sense of latent good inside, achieved by the healthy evolution of early narcissism and subsequent evolution of ego competence, may be able to integrate potentially traumatic experiences without succumbing to them. The individual who can integrate the spectrum of his own inner fantasy with the facts of the real life tragedy and understand that the two worlds of experience, while interrelated, are discrete is able to master the catastrophic event.

An adequate theory of trauma must encompass successful attempts at mastery of situations that objectively appear overwhelming. Such a theory will emphasize the enduring effect of such difficult experiences on the personality of the person who masters them. Even when traumatic situations are successfully weathered, the experience provides an organizing nucleus for the individual's subsequent adaptation. Never forgotten, it can provide a nucleus of experience that serves as the basis of enhanced insight and compassion, leaving some psychological survivors with an enhanced ability to weather hardship, to sustain a satisfying image of themselves, and to sustain a relatedness with others.

Conclusions

The chapter describes the response of a fourteen-year-old girl to personal catastrophe. She was present when her father shot and killed her mother, her grandfather, and himself. With the support of participation in the component groups of AA, she made a surprisingly successful initial adaptation to her loss. Nearly one year after the tragedy, symptoms of anxiety and depression recurred. Her treatment for nine months in psychoanalytically oriented individual psychotherapy is described.

The technical problems of balancing a therapeutic approach that responded to the demands of significant others in her environment as well as of sustaining an intrapsychic focus that helped her understand the unconscious roots of her guilt are considered. The psychoanalytic theory of trauma is summarized as it relates to the life and therapeutic experiences of the adolescent described.

REFERENCES

American Psychiatric Association. 1980. *Diagnostic and Statistical Manual of Mental Disorders*. 3d ed. Washington, D.C.: American Psychiatric Association.

Breuer, J., and Freud, S. 1895. Studies on hysteria. *Standard Edition* 2:3–17. London: Hogarth, 1955.

Figley, C., ed. 1985. *Trauma and Its Wake*. New York: Brunner/Mazel.

Freud, S. 1920. Beyond the pleasure principle. *Standard Edition* 18:7–64. London: Hogarth, 1955.

Freud, S. 1926. Inhibitions, symptoms and anxiety. *Standard Edition* 20:77–175. London: Hogarth, 1959.

Green, B.; Wilson, J.; and Lindy, J. 1985. Conceptualizing post-traumatic stress disorder: a psychosocial framework. In C. Figley, ed. *Trauma and Its Wake*. New York: Brunner/Mazel.

Horowitz, M. J. 1986. *Stress Response Syndrome*. Northvale, N.J.: Aronson.

Mayhew, A., ed. 1971. *Our Bodies/Ourselves*. Boston: Boston Women's Health Book Collective.

Pynoos, R., and Eth, S. 1985. Developmental perspective on psychic trauma in childhood. In C. Figley, ed. *Trauma and Its Wake*. New York: Brunner/Mazel.

Rangell, L. 1967. The metapsychology of psychic trauma. In S. Furst, ed. *Psychic Trauma*. New York: Basic.

Rothstein, A. 1986. *The Reconstruction of Trauma: Its Significance in Clinical Work*. Madison, Conn.: International Universities Press.

Terr, L. 1981. Psychic trauma in children. *American Journal of Psychiatry* 138:14–19.

Wilson, J.; Smith, W. K.; and Johnson, S. 1985. Comparative analysis of P.T.S.D. among various survey groups. In C. Figley, ed. *Trauma and Its Wake*. New York: Brunner/Mazel.

28 DISADVANTAGED ADOLESCENTS SEPARATING FROM HOME AND HOSPITAL: SPANNING THE ANTIPODES THROUGH PARADOX

DEBRA SCHNALL AND JOSEPH YOUNGERMAN

In psychiatric hospitals serving impoverished communities, it is a commonplace observation that the treatment of patients is encumbered by social and economic factors in any number of striking and subtle ways. In treatments spanning charged dichotomies, socioeconomic as well as psychological, how therapists and patients unwittingly participate in and extricate themselves from societal patterns and transferential misperceptions is often elusive. For example, in hospitalizing children from disadvantaged backgrounds, therapists and family members alike may be adversely influenced by the economic and social disparities between the home and the hospital. Such socioeconomic realities may foster the child's adoption by the institution (Palmer, Harper, and Rivinus 1983) with the active collaboration of the rescuing staff and the abandoning family. The structure of inpatient therapy, in which the child patient is intensively treated in a therapeutic milieu while the family is seen only adjunctively (Greenberg 1982; Meeks 1980; Simmel 1929), further reenforces this perceived dichotomy between the depriving family and the providing hospital.

In the traditional psychiatric literature, Rinsley (1965, 1968) has emphasized parents' overt resistance to the hospitalization of their children. Masterson (1972) has urged an initial treatment plan that severely restricts parental visitation of hospitalized borderline adolescents. By contrast, we are reporting the antipodal problems encountered in the hospital treatment of a vastly different population: abused and abandoned adolescents from an inner-city ghetto. Often the broken trail of courts, agencies, foster homes, and residences has left these children virtually orphaned long before they reach our tertiary-care public psychiatric hospital. In many instances, the initial and continuing family approach is the task of simply locating a family or family member that has been or can become connected to the hospitalized child. Even when such a connection can be forged, unwarranted overdetermined dependency on the hospital may persist as a central issue. If the pitfalls of psychologically and socioeconomically prolonged length of stays are to be avoided, the deeply rooted transference and countertransference issues of institutional dependency must be directly confronted (Halperin, Lauro, Miscione, Rebhan, Schnabolk, and Shachter 1981).

In the treatment reported, a family pushed the pathological splitting between provident hospital and destructive family to an absurd conclusion by serially presenting for hospitalization one child after another with psychotic symptomatology. The first child presented without a family. After the second was hospitalized, family therapy was finally able to be initiated, but the considerable therapeutic zeal of the hospital staff became depleted in the family's endless consumption of multiple treatment modalities. When a third sibling requested hospitalization, the staff could no longer ignore the caveat that "the presence of an accepting and cooperative attitude towards hospitalization [is] an ominous sign" (Hendrickson, Holmes, and Waggoner 1959, p. 527). Either the entire family had to be hospitalized, or the fundamental premise of hospital treatment, by which individuals were "rescued" from their family, had to be radically altered.

At this therapeutic impasse, the introduction of a parameter appeared urgently necessary. To protect the directly supportive individual and family interventions from being swamped by the family's symbiotic neediness, paradoxical therapy techniques were introduced. What evolved was a family treatment that employed paradox (Bergman 1980; Papp 1981; Selvini-Palazzoli, Boscolo, Cecchin, and Prata 1978; Watzlawick 1978; Watzlawick, Weakland, and Fisch 1974) to disengage the family from their overly dependent merging with the idealized hospital family (Looney, Blotcky, Carson, and Gossett 1980). The therapists' self-contradictory instruction to the family was to follow not the hospital staff's recommendations but the previous family authority, an absent grandmother who personified the pathological family tradition of incest and abuse. By refusing this paradoxical instruction, the family established its autonomy. An additional aspect of this treatment was that splitting was acknowledged within the hospital staff (Kernberg 1975, 1976) and therapeutically structured (Kolb and Shapiro 1982) to further the independence of the family both from its own past tradition of incest (Gutheil and Avery 1977) and from its new iatrogenic dependency on the hospital. The family was required to accept itself as organized and competent enough to care for its children, while the hospital staff was constrained to accept themselves as less than totally benevolent and omnipotent, as even at times fragmented, furious, and depressed, and yet as still caring and effective. Such strategies severely strained but ultimately strengthened not only the family but the hospital staff as well.

Individual Alliances

A pubertal girl of twelve was hospitalized for suicidal ideation with sexualized auditory and visual hallucinations. She reported men's voices propositioning her and scenes of people having sex. During latency, Jeannette and her older sister had been sexually abused by their mother's boyfriend. They were sent out of state to their paternal grandparents' home. After a year, the patient, though not her older sister, returned home, where the sexual abuse began anew. When she finally told her teacher, she was again removed from the home and placed in a residence. She complained that boys were bothering her sexually and was placed in a foster home, where she enjoyed the foster mother's interest in her grooming and hygiene but began to experience sexual hallucinations and suicidal ideas that led to acute hospitalization. When the symptoms did not remit, she was transferred to our tertiary-care, state-funded hospital for extended treatment.

On her admission, our staff was faced with a common problem: the individual treatment of a seriously disturbed youngster quite separated from her family through multiple placements. In fact, a city-agency caseworker had to sign her into the hospital. Her family, who had no telephone, did not respond to letters or telegrams for months. As the clear alternative to familial abandonment, Jeannette was adopted by the hospital staff and, in turn, adopted the hospital. Aspiring to be a nurse, she walked the ward with a hygiene text under her arm. Though still hallucinating and suicidal, she began attending the hospital school, worked on her personal hygiene with the nursing staff, participated

437

increasingly in art and athletics programs, and attended twice-a-week individual psychotherapy sessions.

For several months, Jeannette lived within the hospital without any contact with her family. Finally, in response to yet another letter, her mother appeared in the hospital lobby, fifty minutes late for the scheduled appointment. Choosing not to criticize but simply to chat with her in the lobby, the therapist made an explicit decision not to pressure the mother to join the hospital treatment of her daughter. One month later, mother and therapist met again at an event for the youngsters and their families. A relationship was now established. Soon weekly sessions began, with the emphasis on practical help with current everyday problems of housing, welfare, and family life.

After several months, the mother's concerns turned more specifically to problems with her elder son, Michael, age eleven, who was reporting terrifying hallucinations, seeing knives and hearing voices telling him to kill his mother. With his mother's consent, a rapid assessment was followed by acute hospitalization. Though Michael welcomed hospitalization because it promised relief from his terror, he desperately missed his mother and indignantly resented any restrictions. Limit setting precipitated attacks of unbearable humiliation, wild rages of cursing and throwing, and confused medleys of threats and fears: his mother was coming to kill the staff; he must be discharged to protect his dead or dying mother. In a panic, he threatened his self-dismemberment with a plastic cafeteria knife. Once he cut himself with broken safety glass and battered himself on the seclusion room wall. Violence to the point of murder toward himself and his mother was the major issue of his treatment, in distinct contrast to his sister's fears of sexual attack. Although the form of their symptomatology was similar (i.e., auditory and visual hallucinations), the content was quite dissimilar (i.e., matricidal and aggressive for Michael, suicidal and sexualized for Jeannette).

In part, this dissimilarity was based on a profound difference in their mother's presence. During Jeannette's acute hospitalization, the mother had been completely absent for months; while for Michael's acute hospitalization, she was erratically present. She continuously announced her visits but arrived unpredictably. Whenever she broke her promise to visit, Michael would pace the ward in mounting agitation, often striking another child. He split the female staff into the good and the evil. With the idealized staff, he found intolerable, and would vehemently deny, any small discrepancy between his expectations and their behavior. With the evil staff, at times he reached the delusional belief that they were deliberately trying to hurt or to kill him and then provocatively precipitated punishment or seclusion. Whenever his mother did visit, she brought sacks of food and was greeted with excited hugs and kisses. This tired, obese woman and solemn, withdrawn child then became lively and animated together, he the charming entertainer, she the warmly responsive and undividedly attentive audience.

Although Michael's hallucinations did somewhat abate, his fantasies and fears of killing first his mother and then himself continued and were enacted in numerous rage attacks on the acute unit. After five months, it proved necessary to transfer him to our extended-care facility.

Meanwhile, at home, the next younger sibling, ten-year-old Tony, became acutely symptomatic one month after his brother's acute hospitalization. He reported auditory hallucinations of his former stepfather telling him to kill his mother or else be killed himself while he slept. Although he had no intention of ever hurting his mother, Tony was terrified by these hallucinations. Matricide clearly persisted as an issue for the sons in this family.

On evaluation, Tony physically looked like a junior version of his mother and interacted with her like his elder brother: he entertained her, bouncing and bubbling in his chair, the comic clown in dramatic counterpoint to her tragic posture. Together, the two of them, detailing their separate hypochondriacal complaints, could amuse each other to the point of tearful laughter, which they were at a loss to explain. Our initial attempts to separate Tony's anxieties and complaints from those of his older brother, and from those of his mother, were not successful. He insisted on the separate reality of his own distress, and his mother insisted she was unable to sleep soundly with any son at home hallucinating murder. To forestall yet another hospitalization, we reluctantly prescribed medication: twenty-five milligrams of thioridazine at bedtime for Tony and a mild anxiolytic for mother, who was complaining of tension and shortness of breath. Fortunately, the pharmacological management of these symptoms did obviate the need for another hospitalization. Several months later, when Tony was seen without his mother for a more extensive evaluation, his affect was appropriate, his focus was his school difficulties, and he comported himself like a mature and articulate fifth grader. As his hallucinations had ceased, his medication was discontinued. His individual problems seemed mild in comparison to the overwhelming difficulties he had displayed in the midst of his family.

Family Alliances

Throughout this period, there were separate individual therapies of the children in varying stages of evaluation and treatment. The boys spoke of their hallucinations of aggression and of their fears of matricide and of being murdered. Jeannette spoke of her sexual hallucinations and of her fantasies of merging with her mother or with her boyfriend sexually.

It was not the individual treatment of the three siblings but the individual work with the mother that was the cornerstone for the subsequent family treatment. The mother grew to realize her multiple needs for help in parenting her children. In her individual sessions, she had begun to question why all her children had problems, to talk about her former boyfriend who had sexually abused her daughters, and, finally, to disclose her own incestuous rape, which had resulted in her first pregnancy. She had never expressed a word of anger about her second pregnancy, which was the result of her mother's locking her in the bedroom with a man, but had accepted her mother's indictment of her as a bad mother. With therapy, she became able to defend herself against her mother's continuing verbal attacks and broke her previous tacit identification with her mother by explicitly telling her daughters not to have sexual relations with their boyfriends. She even brought her own current boyfriend into couples therapy, which was arranged at a local community mental health center.

It was in this context that family therapy was finally able to be initiated. The cotherapists were the individual therapists of Michael and of Jeannette and mother. In the very first session, the family indicated its willingness to organize itself as a distinct unit by deciding that an uncle living in their apartment needed to leave. How the children leave the family then became the central issue in the therapy. It became clear that sons and daughters have distinctly different ways of leaving home. The boys get their push out of the family through real or fantasied acts of aggression; hallucinated matricide or actual fights necessitate their leaving home to haunt either the streets or the hospitals. On the other hand, the girls leave home, on some level under the aegis of their mother, by getting raped or by getting pregnant. These family patterns, first inchoately recognized in the mother's individual sessions, were clarified and expanded within the family meetings. The family was repeatedly asked whether the children would follow these family traditions.

With the family's permission, the sessions were videotaped for supervision. Extensive family resistances then pushed the therapists to introduce a new parameter, following Selvini-Palazzoli et al. (1978): the videotapes would be reviewed by an imaginary team of family therapy experts who would define in writing their own ideas about family dynamics. This strategy allowed the cotherapists to join with the family in opposing the experts' paradoxical instructions, which were simply positive restatements of the family's traditional patterns. For example, when the family began missing sessions, they received a detailed letter (excerpted below) from the imaginary team of experts, paradoxically urging them to continue the tradition of separating the children from the family by sexual, aggressive, and psychotic acts:

Dear Family,

The team has seen the last videotape, and agrees with Tony that the family should not talk bad about Grandmother. She is very smart and very exciting and the whole family can learn from her.

Grandmother knows that a family can survive sex between fathers and daughters but that sex between mothers and sons would break up the family. As Michael and Tony are changing from boys into young men, the family could be destroyed by sex between mother and them. Michael has protected the family against this possibility by leaving home to come to the hospital, and Tony hides his masculine body by keeping his baby fat.

The team thinks that the boys should go on helping mother like this. They should only stop when she has completely learned her lessons from grandmother.

On receiving this letter, the family did not miss their next session. Indeed, they came in an uproar. The girls protested that, contrary to family tradition, they were not going to get pregnant before they were married and that they were going to finish school. Mother applauded and announced further changes at home. She had purchased four separate beds, one for each child; and she had bought new books and magazines for the children, replacing the pornographic magazines she had previously bought to help the girls understand "how to get along with men."

After a period of rapid changes in the family, resistances again intensified to planned changes of staff and transfer from inpatient to day-treatment status. A final paradoxical letter was sent to the family cautioning them further against changing too quickly:

Dear Family,

The team of family experts wants to say goodbye for the summer and to congratulate the family. Once again the cotherapists and the entire hospital staff are pushing too hard for change, as shown by Michael's partial discharge to day treatment. The family is smart to resist the hospital's push for change.

The team feels that it is more important to the family to listen to grandmother than to the staff of the hospital. She is a very good family therapist and the family should take all their problems to her during the summer and follow her directions. She will teach people to avoid jealousy between mothers and daughters and to avoid sex between mothers and sons. Mother and the children have learned their lessons well, and grandmother can continue to help them.

Jeannette can always act crazy again in order to avoid jealousy between herself and mother. Michael can also act crazy to live in the hospital again if things get too sexy at home. Tony can continue to be the baby in the family and stay at home to protect the family from the fact that he is growing up. Mother can avoid jealousy and remain loyal to grandmother by not marrying her boyfriend.

The family can continue to help the hospital staff feel important and useful by letting them know about the family problems and acting like they need to be taken care of all the time. This will keep mother, grandmother, and the hospital staff from getting depressed. Be sure to keep this letter and read it each Friday night at dinner.

In the final stages of hospital treatment, the outrage in the family, which these letters had produced, was matched by an outrage in the hospital. The hospital interdisciplinary treatment teams reacted to the letters of the imaginary expert family therapy team as they had originally reacted to the family: they were inhuman, uncaring, destructive, and flagrantly insensitive to symptoms. The splitting that had occurred between staff and family had become transposed into a split within the hospital staff. While the family had begun to make consistent progress, the staff had begun to argue constantly, and heatedly, about the family. There was scant agreement about what to write in the medical records, let alone how to work in a concerted cooperative way with these patients. Team meetings degenerated from productive task-oriented discussions to extended emotionally overwrought debates. The primary therapists were seen as neglectful parents by the nursing and program staff, who asked how patients could be allowed to live at home when they often come to the hospital school with unwashed hair and dirty, ill-fitting clothes.

In spite of, or because of, this split within the hospital staff, the youngsters were able to manage at home. Both were permitted an extended period of day treatment and then placed in regular public schools for the new school year. The ongoing outpatient couples therapy was transformed into outpatient family therapy that did not require paradoxical parameters, and the youngsters and the family were successfully discharged from the hospital. A year later, mother proudly came to show the wedding pictures of her not pregnant but married eldest daughter. After three years of intensive work, a new family tradition had been forged.

Discussion

To the majority of our patients who live in a socially and economically disadvantaged inner-city area, the grounds and facilities of the hospital, with its swimming pool and polished wood gymnasium floor, may look at first glance like a health club or recreational resort. Burned-out buildings abutting vermin-infested, erratically heated apartments stand in striking contrast to the spacious, semiprivate, well-heated, and even air-conditioned dormitory rooms of the hospital. Only the institutional food, nowhere near the standard of mother's home cooking, tarnishes the idealized image of the hospital. For many deprived youngsters, the initial stage of hospitalization is a wondrous summer camp experience. Not only is the hospital spacious and the staff caring and supportive, but the real problems of teenage life within the family and the city are distant.

For the staff as well, part of the early alliance with the patients may be based on splitting: now that these youngsters are here in the hospital, they are good, and the family is distant and bad. Individual work with the patient, whether in school, on the ward, in art or recreational therapy, or in individual psychodynamic sessions, may perpetuate this view of a tractable child behaving well in an ideal hospital.

These initial cures, or apparent cures, are predicated on an apparent autonomy of the adolescent, which discounts the dependency both on the absent family and on the present hospital staff. Such alloplastic solutions last only until the family becomes engaged. Unfortunately, the family may not put in an appearance for weeks or even months, particularly when their child has been placed by social service agencies rather than by their active, voluntary consent. Labeled abusive, neglectful, or unable to care for their child, the family may not quickly venture to disconfirm these labels.

In this fashion, the developmental process of adolescent separation from the family may easily become confused with, and reduced to, the physical separating of teenager from family. Growing up, then, becomes synonymous with "splitting," in adolescent not psychiatric jargon, where "to split" means simply to exit especially rapidly and irrevocably, with reliance on physical action rather than on complex negotiation.

In this family, the confused process of physically separating the adolescents from their family had begun well before hospitalization. Sexual abuse by the mother's former boyfriend and maternal neglect of this continuing abuse had forced the daughter to separate from her mother through foster-care placement. In this process, the family of origin was deemed bad and the foster family good. Yet the foster family was insufficiently good enough to help Jeannette contain her terror-filled hallucinations. She required hospitalization, with the expectation that the hospital would be omnipotently good enough.

Although that expectation was initially confirmed, too much of a good thing did not prove workable. As an idealized patient in an idealized hospital, she had left her problems back home. Her sexualized separation-individuation struggles were not played out in individual treatment or within the milieu until the family reappeared on the scene. The arrival of the family was heralded by the appearance of the mother, who began to explore her own life history of separations. A multigenerational family tradition of dysfunctional adolescent separations—the females through sex, the males through aggression—was disclosed.

444

When the individual therapists joined together as family cotherapists, the family eventually resisted this approach, not only by missing appointments, but by identifying a new patient, the next younger child, and requesting his admission into the idealized sanitorium, as though the answer to the question of pathological separations was to reunite the entire family within the omniprovident hospital.

To gain control of the therapy, the family cotherapists sought to gain control of the splitting by creating a new split: a team of experts was hypothesized to review the family's and the therapists' progress together. The hypothetical experts then joined the family resistance, paradoxically reframing that resistance as positive: the family was right to resist rapid change, and the family therapists were wrong to push for more family meetings but should meet less and less frequently. The experts enraged the family by speaking openly of, and paradoxically reenforcing, the family tradition of incest and insanity. It was mind boggling for the family to be directed by the experts to listen to the teachings of the grandmother about how teenagers leave their families: daughters leave by getting raped or pregnant, and sons leave by fighting or insanity. The family became engaged in fighting off, or "extrojecting," this old family tradition.

With the full involvement of the family in treatment, the hospitalized adolescents could safely be sent home on weekend passes and, eventually, on day-treatment status. However, this process of separation from the hospital generated a parallel current of pathological splitting within the institution. The line staff shifted the accusations of neglect from the family to the family therapists, blaming them for not addressing the substantive issues of Jeannette's dirty hair and Michael's unkempt clothes. Not the adolescents or the family but the family therapists were at fault. While accepting some responsibility for the adolescents' current state, the family therapists argued that the youngsters were not uniformly neglected and that the family had much to offer. Not all goodness flowed from the hospital to the family. The family itself was a source of emotional attachment, caring, and competence.

The therapists progressively became the mediators of the various splitting processes. For the family, they allied themselves against the bad experts and bad family tradition, yet they did still remain part of the hospital staff, concerned about unwashed hair and ill-fitting clothes. To the hospital staff, the therapists were not just seemingly neglectful but also personally and professionally respected. Unlike the parents, they could not simply be dismissed as incompetent or exiled to another hospital. In this regard, the long-standing hospital tradition of the primary therapist serving as coordinator of all hospital treatment decisions acted as a powerful counterweight to the splitting that might have been reenforced by the more conventional division between a psychiatrist as administrator and a social worker as family case manager. The interdisciplinary team, with some of the egalitarian respect of two decades ago, when the hospital was organized, still intact, could not blithely denounce or disregard any viewpoint. It remains a testimony to the personal and professional cohesion of the staff that this extraordinarily demanding family, and the extraordinarily demanding treatment that it spawned, did not split the hospital asunder.

As the family was discharged from treatment within the hospital, the therapists, under the aegis of the hypothesized experts, delivered a final paradox. They acknowledged that the family had become self-contained and competent and asked the family to acknowledge that the hospital staff had become needy, incompetent, and depressed like a mother who feels bad that she is no longer needed in the care of her children. The experts warned the family not to leave the greater hospital family, not to separate into an autonomous good-enough unit that could function independently, but to continue their own needy complaints and to refer other patients with such needs to the depressed and abandoned hospital.

In these ways, splitting proved useful in the definition of boundary during separation, both for these adolescents from their family and for this family from the hospital. In individual therapies, the adolescents and their mother were each differentiating their own boundaries, leading to a healthy process of adolescent separation from the family. In the family therapy, the family initially defined itself as a nuclear family by splitting off, and pushing out, a parasitic relative who had been living in their apartment. Later, the family was challenged by the question of whether they could create their own boundaries vis-à-vis the hospital. Using paradox, the experts helped push the family to delimit its boundaries from the previous family traditions of incest and insanity and from the hospital standards as well.

Within the hospital, the staff was pushed to realize professional boundaries and therapeutic limitations, too. With the youngsters on extended day-treatment status, teachers had to instruct ill-kempt pupils, nurses had to care for and discipline youngsters not under their total supervision, and coordinating therapists had to work with patients living in real families. No one could become the idealized therapist or represent the idealized profession. Within the interdisciplinary treatment team, each discipline emerged from a fused idealized omnipotence into a separate profession with definable treatment responsibilities and real, though limited, powers.

Conclusions

When socioeconomic disparities between home and hospital reenforce psychopathological splitting in families, therapists may encounter unusually refractory resistances in their work with disadvantaged borderline adolescents. Idealization of the hospital and disparagement of the family promote a symbiotic dependency on the former and an abandonment of the latter that may be mistaken for adolescent growth. To overcome this pathological splitting, transference-countertransference issues at personal, familial, institutional, and societal levels must be directly confronted. Paradoxical family-therapy techniques may also prove warranted to achieve the discharge of young inpatients to their disadvantaged families. However, such techniques severely strain, though ultimately strengthen, both the hospital and the family.

NOTE

The authors gratefully acknowledge the essential contributions and support of Len Handelsman, cotherapist; Judy Morgan, family therapy supervisor; Richard Feinberg, hospital director; and the staff of Bronx Children's Psychiatric Center.

REFERENCES

Bergman, J. 1980. The use of paradox in a community home for the chronically disturbed and retarded. *Family Process* 19:65–71.

Greenberg, H. 1982. *Hanging In: What You Should Know about Psychotherapy.* New York: Four Winds.

Gutheil, J., and Avery, N. 1977. Multiple overt incest as family defense against loss. *Family Process* 6:98–116.

Halperin, D.; Lauro, G.; Miscione, F.; Rebhan, J.; Schnabolk, J.; and Shachter, B. 1981. Countertransference issues in a transitional residential treatment program for troubled adolescents. *Adolescent Psychiatry* 9:559–577.

Hendrickson, W.; Holmes, D.; and Waggoner, R. 1959. Psychotherapy of the hospitalized adolescent. *American Journal of Psychiatry* 116:527–532.

Kernberg, O. 1975. *Borderline Conditions and Pathological Narcissism*. New York: Aronson.

Kernberg, O. 1976. *Object-Relations Theory and Clinical Psychoanalysis*. New York: Aronson.

Kolb, J., and Shapiro, E. 1982. Management of separation issues with the family of the hospitalized adolescent. *Adolescent Psychiatry* 10:343–359.

Looney, J.; Blotcky, M.; Carson, D.; and Gossett, J. 1980. A family systems model for inpatient treatment of adolescents. *Adolescent Psychiatry*. 8:499–511.

Masterson, J. 1972. *Treatment of the Borderline Adolescent: A Developmental Approach*. New York: Wiley.

Meeks, J. 1980. *The Fragile Alliance*. New York: Krieger.

Palmer, A.; Harper, G.; and Rivinus, T. 1983. The "adoption process" in the inpatient treatment of children and adolescents. *Journal of the American Academy of Child Psychiatry* 22:286–293.

Papp, P. 1981. Paradoxes. In S. Minuchin and C. Fishman, eds. *Family Therapy Techniques*. Cambridge, Mass.: Harvard University Press.

Rinsley, D. 1965. Intensive psychiatric hospital treatment of adolescents. *Psychiatric Quarterly* 39:405–429.

Rinsley, D. 1968. Theory and practice of intensive residential treatment of adolescents. *Psychiatric Quarterly* 42:611–638.

Selvini-Palazzoli, M.; Boscolo, L.; Cecchin, G.; and Prata, G. 1978. *Paradox and Counterparadox*. New York: Aronson.

Simmel, E. 1929. Psycho-analytic treatment in a sanatorium. *International Journal of Psycho-Analysis* 10:70–89.

Watzlawick, P. 1978. *The Language of Change*. New York: Basic.

Watzlawick, P.; Weakland, J.; and Fisch, R. 1974. *Change*. New York: Norton.

29   LONG-TERM TREATMENT OF THE
      HOSPITALIZED ADOLESCENT AND HIS
      FAMILY: AN INTEGRATED SYSTEMS-
      THEORY APPROACH

JAMES M. JONES, GLEN T. PEARSON, AND RHONDA DIMPERO

It is axiomatic among providers of psychiatric services to adolescents that certain tensions inhere in the relationship between patients' families and therapists. These tensions are particularly acute when an adolescent is hospitalized. The child, more often than not, is an unwilling patient, brought to treatment by parents whose own unwillingness is exceeded only by their fears for the child and their anger at him.

Admission to inpatient care entails a painful acknowledgment of failure on the part of parents, and the anxiety that motivated them to hospitalize their child is usually followed by feelings of shame and guilt. These feelings are usually experienced in relation to the hospital staff, by whom the parents fully expect to be blamed for their child's problems in living. The adolescent patient further heightens the tension by exaggerating his characteristic symptomatic behavior and by complaining simultaneously to his parents about how he is being treated by the hospital staff and to his treatment staff about how he has been treated in the past by his parents. The treatment team itself usually contributes to this state of dynamic tension. By assuming unilateral responsibility for making decisions concerning the patient's care, the treatment staff reinforces the assumption that parents are blameworthy. In addition, attitudes characterized by aversion, condescension, and criticism toward parents and by protectiveness toward children against their parents are endemic among inpatient direct care staff.

The relationship between treatment team and family, which begins at best in uncertainty and at worst in mistrust, must somehow be transformed into an alliance in which trust and mutual respect provide a context for examining painful problems and for working together for change.

The concept of alliance between individual patient and therapist has been richly explicated in the psychiatric literature over the past three decades; family system and process issues have received increasingly theoretical attention and informed empirical study during the last fifteen years. However, the therapeutic interfaces among patient, provider, and family have been relatively neglected. In this chapter, we propose a conceptual model for integrating the psychodynamically oriented inpatient treatment of the adolescent with the systems-oriented treatment of the patient's family.

The Need for an Integrated Model: Pieces of a Puzzle

Over the past ten years, there have been attempts to synthesize principles of family systems theory with those of psychodynamic theory, in hope of yielding an integrated approach to treatment that would incorporate the best of both bodies of knowledge. As a part of this endeavor, authors who work with hospitalized patients have attempted to develop models for working with the families of inpatients. Their contributions range from the development of a collaborative institutional and therapeutic alliance with families, taking into account the difficulties inherent in engaging severely dysfunctional families in treatment (Hanrahan 1986; Harbin 1979; Stewart 1984; Weitzman 1985), to describing stages of different levels of therapeutic involvement of families in the long-term hospitalization of adolescents (Jones 1985) to a description of the relevant functions of the family therapist as the person on the boundary between the hospital and the family (Hunter 1985).

While these contributions and others have helped to delineate some pieces of the puzzle, the task of developing an integrated family systems model of inpatient treatment remains. Before going on to describe our approach to this model, it is important to mention several other pieces of the puzzle from the family therapy literature that need to be considered in developing this integrated approach.

Hatfield (1979) has discussed the issue of establishing a collaborative relationship with families in treatment. She describes the family's need to derive a sense of confidence from working actively on behalf of their family member and emphasizes the benefit of the family's being involved as a "partner" in the treatment of mental illness. Appleton (1975) has addressed the issue of mistreatment of the families of psychiatric patients, describing situations in which family members either were ignored by mental health professionals or received the impression that they were to blame for their family member's difficulties. Lamb (1983) discusses the need to replace blame with practical assistance to families. Anderson (1986) has spoken eloquently to the issue of how mental health professionals, including some leaders in the field of family therapy, unintentionally convey disrespect to families and leave them feeling blamed and attacked. The National Alliance for the Mentally Ill has become increasingly vocal regarding families' need to receive more information and support from mental health professionals.

There is also a growing body of literature related to the use of educational approaches to the families of psychiatric patients. Anderson (1983) has described a psychoeducational process for families of schizophrenic patients, in which family members are offered information about the illness and are given ideas about how to manage the patient. McFarlane and Beels (1983) describe a decision tree model for determining the nature and level of involvement of families of schizophrenic patients, emphasizing that family therapists need to attend to the interaction between the illness and the family in both causal directions. The establishment of an educational and collaborative context with families can minimize resistance and proves useful in achieving positive long-term outcomes.

Another piece of the puzzle relates to what occurs in the treatment milieu, including the stages of treatment that the adolescent patient goes through, the nature of the therapeutic group process, individualized treatment modalities, and the critical role of the treatment team in the overall process. Many authors (Looney, Blotcky, Carson, and Gossett 1980; Rinsley 1968) have addressed various aspects of the inpatient treatment process. In particular, Rinsley (1980, 1983) has eloquently described the severely disturbed adolescent who requires long-term inpatient psychiatric treatment, conceptualizing symptomatic behavior as a major deviation from the normal process of personality development. He defines the characteristics of a therapeutic

451

milieu that are necessary for the reorganization of the adolescent's intrapsychic structure, outlines the stages of inpatient treatment, and provides a theoretical basis for understanding the adolescent's dysfunctional behavior and procedural guidelines for addressing it.

Unfortunately, Rinsley offers only cursory attention to the role of the parents in the treatment process and says little about the establishment of an alliance with them. He does make passing reference to a concomitant, dynamically oriented casework process with the patient's parents and offers a brief description of the need to engage in a "study of the parents' fantasies during the resistance phase of their child's treatment." In our experience, a great deal of time, effort, and skill are required to engage parents in such an introspective process, which cannot even be undertaken without first establishing a treatment alliance. The psychotherapeutic pursuit of parents' fantasies may be contraindicated when other approaches are less threatening, and, in the long run, they may be more beneficial to the family, including the hospitalized adolescent.

If one conceptualizes the difficulties of the seriously disturbed adolescent as a major deviation in the normal developmental process, it becomes clear that the hospital treatment team and the parents will share a common goal—to help the adolescent get back on the developmental track. The first step in the treatment process requires that the hospital reach an understanding with the parents that they are allies in the endeavor to reach this goal. This lays the groundwork for the establishment of a therapeutic context within which the hospital staff and the family can work in a collaborative fashion. Once this context has been established, the hospital treatment team can proceed to help the family understand and participate in the treatment process, explaining the program philosophy and clarifying what is expected of the parents. In order to do this effectively, there is a need for a treatment model that coordinates the therapeutic efforts of the hospital and those of the family. Critical issues that need to be incorporated into the model include understanding the ways in which the stages of treatment of the individual adolescent fit with the stages of family involvement, recognizing and utilizing the ways in which adolescents re-create their family dynamics within the therapeutic milieu, and recognizing and working with countertransference issues concerning both the child and his family within the treatment team.

Proposal of an Integrated Model:
Assembling the Puzzle

The development of an integrated family systems model for inpatient treatment of adolescents is a task of some complexity. The model requires flexibility in order to respond to the complicated and, at times, apparently contradictory needs of the family and of the treatment milieu. On the one hand, great care needs to be taken to proceed in a manner that leaves families feeling, not blamed for their child's difficulties, but rather engaged in a collaborative relationship. On the other hand, a context needs to be established in which serious problems in living can be addressed interpretively by exploring the possible meanings of interactional processes both within the family and within the treatment milieu.

The focus cannot remain solely on the hospitalized adolescent without contributing to his fixation in the role of identified patient—"the problem." However, owing to the seriously problematic nature of the adolescent's behavior prior to hospitalization, particularly as it has affected the family, it is in precisely such a role with respect to his family that the troubled youngster begins the treatment process. The integrated approach to treatment must offer clear guidelines for engaging the family in a way that does not blame either the adolescent or the family but that strives to establish a context of collaboration with all family members in working toward the shared goal of restoring the patient to optimal developmental functioning. This enhances the level of functioning of the family, both as individual members and as a unit.

The principles of general systems theory, as they have been applied to the family, offer a foundation for the integrated model of treatment (Baker 1969). A human system develops a set of "rules" or guidelines that influence and guide the interaction among various elements of the system (Bateson, Jackson, Haley, and Weakland 1968). In relation to families, these rules spring from a complex combination of sources that include tradition, conscious decision making, habit, and environmental influence. At a given time in a family's life cycle, the rules dictating the interaction of the system components may be adaptive, but, if the family system is not able to change its structure gradually and flexibly in response to the developmental changes of its individual members, dysfunctional patterns are likely to become established. These dysfunctional patterns can then impede the growth and development of those individuals. In an integrated comprehensive treatment approach, the hospital system joins with the family system in a way that promotes adaptive change in the rules dictating interaction in the family system, facilitating conjoint efforts by the hospital and family to help the adolescent get back on the developmental track.

The coming together of a family system and the hospital's treatment team system establishes a larger, superordinate system (therapeutic "supersystem"), composed of the hospital treatment team, the hospitalized adolescent, and the family members who are not in the hospital. Following the principles of general systems theory, this system would naturally develop a set of rules dictating the nature of the interaction among the various elements. By clearly defining these rules from the outset, the hospital treatment team can establish the necessary context for working not only with the adolescent but also with the family in a manner that will have an ameliorative effect on the family system.

Lewis (1980; Lewis, Beavers, Gossett, and Phillips 1976) and others have described a number of characteristics that are typical of family functioning along a continuum ranging from severely dysfunctional to optimal. Among the variables characterizing optimally functioning families are the following: (1) an effective parental coalition, which allows children to participate in the decision-making process but reserves the final say for the parents; (2) boundaries that are clear but permeable, promoting effective communication; (3) a climate in which affect can be shared openly and safely; and (4) respect for subjective views. These characteristics need to be incorporated in the rules of the therapeutic supersystem involving the hospital and family.

There are three major components in the proposed framework for integrated treatment of the hospitalized adolescent and his family. First is the partnership that the hospital treatment team forms with the parents, with the goal of forming an effective executive system. The second is the process that occurs in the therapeutic milieu between the treatment team and the patient. The third component is the ongoing interactional process between the hospitalized adolescent and his family. The manner in which information is shared, both within and among the three subsystems, has a major effect on the functionality of the system as a whole. Each of the components will be described individually, and then the interactional process among them will be discussed.

The first component is an alliance between the hospital and the parents to form an executive coalition for the therapeutic supersystem. Initial efforts to engage the parents must take into account the demoralized and dysfunctional state of the parents' own executive coalition. For some length of time prior to hospitalizing their child, the parents have felt a progressive loss of control of his behavior. Despite their best efforts, they have been unable to curb the adolescent's antisocial or self-destructive acts. That it must be a major goal of treatment to help the parents become more effective in setting clear and appropriate limits for the child is obvious; it is crucial that this goal be approached in a manner that does not strip the parents of their dignity or undermine what remains of their authority in the family. To establish a partnership that models an effective parental coalition, the treatment team must effect a shift in the traditional doctor-patient relationship, in which the physician prescribes treatment for a passively accepting patient. As one arm of the executive coalition, the treatment team needs the authority to make decisions about the adolescent's day-to-day treatment needs. It is imperative that the parents understand from the outset that they must delegate this authority to the treatment team in order for treatment to proceed effectively. Conversely, it is also imperative that the treatment team understand that it is only by leave of the adolescent's parents that they may have this authority. The hospital must begin by respecting the ultimate authority of the family, which is then, and only then, followed by a request that some of it be shared. The treatment team must be empowered to exercise its expertise concerning treatment modalities, including such issues as what privileges are granted and whether and when family visits occur. The degree to which the family is willing to grant this authority will be greatly increased if the treatment team makes efforts to consult the parents concerning major decisions whenever feasible and to inform them after the fact in order to receive their feedback when it is not possible to consult with them prior to making decisions. Obviously, an effective executive coalition will require clear but permeable boundaries that promote two-way communication.

The second component is the process that takes place in the therapeutic milieu of the unit, between and among the members of the treatment team and the adolescent patient group. In order for the milieu to be therapeutic, it needs to be organized along the lines of a healthy family system, with an effective executive coalition—the team—that provides a clear and safe structure in which to encourage growth-promoting participation by the adolescent patients. There are three principal means by which this structure is maintained. First, the members of the treatment team meet regularly in an atmosphere that is conducive to the safe sharing of ideas and feelings about the individual patients, the group as a whole, and the decision-making processes of the team itself. This is similar to the process in a healthy family by which the parents work together. Second, the treatment team meets with the adolescent group on a regular basis to work on problems of living that have arisen within the group. Frequent meetings of the treatment group assure that each child will have the opportunity to examine his own feelings and behavior in relation to significant others. Although the therapeutic emphasis is on the here-and-now on the unit, there is often the opportunity for interpretive reconstruction of the adolescents' psychopathological issues as they are relived in the hospital. Third, there is a clear structure involving the gradual increase of privileges, commensurate with the adolescent's ability to handle the responsibilities of such increases. Adolescents should have ample opportunity to provide input in the decision-making process throughout the daily interaction in the milieu, especially in the group process meetings.

The third component of the therapeutic supersystem is the work that the family does in examining the strengths and problem areas that exist in the interactional process of their family system. They do this with the assistance of their family therapist in the context of family therapy, but they draw on a wealth of material from a variety of sources that extend beyond the confines of the therapy hour. They utilize historical data, educational input provided by the hospital by way of reading material and lectures, discussions in parent groups, and their own experiences together as a family that emerge in the course of therapeutic visits. The family moves at a pace that is dictated by its overall level of functioning and the degree to which it feels threatened by change. It is the task of the treatment team, and particularly the family therapist, to be sensitive to these two factors and to time interventions with the family accordingly.

The therapeutic supersystem can be diagramed to illustrate the elements of the system, where they interface, and how they interact (fig. 1).

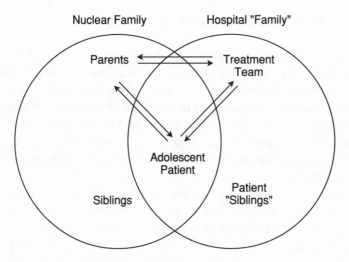

Fig. 1.—The therapeutic supersystem

As in a family system, functioning is enhanced by the maintenance of clear but permeable boundaries and the presence of a coherent and flexible set of guidelines that dictate interaction. One arm of the executive coalition of the system is composed of the parents, who are in charge of their family but open to input from external sources. The other arm of the executive coalition is composed of the hospital treatment team, which is in charge of what occurs in the therapeutic milieu but also open to input from its executive partner, the patient's parents. It should be emphasized that the executive coalition is something more than a treatment alliance with a family. The treatment alliance is a relationship that lays the groundwork for treatment to proceed. The ongoing negotiation of the relationship involved in the executive coalition is a major thrust of the treatment process. An effective parental coalition is modeled for the family through the clear communication and respect for boundaries between these two arms of the system. When something important about the adolescent's interactional process is learned from the work in the milieu, it can be shared, with permission, with the family in the hope that they can use the information in the parallel work that they are doing in family therapy. Conversely, when the family makes discoveries of its own, they can be brought back into the group process on the unit, where they can be incorporated into the work that the adolescent is doing there.

457

Operationalizing the Model: Roles of the Team

An integrated treatment program for seriously disturbed adolescents and their families demands of its leaders that they thoroughly understand and subscribe to the principles of system theory presented. Psychiatrists who are accustomed to treating individual patients in a medical model of intervention may experience tension between their traditional physician's role and the role of coordinator of a complex, process-oriented system. The specific intervention skills and strategies that one has cherished as most important in the therapy of the individual patient must often be subordinated to the need to attend to more pressing process issues within the milieu, within the family, or among one or more of the interacting subsystems. The psychiatrist must retain appropriate medical and legal responsibility for the care of the patient while working collaboratively as a team member with nurses and child-care workers, the family therapist and other team professionals, the adolescent and his peers as a group on the unit, and the family. He or she must be able to negotiate, share power, and deal directly and openly with conflict arising from within or among any of the components of the system. Institutional support for the integrated treatment process and an organizational structure and employment policies that assure reasonably consistent staff commitment to the model are invaluable, if not indispensable.

Other treatment team members must also maintain an awareness of the interactional process within and among the various elements of the supersystem. The family therapist is actively involved in both subsystems, serving as the liaison between the family and the treatment team. The family therapist's functions include not only the assessment and treatment of the family in family therapy but also the facilitation of communication and the maintenance of clarity and permeability in the boundaries between the family system and the hospital system. In collaboration with the adolescent's treating psychiatrist, the family therapist represents the hospital in joining with the parents to form an executive coalition vis-à-vis the hospitalized adolescent and the unit milieu.

Nurses and direct care staff on the unit replace the parents as the primary objects of the adolescent patient's world during hospitalization. By identification with the family process model of the supersystem, the milieu on the unit recreates a family for the adolescent; and,

458

within this network of transference relationships, the adolescent reexperiences his infantile conflicts, displays his primitive pathological defenses, and reenacts his unique manifest behavioral symptoms toward the unit staff. Direct care staff must, therefore, have clear authority to set limits and otherwise to respond to the rapidly changing needs of their adolescent patients. Effective responsiveness requires that the staff possess qualities of flexibility, empathy, respect, and healthy affection for adolescents and that they be proficient in verbalizing their own thoughts and feelings. Spending as they do most of their working day with patients, direct care staff have access to much patient material around issues of daily living and object relationship. Because of this proximity to the adolescent and their responsibility for immediate interventions as needed by the adolescent, nurses and child-care workers are frequently the targets of the child's hostility, the subjects of his conflictual anxiety, or objects for his instinctual wishes. Adolescents often form very close, warmly toned attachments to these team members. For these reasons, a part of treatment can be conceptualized as taking place primarily in the context of relationship between the child and his direct care staff members.

Obviously, the primary focus of the nurses and direct care staff must remain on the process within the milieu. Yet, they, too, must maintain awareness of the process within the family and between the adolescent and the family. Various countertransference reactions toward parents on the part of direct care staff members are common and must be addressed in an ongoing way within the process of the intrateam subsystem. Regular participation in this process by the family therapist facilitates the development of empathy for the family on the part of staff, who will otherwise identify solely with the child.

Traditionally, the psychiatrist unit director and nurse supervisor form an executive coalition for the unit treatment team. If the subsystem is optimally functional, team members will be free to speak openly and directly to address whatever issues they perceive, including problems and conflicts involving the team leadership. Team members may be in a position to detect conflicts of which they are consciously unaware, and, if the staff process is consistently open to self-examination without fear of reprisal, the treatment team itself will represent to the patient group as a healthy family system in which the parental coalition conveys support, leadership, and respect rather than control and dominance. In turn, given that appropriate permeability has been maintained in the boundary between hospital and family, the parents can witness in vivo an example of optimal functioning, both in the executive coalition of the treatment team and in the response of the team to their own child.

Applying the Model: The Case of Brenda

The concept of a hospital-based integrated treatment approach to borderline adolescents and their families emerges from reflection on our experience in working with this population. The case of Brenda, which is presented both from the perspective of the inpatient unit milieu and from that of the family work, illustrates the applicability of this conceptual model.

CASE HISTORY

Brenda, a fifteen-year-old white female from a nearby rural community, was referred for psychiatric treatment because of a five-year history of acting-out behavior, including running away from home, lying, obsessional fantasies about having a baby, sexual activity, and drug abuse. In addition to her severe behavioral difficulties, psychological testing suggested that she had quite limited intellectual and verbal skills. Her parents had divorced when she was an infant, and Brenda, who had already experienced her mother as libidinally unavailable owing to a depressive illness, was left in the care of a grandmother while her mother worked two jobs. She was found to be a slow learner when she began school and was placed in special education. In the classroom, Brenda was difficult to manage; she spent a lot of time either daydreaming or engaging other students and teachers in physical altercations. Throughout her school years, she was afraid of being abandoned. When Brenda was nine, her mother remarried and became able to spend more time in the home. Initially, Brenda was excited about having a "dad," but the marriage was conflicted owing to the stepfather's excessive drinking; and, as Brenda now had more contact with her mother, she experienced her as rigid, critical, and overly moralistic. The marital conflict provided Brenda a fertile ground for splitting, and her behavior problems increased in severity following her menarche at ten. Not only was Brenda able to pit one parent against the other, but she also managed to involve the extended family and neighbors in disputes about parenting issues. On one occasion, she even managed to persuade school officials to contact childrens' protective services regarding alleged abuse by her parents. No evidence of abuse was found, and Brenda later admitted that she had fabricated the story to get attention. Brenda ran away from home and school and was raped on one occasion at age eleven. She developed frequent somatic illnesses, often in conjunction with her menstrual periods. She experienced the loss of a close friend, a peer who was killed in a motor vehicle accident. Brenda's mother finally withdrew her from school and sought psychiatric attention when the school authorities denied the mother's request to attend school with Brenda in order to watch over and, thereby, control her drug use. After psychiatric evaluation, Brenda was admitted to the hospital.

RESISTANCE/REGRESSION PHASE OF TREATMENT

During the early phase of her adjustment, Brenda was demanding with female staff and coy, seductive, and helpless with males. The nurses (mostly women) felt drained and angry at the doctors (mostly men), who they felt were being critical of the nurses for not being more empathic and understanding of Brenda's limitations and physical ailments. The patient group also quickly became frustrated with her bids for attention, not only because of the amount of staff time she consumed with her illnesses, but also because of her directly provocative behaviors in group process meetings. Brenda's response to confrontation was to become enraged and to accuse people of wanting her to die. Her difficulty in comprehending and relating to the psychodynamic and interpersonal issues, which were most often the focus of group meetings on the unit, was a stumbling block to her acceptance by the group. She often looked lost and confused while others were talking, and she became especially uncomfortable when other girls expressed anger toward their parents.

As Brenda became more distressed, she began to focus all her needs and demands onto the unit nurse supervisor. She attempted to use the relationship to keep other staff from setting limits for her, suggesting that she and the nurse supervisor had made deals that did not involve other team members. Fairly soon, the supervisor began experiencing a countertransference reaction in which she felt torn between wanting to meet Brenda's needs and feeling overwhelmed by them, much the same as Brenda's mother had felt. She concluded that Brenda was untreatable on the unit owing to her intellectual limitations and suggested that she be transferred to a less intensive treatment setting. A major split developed in the treatment team, with the rest of the nurses and the direct care staff supporting the idea of a transfer while the psychiatrists and social worker remained adamant that Brenda could be treated on the unit. This conflict was dealt with through repeated discussions, which gradually moved from each "side" trying to convince the other that they were wrong to listening and recognizing that the team was being engaged by Brenda in an interactional process similar to the one that had occurred in her family. This recognition provided the impetus for the team to come up with a compromise that allowed Brenda to remain on the unit. The psychiatrists and social worker developed an appreciation for how difficult Brenda could be to deal with, and, once they felt understood and supported on this point, the direct care staff were able to accept the decision that Brenda would not be transferred. Coincidentally, an administrative reorganization of direct care services was implemented at about this same time. The goal was to streamline the decision-making process by dividing the patient group into smaller subgroups and assigning direct care staff to one group. As a result, fewer people were involved in treatment decisions, which had the effect of drawing a clearer boundary around Brenda's unit "family" and thereby limiting (though not eliminating) her opportunities for splitting and triangulation.

The first few months of Brenda's hospitalization were characterized by the establishment of a reasonably stable executive coalition between her parents and the treatment team. While few, if any, structural changes occurred within the family unit as a result of family therapy, the parents formed a strong alliance with the social worker and seemed to feel confident about decisions made by the staff. They attended a parents' support group, which seemed to help in solidifying their alliance. As this process occurred, assessment data were accumulated that not only formed the data base for future interventions directly in the family but also helped the team understand the dynamics of Brenda's interactions on the unit in this early phase of treatment.

As the split in the team was resolved and the unit "family" was able to take a more consistent and nurturing approach, Brenda began to build some strong attachments to peers and staff. As her acting out decreased, therapeutic visits with her parents were increased. At that point, she began to feel torn between her loyalty to her parents and her feelings of dependency on the hospital staff. She also experienced increasing awareness of her desperate need to be close to her mother and her profound fear of being angry at her. As her ambivalance intensified, she began to regress, demanding increased nursing care for her multiple somatic complaints. She responded to confrontation from peers regarding her hypochondriasis by becoming intimidating and aggressive. Apparently, she experienced their confrontation as an attempt to take away the nurturance she desperately needed, which reawakened the feeling of being abandoned that she had experienced as a small child when her mother was not available to her. Finally, these feelings became intolerable to Brenda, and, when the opportunity presented itself, she ran away from the hospital.

When Brenda left the hospital, she made no attempt to contact her parents but instead sought out other adolescents and young adults who were involved in antisocial behavior. During the sixteen days that she was gone, she was involved in a number of dangerous situations, several of which could have cost her her life. Fortunately, she was discovered by the police, and, when her parents were notified, they had her readmitted to the hospital. She returned in a primitive rage, and, while waiting for a bed to become available on the adolescent unit, she had to be placed in restraints on an adult unit. During this interim period, the treatment team spent a great deal of time talking about feelings related to Brenda's runaway, including anger, anxiety, concern, and relief. Her parents, with whom the hospital had remained in constant touch during the runaway, also had the opportunity to meet with the social worker and psychiatrist to ventilate their feelings and join the staff in deciding how to proceed. Family therapy sessions were suspended temporarily until Brenda's rage at her parents subsided.

WORKING-THROUGH PHASE OF TREATMENT

When Brenda was able to return to the adolescent unit, she was amazed that the primary feeling that the staff and other patients expressed to her was one of concern for her safety and relief that she had returned unharmed. In retrospect, Brenda was able to pinpoint this as the pivotal event that helped her make the decision to begin working actively in treatment. As she began to experience group process meetings as supportive, Brenda began talking about the fact that prior to her runaway, as she had begun feeling closer to her peers, she began to experience sexual feelings toward the other girls. She reported being terrified by these feelings, and this, along with the loyalty conflict she experienced regarding her feelings about the hospital and her family, apparently precipitated her runaway. As she verbalized these feelings, she was surprised to learn that the other girls were supportive and let her know that they struggled with all the same issues. Brenda began to feel more accepted within the group and continued to try to make use of group process meetings to talk about her feelings. She also decided that she was ready to resume family therapy and begin focusing on her relationship with her mother. After spending the first two sessions processing everyone's feelings about the runaway, Brenda began talking with her mother about her early childhood and her feelings of abandonment. Although she had mentioned this issue to her mother previously, Brenda had never shared much affect. On this occasion, however, Brenda expressed a great deal of sadness, at one point sobbing uncontrollably. Her mother was able to respond empathically rather than defensively, and Brenda was particularly surprised when her mother revealed that she, too, had experienced a major loss because she was unable to share this important time in Brenda's childhood. As they talked about this issue over the course of several sessions, Brenda and her mother seemed to experience a new kind of closeness. Significantly absent, however, was any discussion of anger on Brenda's part at what she had perceived as her mother's abandoning her.

As Brenda began to feel closer to her mother, she once again began to feel a loyalty conflict, and, as a result, she began to withdraw from relationships on the unit. This was accompanied by a behavioral regression involving almost infantile behavior and multiple somatic complaints. On an occasion when Brenda and her parents were waiting on the unit for their family therapist to arrive for an appointment, the unit nurse supervisor, whom Brenda had previously idealized, took the opportunity to report Brenda's regression to her parents. Brenda became verbally abusive with the supervisor, and, rather than helping her gain control of her behavior, Brenda's parents reacted protectively and complained bitterly to their family therapist about the supervisor. This event precipitated a crisis in the therapeutic supersystem, both in the executive coalition between the team and the family and within the treatment team itself. By utilizing the foundation of positive relationships that had been established over the course of treatment, the psychiatrist and the social worker were able to help the family and treatment team step back and take a look at what was happening. It became clear that Brenda had transferred her rage at her mother onto the nurse supervisor, making her the "bad mother." Brenda's mother was able to recognize that she had often been in that position, and, because it had been a relief to her for the supervisor to be in that position, she had colluded with Brenda to keep her there. In a joint meeting that included the supervisor, Brenda's mother was able to respond empathically with the supervisor, which helped the supervisor in dealing with her feelings of hurt and anger at being the target of Brenda's rage. As a result of this series of events, the issue of Brenda's need to find an appropriate way to deal with her rage at her mother was clarified for the entire supersystem. Brenda began working on this issue with her mother in family therapy and on the unit with the supervisor. Over the course of several months, she began to develop the ability to feel angry at maternal figures without feeling threatened that they would leave her.

As Brenda continued making progress on the unit and in her relationship with her mother, the balance within the family system began shifting. The stepfather's role in the family had revolved around his helping mother "take care of" Brenda, serving as a buffer during times of conflict. The foundation of the marital relationship was relatively weak, a fact that became obvious and brought matters to a head when the parents went on a vacation trip without Brenda and came face to face with the emptiness in their relationship. They came to the hospital demanding to take Brenda out, although they had difficulty articulating their motivation. The social worker, psychiatrist, and Brenda's individual therapist responded to the crisis by meeting with the parents, again falling back on the foundation of trusting alliance with them. After discussing their wishes at length and recommending strongly that they reconsider, it was suggested that they attend the parents' support group, which fortunately was meeting that same evening. With all this support, they were able to decide to leave Brenda in treatment. Subsequently, Brenda's mother identified some of her concerns about the marital relationship. The parents then met as a couple for several sessions with the family therapist to focus on this relationship, and some progress was made in this area.

One more crisis occurred during the working-through phase of treatment, this time within the executive coalition of the therapeutic su-

465

persystem. Brenda experienced a change of physicians when her psychiatrist left the unit. Brenda worked diligently at separating from her former doctor and attaching to her new doctor, managing to make productive use of this unexpected event in her treatment process. Brenda's parents, however, seemed unsure as to how the new doctor was going to share control of the decision-making process and chose to make a battleground of a shopping trip with Brenda. At this point, with support from her family therapist and doctor, Brenda was sufficiently allied in treatment to be able to reassure her parents about the trustworthiness of her new doctor and get them to back off. Brenda's parents, impressed with her level of trust, calmed down, and, throughout the rest of the course of inpatient treatment, the executive subsystem remained strong.

SEPARATION-TERMINATION PHASE OF TREATMENT

Over the next several months, Brenda continued to work consistently in all areas of her treatment program. She obtained a volunteer job, attended public high school, and began dating while home on visits. Family therapy went well, although Brenda found it difficult to discuss her dependency on the hospital for fear that her mother would think her disloyal. A tentative discharge date was set for several months in the future to coincide with the end of the spring school semester. Not long after this was done, Brenda began experiencing a regression, becoming somewhat defiant and withdrawn, both on the unit and at home on visits. Even with support and confrontation, Brenda was unable to reverse this regressive trend, and, as the spring drew to a close, the treatment team recommended that Brenda's discharge date be postponed to the end of the summer. The strength of the executive coalition was tested at this point, but Brenda's parents were able to stand firm in support of the recommendation, and Brenda was then able to move past her oppositional and dependent posture to a more mature and negotiating one. Over the next several months, she was able to regain the behavioral consistency that she had demonstrated previously and could accept support from peers, the treatment team, and her parents. She was discharged to return to live with her parents after twenty-seven months of inpatient treatment, with plans to continue individual, group, and family therapy.

Discussion

Most workers in the field expect that an individual adolescent will proceed through the course of treatment in three broad phases: (1) resistance/regression; (2) alliance/working through; and (3) separation/ termination. These phases should be conceptualized not as chronologically consecutive segments of time but as overlapping periods, each of which contains all the elements of resistance, regression, alliance, working through, separation, and emergence from the hospital. The features of the treatment process that are characteristic for each of the so-called phases simply reflect which of these ubiquitous themes dominate the foreground of treatment during the early, middle, and late stages of hospitalization: resistance and regression during the early stage; alliance, interpretation, and working through during the middle; and separation and termination issues during the last.

The management of the adolescent's family is also addressed in a series of stages described by Jones (1985) (see fig. 2). In the first two stages of family involvement, corresponding roughly to the phase of resistance and regression in the adolescent, the family therapist moves from establishing an alliance with the family and assessing their treatment needs to providing problem-solving information in a psychoeducational format. In the third stage of family involvement, corresponding roughly to the phase of alliance and working through, a contract is

Adolescent	Family
Resistance/Regression	Assessment/Alliance
Alliance/Interpretation Working Through ("Definitive")	Education/Socialization
	Focus on Relationship
Separation/Termination ("Emergence")	Reintegration

FIG. 2.—Phases of inpatient treatment. For the adolescent phases, see Pearson (1987), and Rinsley (1968, 1980). For the family phases, see Jones (1985).

467

established to study the system of relationships in the family and to explore the meaning of their interactional process. The final stage of family involvement, corresponding to the phase of separation and termination for the patient, involves the active reintegration of the patient into the family system and helping the family consolidate their treatment gains.

The course followed by Brenda, her parents, and the treatment team during her hospitalization illustrates vividly the process of systems interaction among child, family, and staff across the phases of inpatient treatment that have been previously described (Jones 1985; Pearson 1987; Rinsley 1968, 1980).

During an initial phase of passive-dependent, compliant resistance on Brenda's part, her parents are engaged in an extended phase of alliance building and assessment. Historical data and observations concerning the family's interactional process help the team understand Brenda's behavior on the unit and formulate both behavioral and interpretive interventions, thus setting the stage for a more direct behavioral expression of Brenda's psychopathology. Her running away and sexual and aggressive behaviors reflect simultaneously an intensification of resistance (in the active rather than the passive mode) and the emergence of symptomatic acting out as a defense against unconscious conflicts surrounding attachment and abandonment depression.

Once control of the patient has been secured, interpretive work on these issues can begin, providing that the basis for alliance has been established in the initial phase. For the child, this means that she has experienced enough gratification of her infantile dependency needs by staff to have formed a meaningful attachment, so that staff efforts to maintain control during the actively regressive phases are experienced by the patient not solely as punitive and repressive but also as caring and reassuring. For the parents, it means that they must have experienced enough respect for themselves and concern for their child that their confidence in the hospital staff is not fatally shaken either by the behavioral crises that the child precipitates or by the measures used by the staff to respond to them.

As the interpretive work proceeds and the child and family experience more interaction with each other, there evolves a dialectic, in which changes in either the child or the parents evoke unsettling anxiety in the other. This anxiety often precipitates regressive behavior but can also motivate experimentation with therapeutic change. Brenda's mother and stepfather initiate this process by giving her a clear message that they are not going to rescue her from treatment. This provides a context for Brenda to begin working on her relationship with mother; and, as she does so, her rage at her mother comes intolerably close to consciousness and is regressively displaced onto treatment staff, allowing Brenda to enact the same passive-compliant infantile clinging to the mother that she had showed toward staff in the initial phase. Since this situation is gratifying both to Brenda and to her mother, it is necessary to intervene interpretively not only in Brenda's therapy but also in the family therapy. Appropriate permeability in the boundary between the two subsystems is essential to therapeutic progress at this point.

The interactional dialectic continues during a sustained phase of working through. As the child progressively relinquishes her primitive defenses, she relates to her parents on a more developmentally appropriate level, similar to that which she is simultaneously achieving with her treatment staff. Among other things, this means that the patient is no longer unconsciously colluding with the mother in defense against her own unresolved psychopathological issues, which are then reactivated and expressed in the reemergence of conflict in the marriage. It then becomes necessary to address the couple's treatment needs separately from those of the child in order to help them begin establishing a mature parental coalition. In some cases, individual therapy for one or both parents would be indicated at this point.

During the termination phase, at different times, both parents and child experience anxiety and regressive pulls, and both are able to respond adaptively to these threats in each other. Under these conditions, the hospital staff is able to assume a progressively less authoritarian role as the family, including the adolescent, tries its hand at negotiating its own decisions. Optimally, the treatment team will be functioning essentially as a supportive consultant to the family for some period of time prior to discharge and will continue in this role during the aftercare phase.

Conclusions

Several years ago, Looney et al. (1980) suggested that the functioning of an adolescent inpatient treatment unit could be evaluated by reference to the variables of family process first described by Lewis, Beavers, and their coworkers (Beavers 1977; Lewis et al. 1976). Looney

469

makes passing reference to the variable of system openness, which is characteristic of optimal families, and states that openness is necessary for the treatment unit lest it become a "myopic, self-contained microcosm." Our proposal for a conceptual model of inpatient treatment expands and elaborates this notion and attempts to provide both a theoretical and a practical basis for integrating the treatment of the adolescent with that of the family.

In most of the foregoing discussion, we have bowed to convention in using the term "treatment team" as if it were synonymous with "hospital staff." We should now like to correct ourselves by suggesting that a better definition of the "team" would include the patient and the family along with the staff; that is, the superordinate system as a whole should function as a team. Teamwork is encouraged by requiring every person involved in the process of treatment to be aware not only of his or her own internal process and the interactional process between himself or herself and one or two others but also of the ongoing operation of process factors in all the other elements of the interacting systems of unit and family.

In the early phases of treatment, the child and his parents have a very limited awareness of their own process issues, let alone of those of other team members or of interacting systems, and it is the responsibility of the treatment program to monitor and intervene in the system. Across the course of treatment, the child and family should assume progressively more responsibility for monitoring and decision making; the burden of team leadership should shift from the staff to the child and family so that, by the time the patient is ready to leave the hospital, the adolescent and his parents have some experience negotiating and making decisions for themselves, with the staff component of the team in a supportive and consultative role. To the extent that this ideal is realized, the tendency of adolescents and parents to regress after discharge is mitigated.

If, as Looney has suggested, the process of treatment in the adolescent inpatient unit can be studied using measures that have been found reliable and valid in family research, then we suggest that these same measures, with appropriate modifications, can be applied in an integrated way to the evaluation of the treatment process as it effects not only the adolescent patient but also the family. Conceptualizing the treatment process in a systems-theory model thus provides a potential paradigm for research as well as a practical guide for clinical practice.

REFERENCES

Anderson, C. M. 1983. A psychoeducational program for families of patients with schizophrenia. In W. R. McFarlane, ed. *Family Therapy in Schizophrenia*. New York: Guilford.

Anderson, C. M. 1986. The all-too-short trip from positive to negative connotation. *Journal of Marital and Family Therapy* 12(4): 351–354.

Appleton, W. S. 1975. Mistreatment of patients' families by psychiatrists. *American Journal of Psychiatry* 131:655–657.

Baker, F. 1969. Review of general systems concepts and their relevance for medical care. *Systematics* 7(3): 209–229.

Bateson, G.; Jackson, D.; Haley, J.; and Weakland, J. 1968. Toward a theory of schizophrenia. In D. Jackson, ed. *Communications, Family and Marriage*. Palo Alto, Calif.: Science and Behavior Books.

Beavers, W. R. 1977. *Psychotherapy and Growth: A Family Systems Perspective*. New York: Brunner/Mazel.

Hanrahan, G. 1986. Beginning work with families of hospitalized adolescents. *Family Process* 25:391–405.

Harbin, H. T. 1979. A family-oriented psychiatric inpatient unit. *Family Process* 18(3): 281–291.

Hatfield, A. B. 1979. The family as partner in the treatment of mental illness. *Hospital and Community Psychiatry* 30(5): 338–340.

Hunter, D. K. 1985. On the boundary: family therapy in a long-term inpatient setting. *Family Process* 24(3): 339–348.

Jones, J. M. 1985. Stages of family involvement in the residential treatment of adolescents. *Journal of Marital and Family Therapy* 11(4): 381–390.

Lamb, H. R. 1983. Families: practical help replaces blame. *Hospital and Community Psychiatry* 34(10): 893–908.

Lewis, J. M. 1980. The family in the matrix of health and illness. In C. K. Hofling and J. M. Lewis, eds. *The Family: Evaluation and Treatment*. New York: Brunner/Mazel.

Lewis, J. M.; Beavers, W. R.; Gossett, J. T.; and Phillips, V. A. 1976. *No Single Thread: Psychological Health in Family Systems*. New York: Brunner/Mazel.

Looney, J. G.; Blotcky, M. J.; Carson, D. I.; and Gossett, J. T. 1980. A family-systems model for inpatient treatment of adolescents. *Adolescent Psychiatry* 10:499–511.

McFarlane, W. R., and Beels, C. C. 1983. A decision-tree model for integrating family therapies for schizophrenia. In W. R. McFarlane, ed. *Family Therapy in Schizophrenia*. New York: Guilford.

Pearson, G. 1987. Long-term treatment needs of hospitalized adolescents. *Adolescent Psychiatry* 14:342–357.

Rinsley, D. B. 1968. Residential treatment in theory and practice. *Psychiatric Quarterly* 42:611 –638.

Rinsley, D. B. 1980. *Treatment of the Severely Disturbed Adolescent*. New York: Aronson.

Rinsley, D. B. 1983. Theory and practice of intensive residential treatment of adolescents. In A. H. Esman, ed. *The Psychiatric Treatment of Adolescents*. New York: International Universities Press.

Stewart, R. P. 1984. Building an alliance between the family and the institution. *Social Work* 29:386–390.

Weitzman, J. 1985. Engaging the severely dysfunctional family in treatment: basic considerations. *Family Process* 14(4): 473–486.

HELEN A. WIDEN

In the decade of the 1980s, psychotherapists on college campuses have
been confronted more and more with the health- and life-threatening
behaviors of their patients. There has been a general loosening and
disintegration of the external and intrapsychic regulatory structures
that govern behavior. The adolescent and young adult population suf-
fers an increasing incidence of violence, sexual abuse, suicide risk and
actual suicide, accidents, homicide, substance abuse, and eating disorders. In the realm of sexuality, that central developmental concern
of adolescents, there has been a notable increase in teenage pregnancy,
active bisexuality and homosexuality, and sexually transmitted diseases
of all kinds. Not only is the developing AIDS (acquired immunodeficiency syndrome) epidemic the latest threat, but it dwarfs others in the
magnitude of its frightening potential and psychological complexity
(Brandt 1985).

The risk of contracting the AIDS virus in the course of what has
become the somewhat normal and expectable sexual activity on campus
has placed a demand for difficult behavior changes not only on students
but on their psychotherapists as well: "Regardless of one's theoretical
orientation, recent phenomena must be recognized and must result in
a clinician's willingness to modify concepts and theoretical postures"
(Mishne 1986, p. 262).

In 1979, the first case reports of AIDS appeared, and it was recognized as an entity in 1981. Already its effect on our society is and will
continue to be devastating. By the end of 1991, an estimated 270,000
cases of AIDS will have occurred, with 179,000 deaths within the de-

cade since the disease was first recognized (Koop 1987). Our best information is that asymptomatic carriers outnumber patients with AIDS 100 to one (Curran 1985). There is no doubt among writers and researchers that we are seeing a developing epidemic, described variously as "having terrifying potential" (Batchelor 1984, p. 1279), as "going to be a huge medical disaster" (Volberding 1986), and as "a challenge to civilized society" (Keeling, 1986b).

Acquired immunodeficiency syndrome can be controlled only by changes in personal behavior. Behavior change is difficult to achieve, not only in our patients, but in ourselves as well. The demand on psychotherapists is to keep the issue in mind and to make interventions of greater scope and flexibility in the intensely emotion and value-laden area of sexuality. As previously reported (Widen 1987), college psychotherapists have responded to the developing crisis by demonstrating some measure of the same anxieties, resistances, and defenses that their patients have shown in facing this problematic issue. There is a general tendency in both parties to use the defense of disavowal in the interest of doing "business as usual." In order to achieve consensus about what constitutes good practice, there is a need to integrate newer therapeutic interventions into a theoretical framework that includes and yet expands on previous training and experience.

The clinical examples that follow are offered to illustrate the dilemmas that college student psychotherapists face as they confront patients' reports of sexual behavior that has now become life risking. The discussion will offer some ideas about a theoretical frame of reference in which to place technical decisions. First, I offer a brief review of the psychological literature on AIDS as a means of providing a context for the cases and discussion.

The Context

The majority of AIDS cases in the United States have occurred within the risk groups of male homosexuals and intravenous drug users, their sexual partners, and children. The effect on the gay community has been widespread and profound. Gay men have shouldered the emotional burden of a devastating epidemic with few models or guidelines to follow (Morin, Charles, and Malyon 1984). They, in turn, have provided models for others in dealing with the epidemic. For example, fundamental changes have been made in the lives of gay men in San

Francisco, the hardest-hit gay community (McKusick, Wiley, Coates, Stall, Saika, Morin, Charles, Horstman, and Conant 1985). The changes have involved profound personal efforts along with various kinds of psychological and educational interventions. It needs to be added that the development of both more complete psychological insights and appropriate intervention efforts requires a more adequate description of those who are not undertaking particular behavior changes (Joseph, Emmons, Kessler, Wortman, O'Brien, Hocker, and Schaefer 1984). While fear generated by the uncertainties of the disease is a common response for all groups, fear of loss of confidentiality and exposure of sexual orientation is unique to gay men.

Of particular interest to college psychotherapists, heterosexual transmission of AIDS is well documented (Keeling 1986a; Koop 1987; Lederman 1986) and is expected to account for an increasing proportion of those who become infected with the AIDS virus in the future. The size of the sexually active population at risk for sexually transmitted diseases has never been larger and, in 1985, included 69 million sexually experienced persons between the ages of fifteen and thirty-four. A larger number of female teenagers and single adults are initiating sexual activity at an earlier age, having multiple sexual partners, and remaining single for longer periods of time, although the number appears to be stabilizing in the mid-1980s (Parra and Cates 1985). Multiple sexual partners or sex with a person who has multiple sexual partners increases the possibility of acquiring AIDS.

The American College Health Association (ACHA) established a special task force on AIDS in September 1985. The chairman, Dr. Richard B. Keeling, became the editor of a 1986 special report entitled *AIDS on the College Campus*. In the introduction he writes (Keeling 1986a, p. ix):

There have been few cases of AIDS itself among college and university students so far. For that matter, only a small proportion of AIDS cases have occurred in people who fall into the traditional college aged group. On the other hand, the incubation period . . . may be quite long; what someone does now, in college, may not result in recognizable AIDS until long after commencement. Students are commonly experimental; those in college may act out differing elements of their sexuality, exercise inconsistent judgment in their selection of sexual partners, and toy with recreational

drugs. They may not confine their sexual explorations with other
students; they may have relationships with other college and university personnel and with citizens in the surrounding community
as well. AIDS is no longer a disease just located in major metro-
politan areas. . . . Nor is it any longer a disease of gay men.

The central place of sexuality in the emotional lives of college-aged
people brings this issue regularly to the fore in college mental health
centers. Often, the psychotherapist is the only adult who hears about
or knows about current risk-taking sexual behavior of young people.
The U.S. surgeon general reminds us (Koop 1987, p. 5) that "indeed
all adults cannot disregard the responsibility to educate our young. The
need is critical and the price of neglect is high. The lives of our young
people depend on our fulfilling our responsibility." There are calls for
"a comprehensive public education campaign in which psychiatry must
play a vital role" (Rome 1986, p. 140). Most articles, including the
ACHA special report, couple their forecasts of the magnitude of the
epidemic with an urgent call for action on primary prevention through
education about risk, intravenous drug use, and safe and unsafe sexual
behavior. More specifically, American Psychiatric Association president Robert O. Pasnau (1986) accuses mental health administrators of
assuming an "ostrich position" in regard to the AIDS crisis, failing to
prepare their staffs to cope with an epidemic of such magnitude or to
formulate aggressive education and prevention campaigns.

Because of the highly charged and conflict-laden nature of sexual
feeling and behavior in particular, we are really speaking about psychoeducation, that is, an education process that embodies the important aspects of psychotherapy (Gochros 1985). Thus, any effective
education about sexual risk and safety must include steps toward forming an alliance, confronting resistance, working through the integration
of new learning, and supporting cognitive restructuring and behavior
change. It is in the area of education for prevention that the campus
psychotherapist is most frequently confronted with questions of how
to proceed when faced with sexual behavior that carries the risk of
contracting a fatal illness. The case reports that follow illustrate some
of the difficulties in addressing this issue in psychotherapy with adolescents and young adults.

Case Reports

The first vignette is from the seventh session of the time-limited psychotherapy of a female freshman student. It illustrates the kind of intervention around risk of AIDS that therapists are feeling more comfortable to make and for which they are receiving increasing consensual validation from colleagues.

CASE EXAMPLE 1

Most of the seventh session dealt with the patient's contacts with three fellows over the weekend and focused on her defenses against the sexual anxiety that was stimulated. It is an area in which she feels somewhat retarded in her development. With one young man, she was led on the first date from a kiss directly into sexual intercourse. In discussing this, what became revealed were the maladaptive defenses of disavowal and dissociation that result in a sense of depersonalization when she becomes sexually active. She easily explored the various functions of her defenses and connected them to her inability to talk about sex and to her fears of rejection. Furthermore, she exhibited rigid dichotomous thinking, putting sexual content into either/or, right-or-wrong, all-or-nothing categories. She spoke of how "being on the pill" supports this kind of disavowed action because she does not "have to think about pregnancy." I told her that one of the things she does have to think about is AIDS and the risk she incurs with each new partner. She replied that the fellow was "a clean-cut guy."I picked up on my former statement that a kiss is only an experiment and told her that even clean-cut people experiment with many forms of sexuality. Although guilty conflict was recognized, we focused mainly on a deficit in thinking and verbalizing about sex and explicitly made therapy a place for such functions. She said that she listens to what I say, but not all of it sticks with her, and I affirmed her honesty about her response.

As follow-up, the next two sessions saw a wholesome development in her relationship with the young man, with whom, at my suggestion, she risked opening up verbal communication about their sexual interaction. They mutually decided on more restraint, at least until the relationship developed further. She was happy that now she could talk to him not only about sex but about many other things as well and felt more resourceful and masterful in the arena of relations with men.

There is no question that in introducing the consideration of the risk of AIDS when young people speak about their sexual behavior, therapists move beyond a neutral, reflective, interpretive stance and assume functions that are clearly liable to be perceived as parental. The following case illustrates how, rather than creating resistance, this stance actually facilitated the process of treatment.

CASE EXAMPLE 2

This male college student was referred for private, long-term therapy. He was very anxious and was experiencing a current exacerbation of obsessive and compulsive symptoms and psychosomatic complaints that impaired his capacity for academic work. A long and close relationship with an older female student was disintegrating because he was not able to have sexual intercourse with her. He also had difficulty creating and maintaining friendships with other men. For several years, he had been engaging in sporadic visits to gay bars, and some of the long conversations he entered into there led to homosexual activity. He saw himself as bisexual and had some sustained contact with two older bisexual men, whom he took as models for identity formation. His homosexuality was ego dystonic, and his visits to gay bars were currently becoming more compelling, driven, and conflict producing.

The beloved mother of this young man had died when he was thirteen. His relations with his father and stepmother were strained and conflictful. He had instituted massive defenses early against the traumatic effect of his mother's illness and death. He had never mourned but instead had become hypermature and grandiosely self-sufficient. Early in treatment, when defenses against mourning were stubbornly clung to, he told me about recent homosexual activity. I brought up the question of protecting himself from AIDS, and he responded by engaging with me in a lengthy discussion that included consideration of going for HIV antibody testing, which he later did. Throughout the treatment, he continued to feel comfortable in discussing his homosexual feelings, thoughts, and activity, acknowledging in various ways our mutual concern for his health and safety. I gave positive reinforcement to these self-protective communications. It was through the intimacy we established, by my actively providing for him in this way, that it became possible for him to let go of his defenses gradually and to enter into the mourning that was essential for his development. He terminated treatment with a great deal of angry ambivalence, along with readiness to face and master his anxieties about intimacy and heterosexuality. On a chance meeting on the street two months later, he told me that, surprisingly to him, he was doing well.

CASE EXAMPLE 3

The next example illustrates a less clear-cut indication for an AIDS intervention because a firm therapeutic alliance was not established. When the case was purposely chosen for presentation to colleagues at a staff case conference, the intervention met with considerable controversy and divergence of opinion.

The patient is a first-year graduate student who was referred for the time-limited psychotherapy we offer at the Student Health Service, with an understanding that she might be referred outside the college for ongoing treatment. I was the fourth psychotherapist she consulted since graduation from college. A person with a histrionic character disorder, she gave a history of flight after a year or two from her therapists and also from a series of relationships with men. Her needfulness, dependence, and vulnerability to narcissistic injury were evident from the start, and these characteristics made it difficult to refer her immediately.

We began to work together on a temporary basis. She had made a successful adjustment to the campus and was doing well in her program. She said that now she wanted to work on her maladaptive patterns with men and "on my sexuality." She told me that this was the first time in ten years that she had been without a man and the first time that she was trying to keep herself from "jumping into sex too soon." I learned from the medical chart that she had a history of condylomata, chlamydia, and possible herpes infection.

Sexual concerns and a current frustrating infatuation were the manifest focus of the first four sessions, but there was a quickly established preoedipal maternal transference to me. After the fourth session, she canceled, rescheduled, and failed to come, thus missing two weekly appointments. She arrived for the fifth session and told me that, the night she saw me three weeks ago, she met a twenty-two-year-old, attractive, but "off the wall" young man and immediately became sexually involved in a most pleasurable way. She said that the involvement was "safe" because she felt autonomous and does not look to him for dependent gratifications. She said that it was difficult for her to come in to tell me about it, and then she expressed a fearful wish and need for me to tell her what my opinion was about this relationship. Being "therapy-wise," she said that she knew I could not tell her, and she anticipated disappointment and frustration even though she acknowledged ambivalence about "submitting" to me. I told her that, contrary to her expectations, I would tell her what I thought and would talk to her admittedly like a mother. I questioned why she avoids her wish to settle down with an appropriate partner, whether she is wasting her time, energy, and interest, and, also, whether she had thought about the risk of AIDS she incurs with each new partner. After all, she had contracted other sexually transmitted diseases. She appeared tearfully relieved and grateful as we discussed these issues at length. However, she canceled the next few appointments and did not reappear for five more weeks, then in a state of depression after she stopped seeing that man. The therapy resumed on a more continuous basis at that point, and she was referred at the end of the school year.

In the discussion in the case conference, two colleagues told me I should have interpreted the acting out instead of "lecturing the patient." Another countered with the thought that it would be like making an interpretation when someone is jumping off a bridge. Others also agreed with the intervention. Our director observed that the therapeutic issues in responding to AIDS-risking behavior are similar to the issue of alcoholism twenty years ago, when psychotherapists were trying and often failing to deal with it by interpretation only.

The following two cases were reported previously (Widen 1987) and are again presented with the addition of follow-up data that was obtained when the patients subsequently returned to treatment. Case Example 4 shows that the therapist's fears that she had disrupted the therapeutic alliance were unfounded.

CASE EXAMPLE 4

A nineteen-year-old male sophomore came for "a few sessions" under the pressure of becoming deeply injured and "upset" about being excluded from a relationship between two other male students, who seemingly rejected him. There was acknowledged ambivalence about coming for treatment; the therapy threatened adolescent defenses of distance and self-sufficiency. These reactions were addressed. He had full catharsis about the incident, and exploration revealed a pattern of feeling excluded from relations between others that he longed to share. This was traced back also to his childhood relations with his family. He was amazed and gratified by how helpful and enlightening therapy was, and he gradually revealed his homosexuality. One of the two young men had been his first lover. Although he had "known" he was homosexual since early adolescence, he was struggling to achieve a comfortable integration of his sexual identity. His sensitivity to the "stigma" of therapy reflected the anxiety of coming out of hiding (Martin 1982). The revelations of his homosexuality became easier as he approached termination at the end of five sessions of what could be called crisis intervention. He said he would return in a few months for another session of "housecleaning," and he did.

In the single session in the spring, this patient picked up where he left off and told about academic successes and a developing intimacy with another male student. He seemed to be increasingly comfortable and integrated with his homosexuality. This was recognized, and then the therapist felt compelled to bring up the question of concern about AIDS. The patient reacted with discomfort, and he moved to brush off further discussion. As the session ended, the therapist felt as though she had intruded on and disturbed the therapeutic alliance that had been established. It is not easy to join those "therapists trying to maintain a delicate balance: to remain sex positive and gay affirmative while at the same time working toward an education model of safe sex" (Morin, Charles, and Malyon 1984, p. 1291). Therapists must scrutinize themselves to avoid being like those in a study of health professionals whose attitudes toward gays have become more negative since the AIDS epidemic began (Douglas, Kalman, and Kalman 1985).

The young man returned the following November for another comfortable single session in which he reported his developmental progress and further character consolidation. He elicited and received my mirroring confirmation and validation, and he said a more final good-bye.

The last case demonstrates an eventual positive outcome to AIDS interventions, which had been made or withheld with a great deal of countertransference anxiety because of the negative parental transference reactions they stirred up.

CASE EXAMPLE 5

A female undergraduate with unusual acknowledgment and motivation came for help with her compulsive alcohol and oral drug abuse. After psychotherapy alone failed to help her, she was referred to Alcoholics Anonymous, to which program she committed herself fully, while remaining in therapy until she left at the end of the year. She was well structured enough also to be concerned about her lack of restraint in handling money and cutting classes. With a great deal of shame and sensitivity to criticism, she gradually revealed how she had abused herself sexually by being compulsively promiscuous. Following one long high school sexual relationship, she had engaged in about eighteen very short-term sexual contacts; many of them were one-night stands under the influence of alcohol or drugs. I mentioned AIDS, but this was disavowed or ignored. The therapy focused on self-knowledge, self-mastery, and impulse control. Her growing self-esteem more than compensated her for the anxiety and depression she was learning to tolerate.

At one point, I actively intervened by directing her to stop cutting classes and to do her work, thereby supporting a strong motive to achieve academic success. The patient was delighted and grateful when she received her first A at college.

The last months of the therapy were filled with the development and viscissitudes of a current sexual relationship. That one came to an end as she was getting ready to leave town and to terminate therapy and Alcoholics Anonymous for a while. Another man, older, attractive, described as a "scum bag," and recognized as a womanizer, appeared on the scene. She was tempted to have a short sexual fling before departure and not to tell her therapist. She decided not to act out and told her therapist the suspenseful tale. In listening, I was again struck by the risk of AIDS in this young woman's possible behavior. I struggled silently with the question of whether to bring up the issue. I also "decided not to," that is, I refrained from that action. There was possible countertransference compliance in that decision.

I felt regretful for not having spoken up again about AIDS when the patient returned for a single reporting session the following fall quarter. Among other things, she told me that the promiscuous man had come to visit her over the summer for a weekend they spent almost entirely in bed. After that, she had become more committed to the program at

AA that included support for sexual abstinence. She recently returned, and therapy has now resumed on a regular basis. Another relationship with a man was slowly developing with mutual caring, consideration, and restraint. The two were planning eventually to become fully sexually involved, but not until my patient was certain that the act would be in her own best interests. She told me that, in preparation, she wanted to have an HIV antibody test and asked for information about where to go. She followed through to make an appointment and later reported that her prospective partner would come with her to have one himself. A few weeks later, she reported that they had gone together to get the results of the test and celebrated after learning that both tests were negative. I mirrored her pleasure and responsibility.

Discussion

Along with the current rapid changes in the social order that have resulted in changing behavioral phenomena, there has been an explosion of research in the neurosciences, linguistics, and information theory and in theories of social structures and processes. Recent observations and studies of infants and their care givers (Emde 1981; Lichtenberg 1983; and Stern 1985) have made an effect on theories of psychological development and have resulted in a deeper understanding of the therapist-patient dyad. While all this impinges on psychotherapy, what remains central to our work is the intrapsychic perspective on emotional development and an empathic understanding of transference and resistance phenomena in the therapeutic relationship. However, in meeting the newer demands placed on therapy, it is necessary to consider how the brain works in processing information and in what ways perception, cognition, affect, learning, and communication are components of behavior and of that internal behavior we call thought.

The organization of the human being is so complex that both structural arrangements and various types of functional processes can be recognized at many levels, ranging from the intracellular to the societal. If we place psychodynamic theory and practice into the disciplines and methods of structuralism and general systems theory, we can broaden our repertoire of response. Menninger, Mayman, and Pruyser (1983) write that "practically all authors who are concerned with systems theory call attention to the distinction between closed and open systems, the latter being characteristic of living systems. The open system exchanges energy with its environment, its components are materially in flux, and not only does it maintain itself as a whole with a relative degree of constancy, but it may change to different levels of organization, as an organism does when it grows" (p. 92). M. R. Basch (1987, personal communication) states that patients come to therapy with impaired capacities to create order within change and that this results in the closed system of symptomatology. He adds that, in therapy, we transform closed into open systems by adding new information and by bringing to bear one's adult cognitive capacities on maladaptive patterns of expectation.

As a current impediment to growth and behavior change, adolescents and young adults have resorted to an increasing reliance on the defense of disavowal as their world has become more dangerous, their social supports more tenuous, and their psychic structure more fragile. Disavowal helps maintain the aura of invincibility that accompanies youthful attitudes of risk taking and sexual experimentation. It is the mechanism that defends against traumatic anxiety by separating the personal meaning and affective response from the perception of eternal reality. The "ego split" that occurs permits two currents to coexist: an acknowledgement of reality on the one hand along with a belief in the desired situation on the other. That is how students can "know about" the potential risk of AIDS but not feel personally threatened or motivated to change their behavior.

Because what is disavowed is not talked about, psychotherapists have had to become increasingly active. However, therapeutic activity of any kind depends on a strong and empathic therapeutic alliance that reduces the need for defense and on the soothing and expressive function of psychotherapy. Adequate therapeutic engagement can begin to promote "inner speech" and the making of connections. The kind of cognitive interventions that include observing, explaining, and instructing and that are particularly appropriate in college student psychotherapy (Love and Widen 1985) can undo disavowal by permitting the function of speech to transform a primarily factual into a personally meaningful experience (Basch 1983). Therefore, psychotherapists should consider the option of bringing up the subject of AIDS when confronted with risk-taking behavior that has this life-threatening aspect.

The inclusion of the instructive function in the repertoire of psychotherapy poses technical dilemmas. Along with maintaining a good working relationship, when and how does a therapist decide to move from any intrapsychic to a behavioral focus, from a receptive-empathic to an active-instructive position, and from an interpreting to a confronting stance? As the therapist discovered with the woman in case example 5, it is a very frustrating experience for a clinician to see a client engaged in life-threatening activities: "As difficult as it is to be empathic in these situations, it is imperative for the therapist to do so, because moving too quickly with clients who are not ready to face the reality of AIDS can alienate them so that the opportunity to intervene later is lost" (Morin et al. 1984, p. 1293).

While grappling with these technical dilemmas, psychotherapists confront their own discomfort and their own tendencies to disavow the anxiety of this difficult, value-laden issue. The kind of sharing that occurs during in-service training and case conferences can be helpful in working through these technical and personal issues so that the opportunities for helpful interventions are not lost. An active educational campaign on the larger campus and in the community (the recommendation of every writer on the subject of prevention) can aid psychotherapy by providing students with the information, words, and ideas that may later become internalized.

Conclusions

In the mid-1980s, college mental health professionals took the first steps in responding to the unique and unprecedented phenomenon of AIDS: "At no time in history has a public health crisis and our response to it been so interwoven with human values and attitudes; never have the social ramifications of our actions been so problematic" (Silverman and Silverman 1985, p. 21). It seems safe to say that every psychotherapist eventually will feel the effect of the AIDS crisis in their sessions and will observe it in its technical, ethical, and personal aspects. This chapter is a contribution to the communication and sharing of information that are the tools that psychotherapists have in adapting to the uncertainties and anxieties of their work. As time goes on, the decision about when and how to intervene when faced with risk-taking sexual behavior might be made with greater assurance that it has a sound theoretical basis.

REFERENCES

Basch, M. R. 1983. The perception of reality and the disavowal of meaning. *Annual of Psychoanalysis* 11:125–154.

Batchelor, W. F. 1984. AIDS: a public health and psychological emergency. *American Psychologist* 39:1279–1283.

Brandt, E. N. 1985. Implications of acquired immunodeficiency syndrome for health policy. *Annals of Internal Medicine* 103(5): 771–773.

Curran, J. W. 1985. The epidemiology of AIDS: current status and future prospects. *Science* 229:1352–1357.

Douglas, C. J.; Kalman, C. M.; and Kalman, T. P. 1985. Homophobia among physicians and nurses: an empirical study. *Hospital and Community Psychiatry* 36(12): 1309–1311.

Emde, R. N. 1981. Changing models of infancy and the nature of early development: remodeling the foundation. *Journal of the American Psychoanalytic Association* 29:179–219.

Gochros, H. L. 1985. Overcoming client resistances to talking about sex. *Journal of Social Work and Human Sexuality* 4:1–2.

Joseph, J. G.; Emmons, C.; Kessler, R. C.; Wortman, C. B.; O'Brien, K.; Hocker, W. T.; and Schaefer, C. 1984. Coping with the threat of AIDS. *American Psychologist* 39:1297–1302.

Keeling, R. P. 1986a. *AIDS on the College Campus: Special Report.* Rockville, Md.: American College Health Association.

Keeling, R. P. 1986b. Institutional response to AIDS: current status and future prospects. Paper presented to the annual meeting of the American College Health Association, New Orleans, May 27.

Koop, C. E. 1987. *Surgeon General's Report on Acquired Immune Deficiency Syndrome.* Washington, D.C.: U.S. Department of Health and Human Services.

Lederman, M. M. 1986. Transmission of acquired immunodeficiency syndrome through heterosexual activity. *Annals of Internal Medicine* 104(1): 115–116.

Lichtenberg, J. D. 1983. *Psychoanalysis and Infant Research.* Hillsdale, N.J.: Analytic.

Love, R. L., and Widen, H. A. 1985. Short-term dynamic therapy: another kind of learning on the campus. *Adolescent Psychiatry* 12:327–335.

486

McKusick, L.; Wiley, J. A.; Coates, T. J.; Stall, R.; Saika, G.; Morin, S.; Charles, K.; Horstman, W.; and Conant, M. A. 1985. Reported changes in the sexual behavior of men at risk for AIDS, San Francisco, 1982-84—the AIDS Behavioral Research Project. *Public Health Report* 100(6): 622–629.

Martin, A. D. 1982. Learning to hide: the socialization of the gay adolescent. *Adolescent Psychiatry* 10:52–65.

Menninger, K.; Mayman, M.; and Pruyser, P. 1983. *The Vital Balance*. New York: Viking.

Mishne, J. M. 1986. *Clinical Work with Adolescents*. New York: Macmillan/Free Press.

Morin, S. F.; Charles, K. A.; and Malyon, A. K. 1984. The psychological impact of AIDS on gay men. *American Psychologist* 39:1288–1293.

Parra, W. C., and Cates, W., Jr. 1985. Progress toward the 1990 objectives for sexually transmitted diseases: good news and bad. *Public Health Report* 100(3): 261–269.

Pasnau, R. O. 1986. Personal reflections on the syndrome known as AIDS. *Psychiatric Annals* 16(3): 139–140.

Rome, H. P. 1986. Personal reflections on the syndrome known as AIDS. *Psychiatric Annals* 16(3): 139–140.

Silverman, M. F., and Silverman, D. B. 1985. AIDS and the threat to public health. *Hastings Center Report Special Supplement* (August), pp. 19–22.

Stern, D. N. 1985. *The Interpersonal World of the Infant*. New York: Basic.

Volberding, P. 1986. AIDS: overview and current status. Paper presented to the annual meeting of the American College Health Association, New Orleans, May 27.

Widen, H. A. 1987. The risk of AIDS and the defense of disavowal: dilemmas for the college psychotherapist. *Journal of American College Health* 35:269–273.

PART V

TRAINING PRIORITIES IN ADOLESCENT PSYCHIATRY

31 A MODEL CURRICULUM FOR TEACHING ADOLESCENT PSYCHIATRY

LOIS T. FLAHERTY

In recent years, there has been increasing interest in training in adolescent psychiatry. This increased interest is related to several trends. There has been a growth in the scientific interest in adolescence and an expansion of the knowledge base of adolescent psychiatry (Hodgman 1983). Increasing numbers of adolescents are presenting as psychiatric patients, and problems of adolescence, such as pregnancy, suicide, drug abuse, and delinquency, are having a major effect on society. Between 1980 and 1984, the suicide rate among fifteen- to twenty-four-year-olds increased from 5.2 to 12.5 per 100,000, an increase of 140 percent (*Mental Health, United States* 1985). In 1955, 6 percent of psychiatric hospital inpatients were under age twenty-one; by 1960, this percentage had increased to 18 percent of all admissions. Between 1980 and 1984, admissions of adolescents to private psychiatric hospitals rose from 10,764 to 48,375, an increase of 350 percent (Weithorn 1988). The rate of psychiatric admission for individuals under age eighteen to all inpatient facilities rose from approximately 111 per 100,000 in 1971 to approximately 128 per 100,000 in 1980. There was a concomitant shift from public to private facilities, with a 52 percent increase in admissions to private facilities at the same time as there was a 39 percent decrease in admissions to public-sector facilities (Weithorn 1988). These numbers include only those adolescents who received psychiatric treatment. Epidemiologic studies have shown that only a minority of adolescents who require diagnostic and treatment services actually receive them (Offer, Ostrov, and Howard 1986; Offord 1985).

General psychiatrists, not child psychiatrists, provide most of the psychiatric care for adolescents. This has to do with the fact that there are roughly ten times as many general psychiatrists as there are child psychiatrists (30,000 compared to 3,000) and also with the fact that not all child psychiatrists treat adolescents. A recent survey indicated that there are approximately 3,000 child psychiatrists in the United States who spend 28 percent of their time treating adolescents; the approximately 30,000 general psychiatrists spend an average of 10 percent of their time treating adolescents (Enzer, Yager, Bezek, Kestenbaum, and Hendron 1986). Assuming that both groups of psychiatrists devote an average of forty hours per week to clinical care, this means that nearly twice as much care for adolescents is delivered by general psychiatrists (150,000 hours compared to 84,000 hours). This trend is likely to continue as more and more adolescents become psychiatric patients, but the pool of child psychiatrists remains relatively constant, as it has for the past several years. The current pool of residents is about 5,300, with approximately 500 of these in child and adolescent psychiatry residency programs. Although experience in child and adolescent psychiatry is required in accredited residency programs, the amount of time devoted to this is quite variable in both duration and percentage of time; a recent survey of ninety-six general psychiatry programs indicated that the most common rotation in child and adolescent psychiatry was three to four months (Tasman and Kay 1987). There are no data about how much time is devoted to adolescents. Similarly, although presumably all accredited training programs in child and adolescent psychiatry offer training in adolescent psychiatry since it is required, there is not a uniform emphasis on adolescent psychiatry in all programs. It would be accurate to say that the proportion of time allocated to training in adolescent psychiatry as part of general psychiatry residency training programs has generally not been adequate to prepare psychiatrists to diagnose or provide care for this growing patient population and that there may be a problem in child and adolescent psychiatry training programs as well.

One of the major foci of the American Society for Adolescent Psychiatry (ASAP) since its inception has been on training in adolescent psychiatry. In the first volume of the ASAP's *Annals,* a position statement was published on training in adolescent psychiatry that emphasized the need for training of general psychiatry residents in adolescent psychiatry and that recommended that specialized training in adolescent psychiatry be offered as an elective during the final year of residency as well as an option during the first year of child psychiatry fellowship (American Society for Adolescent Psychiatry 1971). In the same year, *Teaching and Learning Adolescent Psychiatry* was published, edited by two founding members of the ASAP (Offer and Masterson 1971). This book included papers on many key issues relevant to the training of general psychiatry residents. In 1980, an ad hoc committee on training standards was formed, and this committee subsequently became a standing committee. In 1985, Looney, Ellis, Benedek, and Schowalter identified key elements of a model curriculum. In 1984, the ASAP convened a Future Directions Task Force to study a variety of issues facing both the society and the field of adolescent psychiatry. The recommendations of the task force emphasized the need to define the expanding body of knowledge of adolescent psychiatry and to address the quality of adolescent treatment, training, research, and continuing education (American Society for Adolescent Psychiatry 1986).

This position paper is an outgrowth of my work as chair of the Committee on Training Standards and as a member of the Future Directions Task Force. In it, I will attempt further articulation and clarification of goals and objectives in training in adolescent psychiatry for the general psychiatrist and will address the development of a model curriculum in adolescent psychiatry for general psychiatry residents.

What Is Adolescent Psychiatry?

A definition of adolescent psychiatry cannot be made without attempting to define adolescence. Historically, the concept of adolescence as a distinct period of development is a relatively new one, following on the recognition of childhood as distinct from adulthood (Keniston 1971). The essence of the period of adolescence is that it is a transition between the time of puberty, the heralding of the attainment of physical maturity, and the assumption of full adult roles and responsibilities, signifying mental and emotional maturity. The fact that the two kinds of maturity are not synonymous holds true only in societies in which a prolonged period of preparation is necessary before the assumption of adult status, that is, in a technologically advanced society, in which advanced education and training are necessary to acquire the skills needed to compete for jobs. It follows then that, while it may be relatively easy to pinpoint the beginning of adolescence, it is difficult to say precisely when it ends. For many reasons, the transition from adolescence to young adulthood may be prolonged, lasting many years, and can take place along with marriage and child rearing. Society's confusion over when adolescence ends is reflected in laws that grant the right to vote and the obligation for military service to individuals over eighteen, provide for free and appropriate education for all handicapped children up to age twenty-one, and prohibit drinking by persons under twenty-one. Adolescence ends for different individuals at different times, and not all adult functions are acquired simultaneously. Indeed, it is now generally recognized that adulthood itself is not a single developmental period but an enormously complex process of continual change.

Nevertheless, adolescence is commonly defined as the teen years, or ages thirteen to, and including, nineteen. Physical parameters of adolescent development include the attainment of adult sexual characteristics and reproductive capacity as well as brain growth and skeletal and muscle development. Psychological parameters include the cognitive development of adolescence as well as psychosexual and social development. For purposes of understanding adolescent development, the adolescent period is commonly considered to comprise three stages—early, middle, and late adolescence. Each of these parameters has unique features that change throughout adolescence.

Having defined adolescence, adolescent psychiatry can be defined as the field of study and clinical practice that concerns itself with the understanding of the developmental period now recognized as adolescence and with the diagnosis and treatment of disorders that arise during this period. Adolescent psychiatry is distinguished by the importance given to development, its influence on psychopathology, and vice versa.

Training in adolescent psychiatry closely parallels the development of the field as a whole, which grew out of clinical observation, theoretical understanding, and a practical need to develop services for disturbed and disturbing youths. The body of knowledge in adolescent psychiatry is far from complete and lags behind that in adult and child psychiatry (Looney et al. 1985). However, it is steadily increasing, and there is now a substantial number of books and periodicals devoted to adolescent psychiatry.

The history of adolescent psychiatry has been well summarized by Slaff (1981). Adolescent psychiatry, as it exists today, has its origins

494

in psychoanalytic theory, which, with its emphasis on development, provided a natural impetus to the understanding of the adolescent period. Freud (1905) and his students explored the far-reaching implications of his work for the understanding of many aspects of the human experience and problems of society. Among these students, his gifted daughter, Anna, contributed greatly to the understanding of adolescent development and psychopathology (Freud 1958). Others—such as Blos, who introduced the concept of adolescence as a second separation-individuation period (Blos 1967); Aichhorn, who provided a way of understanding and approaching delinquent behavior (Aichhorn 1935); and Erikson, with his concept of the identity crisis as a normative phase of adolescent development (Erikson 1950)—continued the strong psychodynamic orientation of the psychology of adolescence. Piaget (1969), studying cognitive development, identified abstract thinking as coming into existence for the first time during adolescence, and Mead (1928), with an anthropological perspective, identified adolescence as a unique period accompanied by rites of passage in the societies she studied.

The increased understanding of the importance of child and adolescent development to the formation of the adult personality led naturally to concerns about how to enhance healthy development and how to counteract or reverse noxious influences on development. By guiding development, one could, theoretically at least, promote healthy outcomes. Hence, the child guidance clinics, which were the first formally organized services for troubled children and adolescents. The juvenile justice system arose out of a similar concept, as did the training schools. In a somewhat separate manner, college and university health services were developed in recognition of the unique needs of the older adolescent and young adult population. More recently, interest has been focused on the transition from adolescence to young adulthood and on the particular problems of the young adult chronically mentally ill population as well as of the homeless, many of whom are adolescents and young adults. Our current era has seen a swing away from an exclusively psychodynamic orientation toward more descriptive, phenomenological approaches and recognition of the importance of incompletely understood genetic and biochemical factors in psychiatric disorders. There is much that is not known about the mechanisms of physical and psychological development in adolescence and about how these affect each other. The field still struggles to define what constitutes normative

495

development and to avoid the pitfalls of over- or underestimating psychopathology in adolescents. It seems likely that the future will see attempts to integrate the rapid advances in the neurosciences with what has been learned from decades of clinical experience.

In 1958, the American Psychiatric Association recognized the field of child psychiatry as a subspecialty and approved training standards for child psychiatrists. This led to the formation of a formal process of certifying examinations given by the Committee on Certification in Child Psychiatry of the American Board of Psychiatry and Neurology (ABPN) and, concomitantly, a process of accreditation of training programs in child psychiatry by the Accreditation Council on Graduate Medical Education, a branch of the American Medical Association. The role of training in adolescent psychiatry as part of child psychiatry training has never been clearly defined. The requirements for accreditation of child and adolescent psychiatry residency programs do not specify the amount of time that should be devoted to adolescent psychiatry in either the didactic curriculum or the experiential component of the training. The certification process, as does that in general psychiatry, involves a written and an oral examination. There is no absolute requirement that a given percentage of the written examination questions deal with adolescence, but approximately 25 percent do. One-third of the oral examination consists of a live interview of an adolescent patient by the candidate, followed by oral examination of the candidate. The ASAP's New Directions Task Force undertook an intensive look at the field of adolescent psychiatry and recommended that both training standards and some kind of certification process for psychiatrists specializing in work with adolescents be developed. The ASAP has taken the position that the completion of child psychiatry fellowship training need not be a prerequisite for competence to work with adolescents. One of the key issues for training is whether, in fact, a large number of residents in general psychiatry would be attracted to training programs in adolescent psychiatry that did not require work with young children beyond that required as part of the general psychiatry training program. It has been suggested that a substantial background in adult work may enhance ability to work with adolescents because of the retaining of the focus on disorders of older adolescents, which in many cases have more in common with adult psychiatric disorders than with those of childhood (Parry-Jones 1984).

496

LOIS T. FLAHERTY

Basic Principles of Training in Adolescent Psychiatry

Minimum competency in adolescent psychiatry should be required for all general psychiatry residents, and a higher level of competency should be required for those who wish to specialize in the treatment of adolescents. Many general psychiatrists may elect not to treat adolescents. However, because of the large numbers of adolescents in various mental health care systems, it is unlikely that the general psychiatrist can avoid having some involvement with adolescent patients, and he will, most likely, be called on to give opinions as to diagnosis and treatment recommendations. For this reason, it is important that all general psychiatry residents develop the ability to perform diagnostic evaluations of adolescents. In addition, they should be sufficiently aware of the currently used and accepted treatment modalities and their indications in order to assist in treatment planning and recommendations. As the kinds of therapeutic interventions available for adolescents have increased, so has the importance of determining the treatment of choice for a given adolescent. Particularly important is the need to determine when more intensive forms of treatment, such as intensive outpatient psychotherapy or hospitalization, are indicated. Recently, much attention has been focused on what is described as inappropriate overuse of psychiatric hospitalization of adolescents (Weithorn 1988). There can be no doubt that there is sometimes a tendency for adolescents to be hospitalized indiscriminately, which can have long-lasting and harmful effects on their development of autonomy and independence. Equally harmful can be the failure to recommend intensive long-term treatment when it is indicated. Both the inappropriate use and the insufficient use of various treatment modalities underscore the need for better training for psychiatrists who treat adolescents so that treatment recommendations are based on recognized clinical indications. The need for improved diagnosis and treatment for adolescents constitutes one of the major problems in adolescent psychiatry.

The Importance of Research Training

There is a tremendous need for research in adolescent psychiatry, and few psychiatrists have the training to do it. Research training is difficult to provide without a cadre of researchers who are themselves trained in research methodology. However, opportunities exist for collaboration between those who have clinical expertise and interest in adolescence and researchers whose primary interest may be in adult psychiatry and who have expertise in research in epidemiology, genetics, phenomenology, or biological psychiatry that could be applied to the study of adolescent psychiatric disorders. In many other medical subspecialty areas, research is an integral part of specialized training; the fact that this has not generally been the case in psychiatry may have played a role in perpetuating the inadequate scientific knowledge base in the field as a whole. It is likely that increased research activity in adolescent psychiatry would stimulate more interest in training among medical students and residents. Whether adolescent psychiatrists become researchers or not, it is important that they develop the ability to review critically the literature, evaluate claims for efficacy (or lack of it) of treatment modalities, and question and wonder about what they read, see, and hear.

Designing a Curriculum

Training in the generic sense can be understood as involving four basic components: *knowledge,* a body of information germane to a specific field or subject; *understanding,* the ability to apply knowledge in useful ways; *skill,* behaviors that are demonstrated as a result of acquisition of knowledge and understanding; and *attitudes,* propensities toward certain behaviors. The development of a specific curriculum in adolescent psychiatry can be conceptualized in terms of these four components; one can begin to think about curriculum development by defining the specific knowledge, understanding, skills, and attitudes that are to be taught.

In a general sense, training programs can be conceptualized both in terms of content, that is, what is to be taught, and in terms of form, that is, how the content is taught. The first step in developing a model curriculum is to decide what should be taught; the second step is to design a program in which it can be taught. In general, it is easier to conceptualize the former than the latter. Different problems are involved in each task. With respect to the content of the curriculum, there may be widely varying views among experts in the field about what should be taught and what are essentials, as opposed to electives.

498

Any model curriculum is likely to be criticized for failing to emphasize one area sufficiently or for giving too great an emphasis to another area not considered important. A curriculum that attempts to be very comprehensive risks superficiality; one that emphasizes one area in depth is in danger of being too narrowly focused. The whole field of psychiatry has undergone and continues to undergo massive expansion in its knowledge base and, at the same time, to extend its scope of interest to a wider spectrum of patients, for example, the homeless mentally ill and young chronic patients. This is no less true for adolescent psychiatry than for psychiatry as a whole. In medicine, it is not, strictly speaking, possible to separate the process of acquiring new knowledge from the process of carrying out clinical responsibilities; that is, to a great extent, one learns as one does. Complete training requires both a comprehensive didactic curriculum and carefully designed practical experiences. These two essential components of training need to be well integrated with each other. For example, if psychoanalytic developmental theory is taught, clinical supervision of diagnostic and therapeutic work with patients should emphasize the understanding of the individual patient from this perspective. The same is true with respect to the teaching of psychopharmacology, family dynamics, and other areas.

With respect to the form of the curriculum, the chief problems faced are twofold: how to fit a specialized curriculum within the confines of an existing general psychiatry residency program, and how to best utilize existing resources. Residency training programs are becoming increasingly constrained by major changes in the health care delivery system that are drastically altering methods of patient care. The question of who pays for the training of new physicians does not at this time have a firm answer (Nadelson and Robinowitz 1987; Sharfstein, Goldman, and Stein 1987). Teaching hospitals are particularly squeezed by cost-cutting measures; whether private, for-profit hospitals will in the future assume a major role in training is not certain. Outpatient clinics, never well supported, although they have traditionally been important teaching sites, are being closed in many teaching centers because of their lack of income-producing power.

Residency training programs, in addition to being influenced by economic forces that influence clinical service assignments, are also being challenged to incorporate more and more specialized areas into the training of all residents. Thus, such areas as geriatric psychiatry, forensic psychiatry, and family therapy, which may have been viewed in the past as specialized areas, are now considered essential to training in general psychiatry. In many of the recent discussions about trends toward increasing subspecialization in psychiatry, concern about losing the role of the psychiatrist as a generalist has been expressed (Reider 1988; Yager, Langsley, Peele, McKegney, and Fink 1987). In this continuous strong support for the generalist, psychiatry differs from most other specialties. The attempt to introduce yet another new area into what is usually already a very crowded curriculum is likely to be met with considerable resistance from both faculty, who see it as competing with residents' involvement in other activities, and residents, who see themselves burdened with additional responsibilities. It is important, therefore, to try to design the curriculum in a way that tends to (1) utilize existing resources and (2) incorporate it into the existing training program as much as possible. By emphasizing the continuities between adolescent and adult development and psychopathology and the commonalities of many basic treatment approaches, a curriculum that is truly integrated into the total curriculum for residents in general psychiatry can be developed.

Accreditation Requirements Relevant to Teaching Adolescent Psychiatry

The Residency Review Committee (RRC) for Psychiatry of the Accreditation Council for Graduate Medical Education defines standards that training programs in all recognized medical specialties must meet in order to be accredited (American Medical Association 1988). These standards, known as the *Essentials,* are revised periodically to reflect changes and developments in the various specialties and subspecialties. Both the general psychiatry and the child psychiatry standards have recently been revised. Significantly, the term "child psychiatry" was replaced by "child and adolescent psychiatry" in 1988. Although the *Essentials* define neither the nature of expected experience in adolescent psychiatry nor the amount of time that must be devoted to work with adolescents, they do specifically mention adolescents. The curricular requirements for training in general psychiatry specify that programs must teach residents about development and to do diagnostic assessments of patients of all ages and provide experience in treatment of adolescents. The requirements are not specific in terms of actual time commitments or numbers of patients. Although the recent changes in the *Essentials* reflect a tendency toward increased specificity, there is also a reluctance to become overly specific, so as to allow some degree of flexibility to be retained by training programs. Implicit in the *Essentials* is the expectation that the general psychiatrist should have the ability to diagnose and at least formulate treatment plans for patients of all ages and with all kinds of psychiatric disorders.

Many of the requirements spelled out in the *Essentials* are relevant to adolescent psychiatry training. Requisite knowledge for general psychiatry residents is defined as including the following: "Understanding of the biological, psychological, social, economic, ethnic and family factors that significantly influence physical and psychological development in infancy, childhood, *adolescence* and adulthood" (p. 98, B.1.b.; italics added). "Comprehension of the etiologies, prevalence, diagnosis and treatment of *all* of the psychiatric conditions in the current standard diagnostic statistical manual as well as of the diagnosis and treatment of neurologic disorders relevant to psychiatric practice" (p. 98, B.1.c.; italics added). "Understanding of when and how to refer" (p. 98, B.1.h.). Curricular requirements include the following: "The curriculum must include 'adequate and systematic instruction in child and adult development' " (p. 98, C.1.f.). "Each resident must have supervised experience in the evaluation and treatment of patients of both sexes, of various ages from childhood to old age, and from a variety of ethnic, racial, social and economic backgrounds" (p. 99, C.2.b). And, in a restatement that specifically refers to adolescents, the *Essentials* also state that specific clinical experiences must include "supervised clinical experience in the evaluation and treatment of children, *adolescents, couples and families*" (p. 99, C.3.c.[3]; italics added).

Application of RRC Goals and Objectives to Training in Adolescent Psychiatry for General Psychiatry Residents

Extrapolating from the RRC requirements for all general psychiatry residents to develop knowledge and skills in psychiatry for all age groups, goals for training in adolescent psychiatry can be summarized as follows: (1) an understanding of adolescent development; (2) the ability to do diagnostic assessments of adolescents; (3) the ability to formulate treatment plans for adolescents; and (4) the ability to refer adolescent patients for appropriate services. Objectives for each of these goals might include the following. (1) The resident should be able to describe the stages of development during adolescence and be familiar with the physical, hormonal, cognitive, and psychodynamic changes that characterize the period of puberty through young adulthood. (2) The resident should be able to gather and synthesize appropriate data from adolescent patients by interviews with patients and families and to collect additional necessary information from other sources (such as schools, psychological tests, etc.) in order to formulate a diagnosis. The resident should demonstrate the capacity to establish sufficient rapport with adolescent patients to gather necessary information from them and should be aware of and sensitive to the adolescent patient's need for confidentiality and to the degree of difficulty in establishing trust. (3) The resident should be able to develop a treatment plan that is relevant to the patient's needs. The resident should be familiar with the role of individual, family, and group psychotherapies in the treatment of adolescents, as well as special considerations that apply to hospitalization of adolescent patients and use of psychopharmacologic agents in adolescents. (4) The resident should be able to refer adolescent patients for necessary treatment services. This implies knowledge of available resources and the ability to communicate with the adolescent patient and family as well as with the diagnostic or treatment provider to whom the referral is being made.

Enabling objectives are basically the ways in which the objectives can be attained. Specific recommendations for general psychiatry residency programs to enable residents to achieve essential knowledge, understanding, and skills for diagnosing and recommending treatment for adolescent patients include the following. (1) Adolescent development should be taught as a significant part of the curriculum on development. (2) Manifestations of psychopathology that are unique to adolescents should be taught, either as part of a course on child and adolescent psychopathology or integrated into the curriculum on psychopathology. (3) Each resident should be responsible for completing full diagnostic assessments on at least three adolescent patients, including one patient from each of the three stages of adolescence. (4) Programs should provide all residents with a minimum experience of treating one adolescent patient in individual therapy for at least six months. (5) Opportunities for elective experiences in adolescent psychiatry should be provided. These can vary and can include group and/or family therapy with adolescents, work in inpatient settings, or consultation to pediatric wards, clinics, schools, and other community settings. (6) Opportunities to participate in clinical research in adolescent psychiatry should be provided.

Essential Resources

FACULTY REQUIREMENTS

There should be least one faculty member who has a primary interest in adolescents and whose major focus is on working with them. While this person may not be the one who provides all the teaching and supervision for residents in adolescent psychiatry, he or she should assume responsibility for overseeing and organizing the residents' experiences. This may include arranging for adequate supervision for all the residents by full- and/or part-time clinical faculty.

CLINICAL EXPERIENCES AND SUPERVISION DURING THE FIRST AND SECOND POSTGRADUATE YEARS

Adolescent psychiatry should not be taught only during the child psychiatry block rotations. In most residency training programs, residents will encounter adolescent patients in many clinical settings, beginning during the first year. These will include their on-call experiences and work in the emergency rooms, on the consultation liaison service, and on adult inpatient services. In many settings, adolescents sixteen years and older are admitted to adult psychiatric wards, and the age group from seventeen to twenty-four is well represented in inpatient populations. Many psychiatric disorders first become apparent during the late adolescent–early adult period. One way in which the residents' learning about adolescent psychiatry can be enhanced is through the making of rounds by the faculty member knowledgeable about adolescent psychiatry on the adult wards to discuss the adolescent and adult patients with a particular focus on developmental aspects. The availability of suitable faculty members for supervision of the treatment of adolescent patients hospitalized on adult wards is also important. Faculty in adolescent psychiatry can be invited discussants at grand rounds

503

and case conferences when adolescents are being presented. The idea that adolescent patients are part of the resident's caseload, but at the same time do have unique treatment needs, can be emphasized in this manner. In this manner, learning about adolescent psychiatry can be integrated into the residents' clinical experiences from the beginning of training rather than delayed until the child psychiatry rotation.

EXPERIENCES DURING THE CHILD PSYCHIATRY ROTATION

In many programs, child and adolescent psychiatry is taught as a block rotation of six months or longer, often during the third year of residency. Experiences during this rotation may include outpatient evaluation and treatment and possibly inpatient work as well. Care should be taken to ensure that residents see a proportionate number of adolescents along with younger children. If the experience during the first two years of residency has been primarily with older adolescent patients, then residents should focus primarily on the younger and middle adolescents during this time. Case conferences given during this rotation should devote a substantial portion of time to adolescent patients. On the whole, the amount of emphasis given to adolescent psychiatry during the child psychiatry rotation should be determined in part by how much emphasis has been given to integrated experiences in adolescent psychiatry during the earlier years of the residency. If the program has provided substantial supervised clinical experience with adolescent patients during the first two years of the residency, then it may be appropriate for the child psychiatry rotation to emphasize the younger age group. However, if there has been little emphasis on adolescent psychiatry outside the child psychiatry rotation, then it is crucial that adequate time be devoted to teaching adolescent psychiatry during this period.

DIDACTIC CURRICULUM

A list of suggested areas to cover in a lecture or seminar format is provided in the Appendix. This list is not meant to be exhaustive. The way in which these topics are taught can vary. They do not have to be combined in a single lecture series on adolescent psychiatry, although that is one way that they could be presented. The teaching of adolescent psychiatry in the didactic seminars can be incorporated into sections of other seminars during all years of training. For example, legal issues with adolescents could be covered in a series on forensic psychiatry. Integration of the teaching on adolescent psychiatry with the overall teaching program offers many advantages, including economy of time (of the residents as well as of the faculty) and the opportunity for residents to utilize their understanding of general principles in their work with adolescent patients. Some topics will be best taught in the context of case conferences, with case presentations and/or live interviews of patients. In contrast to the difficulty in teaching psychotherapy of adolescents, it is easier to teach in didactic format the general developmental issues of adolescents and aspects of differential diagnosis and treatment. One major advantage in teaching many aspects of adolescent development is that, insofar as they can be grasped and understood intellectually, they are fairly accessible to the residents in terms of memories of their own experiences during their adolescent years. Further suggestions on the teaching of these topics follow.

CHILD DEVELOPMENT SEMINAR

In most programs, some teaching on development occurs during the first two years. This should include both normal and abnormal development and feature sections on pregnancy, infancy and early childhood, middle childhood, and various phases of adolescence. Including a fairly extended period on adolescent development in this seminar has the advantage not only of teaching about adolescents but also of providing for a more complete treatment of early development, as development during adolescence is in many ways a reworking of earlier developmental phases. Such a seminar should include older adolescent and young adult development and possibly continue into the adult developmental stages. It should include such things as psychosexual development, object relations, ego and superego development, and the effect of cultural and environmental factors on development. The use of videotapes such as those from *The Electronic Textbook of Psychiatry* (Kestenbaum 1974, 1976) dealing with normal development through adolescence can be particularly helpful.

PSYCHOPATHOLOGY

A seminar on psychopathology can include a section on manifestations of adult psychiatric disorders in adolescents, including schizophrenia, affective disorders, neuroses, mental retardation, and others. Similarly, the manifestations during adolescence of the child and adolescent disorders, which include such things as developmental disorders and conduct disorders, should be taught. In each instance, care should be taken to distinguish the adolescent manifestations of these disorders from either the childhood or the adult manifestations. For example, separation anxiety disorder in adolescents is different from that in younger children, and the manifestations of affective disorders in adolescents differ from those in adults.

ASSESSMENT

This includes interviewing techniques, the collection of relevant data, and the synthesis of available information in order to make a diagnosis and to plan treatment. Although lectures and reading can be helpful, interviewing must be learned by experience. Residents should have ample opportunities to observe faculty interviews and to have their own interviews with patients observed by faculty supervisors.

LEGAL ISSUES

A series on legal issues in psychiatry can include discussions of legal rights of adolescents, laws pertaining to voluntary and involuntary treatment of adolescents, the legal status of emancipated minors, and informed consent. The issues of competency to stand trial, waiver to adult criminal court, and rights of juveniles charged with crimes should be discussed. Laws pertaining to adolescents' rights to refuse treatment versus parents' rights to obtain treatment for them are quite complex and vary from state to state. Knowledge of these laws is of great practical importance for residents who are responsible for obtaining emergency hospitalization for adolescents whom they may see in the emergency room.

PSYCHOPHARMACOLOGY

A didactic series on psychopharmacology can include a special section on issues of drug treatment in adolescents. Discussion of various drugs, such as antidepressants and neuroleptics, should include some mention of whether the effectiveness of these drugs has been studied in adolescents and what the findings have been. It is also important to include discussions of the meaning of psychopharmacological treatment to the adolescent, developmental aspects of resistance to taking medication, and practical ways of handling resistance and noncompliance to taking prescribed medication.

THE TEACHING OF PSYCHOTHERAPY WITH ADOLESCENTS

It is the ability to do effective psychotherapeutic work with adolescents, whether this be long-term individual therapy, crisis intervention, or group or family therapy, which is the sine qua non of the adolescent psychiatrist. Of course, a thorough knowledge of cognitive, emotional, and physical development is essential for this to occur. But good adolescent psychiatrists have a special ability to understand and communicate effectively with their patients, to set limits appropriately, to hold on and to let go when indicated—in short, to develop, maintain, and eventually, to terminate what has been so eloquently described by Meeks (1980) as "the fragile alliance." It is the task of the residency training program to foster this skill in residents. Obviously, not all residents have an aptitude for working with adolescents. Many are "turned off" by emotionally disturbed adolescents and may find that the reactivation of their unresolved adolescent conflicts engendered by exposure to adolescent patients is too disruptive for them to work effectively with adolescents. While these residents will not become adolescent psychiatrists, they should acquire the basic knowledge and skill essential to diagnosis and treatment planning.

The particular transference and countertransference problems that arise in the psychotherapeutic treatment of adolescents are complex and have been well described by writers such as Masterson (1971) and others. Adolescents tend to engender strong emotional responses in adults. These responses include overidentification with the adolescent struggle for autonomy and vicarious gratification from, as well as reaction formations against, sexual and aggressive drives that are seen as being directly expressed in adolescent behavior. The rebelliousness and hostility of many emotionally disturbed adolescents makes them unpleasant to deal with. The need for nonpunitive limit setting is difficult to respond to appropriately, even for an experienced therapist. These issues can best be handled in the context of individual supervision of the resident that allows the careful and nonjudgmental exploration of the resident's experiences with his adolescent patients and may also be discussed as a general issue at ward staff meetings, case conferences, and grand rounds. The continuous case seminar is another format that can combine some of the aspects of individual supervision with didactic teaching and discussions of relevant articles from the literature.

CLINICAL SERVICE ASSIGNMENTS

Clinical service assignments provide the substrate for the experiential component of training in adolescent psychiatry. A variety of different settings can be utilized for training purposes. The settings should provide patient populations of adolescents with a variety of psychiatric disorders and the full spectrum of levels of impairment, from mild to severe. Residents should have the opportunity to work with adolescents of different ages and from different socioeconomic levels and ethnic backgrounds. One way of beginning to think about appropriate settings for training in adolescent psychiatry is to look at what institutions and facilities currently assume responsibility for mental health needs of adolescents. This not only gives an indication of where psychiatric consultation and treatment services are needed but also suggests many opportunities for training via placement of residents or fellows in these facilities as part of their residency or fellowship experiences. This list includes the following: psychiatric outpatient clinics; adolescent inpatient units; general psychiatric inpatient units that accept adolescents; group homes; schools; courts; adolescent medicine clinics; and adolescent inpatient medical wards.

Most residency training programs in general and child psychiatry have ready access to one or more of these facilities. Not infrequently, a training program is developed around a specific clinical setting, such as an adolescent inpatient unit that provides funding for stipends for residents.

There should be a set of experiences that are required of all residents and also elective experiences that are available to interested residents who have already fulfilled the core requirements. As a minimum, experience with adolescents who are hospitalized on adult wards or general psychiatry wards, together with at least one long-term outpatient psychotherapy with individual supervision, should be required. The inpatient experience should be at least six months long and the outpatient therapy experience should be at least one year. Each of these experiences should be supervised by psychiatrists knowledgeable about adolescents. The goals of these experiences include the teaching of fundamental knowledge, skills, and attitudes important in working with adolescents.

In addition to the core experiences, it is desirable to offer elective experiences. These can be taken during the child psychiatry rotation, if time allows, or during the elective portions of the residency. Some possible elective experiences include the following.

Family therapy with adolescents has increasingly been recognized as an important therapeutic modality. There are many unique aspects to treating families with adolescents, with the adolescent's struggle for emancipation from the family counterbalanced by his need to integrate himself into it. The availability of live supervision for the resident greatly enhances the quality of the experience.

Group therapy is recognized as an important treatment modality for adolescents and is frequently offered in inpatient and residential settings. A resident can function as a cotherapist with a more experienced therapist. This experience can provide the opportunity to learn group therapy techniques with adolescents as well as a more thorough understanding of adolescent group process and peer interactions.

Consultation liaison experiences afford the resident the opportunity of learning about the effect of chronic illnesses on adolescents as well as on their families. Adolescents hospitalized on medical wards or seen in outpatient medical clinics offer an opportunity for residents to understand the interaction of somatic, psychological, and social variables. A high proportion of these adolescents have psychological problems that are presenting as physical complaints and/or illnesses in which psychological factors play a major role. Adolescent trauma victims offer another population in which to study the effect of stress on the adolescent's growth and development. Adolescent pregnancy, and its associated psychopathology, is another area to which residents can be exposed during these experiences. Finally, adolescents who attempt suicide are often hospitalized on medical services. As requests for consultation frequently are related to the difficulty primary care physicians experience in dealing with adolescent patients, it is important for supervision to be provided not only to help the resident understand the adolescent's health care and psychological needs but also to help the psychiatry resident assist the primary care physician in providing for these needs. Psychiatric aspects of mental illness with adolescents can be taught in the context of psychiatric liaison experiences during the general psychiatry residency, which can be designed to provide experience consulting on adolescents hospitalized in medical wards. If residents do not see adolescents during their adult consultation/liaison experiences, then this opportunity can be provided as part of the child psychiatry rotation.

Community consultation experiences also offer many opportunities for learning adolescent psychiatry. These may include special education and day treatment programs for adolescents, which may or may not be hospital based. Additional opportunities are provided in juvenile courts, many of which have some kind of psychiatric services associated with them. Group homes and residential treatment centers for adolescents are other possible consultation sites. In connection with each of these experiences, it is important that adequate supervision (preferably on site) be provided.

Goals for Residents Who Wish to Specialize in Adolescent Psychiatry

While the resources outlined can be considered essential for all psychiatrists, additional competency is needed for the general psychiatrist who wishes to treat adolescents. In terms of knowledge, the goals include mastery of the psychopathology of adolescent disorders as well as of adolescent development and other aspects of general psychiatry as they apply to adolescents. To be able to treat adolescents effectively, one should be able to carry out individual, family, and group therapy in inpatient and outpatient settings and on both a long-term and a short-term basis. In terms of skills, which are behaviors, goals include such things as the formation of a therapeutic alliance with adolescent patients, communication with parents and handling of issues of confidentiality, limit setting, and termination with adolescents. Skill in crisis intervention techniques, psychopharmacological treatment, and design and management of a therapeutic milieu is also important. Finally, it is desirable that there be an ability to provide effective consultation to schools and community agencies that serve adolescents. To acquire this level of competency, additional training is needed beyond what can be obtained in the usual psychiatric residency. This additional training can be undertaken during the last year of residency, in the form of an elective experience or as a postresidency fellowship.

Some general psychiatrists may elect to treat certain kinds of adolescent patients without necessarily assuming responsibility for the full range of adolescent patients with all degrees of severity of psychopathology. A general psychiatrist may see a few adolescent patients in individual psychotherapy, for example. The psychiatrist may see only outpatients or only older adolescents. In addition to the basic knowledge and skill areas identified as essential for all psychiatrists, the psychiatrist who provides treatment for adolescents should have skill in the particular treatment modalities used, sufficient understanding of adolescent psychiatric disorders, and the ability to diagnose adolescent patients so that the treatment modality is being used in an appropriate manner, is appropriate to the adolescent's needs, and is applied to the adolescent patient in keeping with generally accepted standards. For example, in order to do effective group therapy with adolescents, one must understand the indications for use of this treatment modality with adolescent patients, be able to evaluate the suitability of particular adolescent patients for group therapy, and then carry out group therapy in a way that uses particular modifications of technique that are necessary for effective group therapy with adolescent patients.

Some psychiatrists may wish to devote a significant part of their professional careers to working with adolescents. They may not be interested in working with children and, therefore, are not likely to enter fellowship programs in child and adolescent psychiatry. If one extrapolates from data about the ASAP members who are not trained in child psychiatry, this group of psychiatrists typically retains a strong focus on adult psychiatry, particularly the problems of young adulthood, and is interested in the manifestations of adult psychiatric disorders in adolescents.

Elective Experiences and Fellowships in Adolescent Psychiatry

Elective experiences are those taken during the regular residency program; fellowships involve training beyond the fourth postgraduate year of residency. There is some confusion about the term "fellowship" because in many programs "fellowships" have been offered to fourth-

511

year residents, and residents are allowed (by ABPN rules) to enter child and adolescent psychiatry training programs after completion of the third postgraduate year. In many psychiatry residency programs, the fourth year is wholly or partly elective. This offers an opportunity for the resident who has an interest in adolescent psychiatry to focus on this area. The majority of training directors of child and adolescent psychiatry training programs surveyed in 1986 stated that they offered elective experiences in adolescent psychiatry for residents (Flaherty 1986). These ranged from additional outpatient experiences to rotations on inpatient adolescent units. Special one- or two-year concentrated programs in adolescent psychiatry have been developed at a few centers. The one best known is the Clinical Research Training Program in Adolescence sponsored by the Michael Reese Hospital and the University of Chicago. This is a two-year program designed to provide advanced interdisciplinary skills for the study of adolescence and to promote research and scholarship on the adolescent age period. The program includes a clinical research project, research seminars, and individualized clinical experiences designed to develop or enhance skills relevant to the fellow's research training. A program has been developed at the University of Maryland that combines clinical experiences, didactic seminars, and research opportunities. This program is under the direction of the Division of Child and Adolescent Psychiatry and involves faculty of the division who have a special interest in adolescents. The program can be taken for either one or two years. The first year consists of clinical rotations. Clinical experiences include inpatient and outpatient work with adolescents and with consultation to the juvenile court and to a day school for emotionally handicapped and learning-disabled adolescents. The inpatient and community consultation experiences are each six months long; the outpatient therapy is for one year and is taken concurrently with the inpatient and community consultation experiences. The second year consists of a full-time research experience in the area of adolescent substance abuse. There is no clinical work with children during this program; residents are expected to have completed the required child and adolescent psychiatry rotation during their third postgraduate year in the residency program. Residents in the adolescent psychiatry program take many of the same seminars as the residents in the two-year child and adolescent psychiatry training program; thus, they are taught extensively about child development and psychopathology. In addition, they have a special continuous case seminar on adolescent psychotherapy.

Programs can be designed to provide a range of experiences in working with adolescents and can be integrated with child psychiatry fellowship training with respect to some of the clinical and didactic experiences. In the event that a resident decides to continue on into full child and adolescent psychiatry training, the second year of the program can be designed to provide didactic and clinical experience with children, with the year of adolescent psychiatry counting toward one year of child and adolescent psychiatry residency.

It is crucial for the psychiatrist who wishes to specialize in work with adolescents to have an understanding of the problems and issues facing researchers in adolescent psychiatry and to be familiar with the current literature as well as that which has made important past contributions to the field. Opportunities for residents to become involved in clinical research projects in adolescent psychiatry should be provided. These projects may include participation in a data-based study but could also consist of scholarly reviews of the literature, clinical case studies, and theoretical papers.

Evaluation

Evaluation of the training program and the trainees is an essential component of training. It provides a crucial method of documenting whether the goals of the program are being met, and it is one of the requirements of the Accreditation Council for Graduate Medical Education's *Essentials* for approved psychiatry residency programs.

The most commonly used method of evaluating trainees is through standardized rating forms. Most residency programs are using forms they have developed to evaluate residents. These forms can be modified to include specific questions about ability to work with adolescents.

A second method of evaluating performance of psychiatric residents is through the use of cognitive examinations. Cognitive examinations are required under the new *Essentials*. Currently, the most widely used example of such an examination is the Psychiatric Residents In-training Examination (PRITE), a national examination given annually to all residents in participating programs. The examination includes several sections, and scores are reported for each section, in terms of both an absolute score and a percentile compared with all residents who took the exam. A proportion of this examination is devoted to child and adolescent development and psychopathology. Although there has been some discussion of developing a separate PRITE exam for use in child and adolescent psychiatry residency programs, it appears that the resources involved in mounting such an effort would be prohibitive, given the relatively small number of trainees in such programs. For the present, rather than develop a separate examination, efforts are being directed toward increasing the emphasis on child and adolescent psychiatry in the PRITE.

A third evaluative technique that has been gaining favor in residency programs is the use of "mock boards." These have been felt to be very useful by programs that have participated. It is often possible for several programs that are geographically situated near each other to pool their resources in organizing such exams. These examinations are modeled after the APBN examinations and include oral examinations based on videotapes, clinical vignettes, and live patient interviews.

Given the difficulty inherent in assessing residents' performance with any of the described methods, it would seem advisable to use a combination of all three methods. It seems likely that, as emphasis on evaluation of training experiences increases, there will be more emphasis on assessment of trainees' knowledge and skills in all areas considered critical to residency training. Those assuming responsibility for developing a curriculum in adolescent psychiatry should work closely with residency training directors at their institutions to make sure that assessment in adolescent psychiatry is incorporated into whatever methods are used to assess residents' performance.

A fourth method of evaluation of trainees and programs is the use of case logs. This is now mandated for general psychiatry programs. The use of case logs can be helpful in monitoring the trainees' patient contacts. Case logs should reflect the varying ages of the patients seen; this will provide a way of monitoring the experience with adolescents.

Recommendations for the Development of National Standards

The notion of evaluation of training carries with it the idea that training should meet certain objectively defined standards that lend themselves to assessment. Given that such standards exist, both trainees and programs can be evaluated. Trainees can be tested to see if they are able to demonstrate the knowledge and skills deemed essential for the practice of a medical specialty. Training programs can be evaluated against standards that are developed for them to help ensure that they will provide their trainees with the opportunities to acquire the requisite knowledge and skills. This process of evaluation, or credentialing, is important in that it allows for some measure of objectively defined standards to be applied in a uniform manner. In spite of the fact that the application of the process of credentialing is an extraordinarily difficult one in psychiatry because of both the controversies and fragmentation that still exist in the field and the fact that clinical competence is incompletely assessed in the format of the written and oral examinations, there is widespread acknowledgment, both within and outside the profession, of the importance of the credentialing process. Credentialing has two major effects: it protects the quality of care given to the public, and it enhances the ability of those who are credentialed to compete in the economic marketplace.

In 1986, the ASAP petitioned the ABPN to establish a separate category of subspecialty certification in adolescent psychiatry. The response of the ABPN at that time was that there was not a need for a separate subspecialty certification process. Factors cited in the board's decision were the existence of subspecialty certification in child psychiatry that included adolescent psychiatry and the lack of a clear definition of adolescents as distinct from children. The board recommended that the ASAP work with the then American Academy of Child Psychiatry to increase the emphasis on adolescent psychiatry in training programs and in the credentialing process. The push for recognition of adolescent psychiatry as a separate subspecialty was controversial, as it was seen by some child psychiatrists as a threat to their field. At the same time, the change in name of both the American Academy of Child Psychiatry and the Committee on Certification in Child Psychiatry from "Child" to "Child and Adolescent" reflected an implicit acknowledgment that these organizations needed to recognize adolescents and adolescent psychiatry as distinct from children and child psychiatry.

It may be helpful to review the requirements of the American Board of Medical Specialties (ABMS), the parent organization of the ABPN, for recognition of a field within medicine as constituting a subspecialty. The ABMS allows for its member boards, subject to its approval, to develop a process whereby physicians who are already board certified

515

in a specialty can have their certificates modified to reflect so-called added qualifications in a subspecialty area. The requirements for added qualifications include (1) completion of at least one year of full-time formal training and (2) satisfactory completion of an examination in the subspecialty field given by the ABMS member board. The training must be a program accredited by the Accreditation Council for Graduate Medical Education.

If the ABPN and the ABMS were to approve a category of "added qualifications in adolescent psychiatry," this would mean that persons who were already board certified in general psychiatry could have their certificates changed to add the phrase "with added qualifications in adolescent psychiatry" if they meet the conditions for this. The conditions would be the completion of one year of training beyond residency plus the passing of an examination in adolescent psychiatry given by the ABPN.

According to the bylaws of the ABMS, recognition of a field as constituting a subspecialty is contingent on the demonstration of the following factors: (1) a body of knowledge distinct from or more detailed than that of other areas in which certification is offered; (2) a group of physicians concentrating their practice in the proposed area (information about rates of increase in their numbers for the past decade and geographic distribution of these physicians is required); (3) national societies focused on the field; and (4) medical school departments or divisions devoting their principle efforts to education in the subspecialty field.

Conclusions

At the present time, there can be no doubt that a body of knowledge about adolescent psychiatry does exist and is growing. There is also a substantial number of physicians who devote the major portion of their practice to adolescent psychiatry. There is a national society, the ASAP, devoted to this field. As a rule, clearly defined academic units devoted to adolescent psychiatry do not exist within medical schools. The task of defining essential training requirements, therefore, must fall to the ASAP and its members.

Evaluation of training and of competency in adolescent psychiatry is difficult without the existence of consensus among training programs or accrediting organizations about what constitutes adequate training and competency in this field. Although it is beyond the scope of this document, there is a need to develop national standards. This issue goes beyond the concern with the quality of training in adolescent psychiatry in our general psychiatry residency programs but also encompasses the question of how to define the area of expertise of those who practice adolescent psychiatry. It has implications in terms of the continuing medical education functions of the ASAP and also of the organization and development of programs at the national and local meetings. Currently, the ASAP is taking an active role in developing and promulgating standards of training and education of both psychiatrists in training and those in practice.

Appendix

Suggested Didactic Curriculum in Adolescent Psychiatry

I. Normal development.
   A. Developmental tasks of adolescence.
   B. Psychosexual development.
   C. Object relations.
   D. Moral development.
   E. Cognitive development.
   F. Social and cultural influences on development.
II. Assessment.
   A. The psychiatric interview of the adolescent.
   B. Family interviewing.
   C. Psychological testing.
III. Psychiatric disorders in adolescence.
   A. Adjustment disorders.
   B. Neuroses.
   C. Depression and suicide.
   D. Schizophrenia and other psychotic disorders.
   E. Concepts of borderline disorders.
   F. Learning disabilities and attention deficit disorders.
   G. Conduct disorders.
   H. Developmental disorders, including autism and mental retardation.
   I. Substance abuse.

IV. Violence and abuse.
V. Sexuality.
    A. Normal sexual development.
    B. Sexual problems.
    C. Sexual abuse.
    D. Pregnancy and parenthood during adolescence.
VI. Effect of divorce and parental death.
VII. Legal issues.
    A. Emancipated minors.
    B. Confidentiality.
    C. Consent for treatment, hospitalization.
    D. Juvenile delinquency and the juvenile justice system.
VIII. Psychiatric aspects of medical illness.
    A. Trauma.
    B. Chronic illnesses.
    C. Death and dying.
    D. Noncompliance with medical treatment.
IX. Psychotherapy.
    A. The therapeutic alliance.
    B. Transference and countertransference.
    C. Communication with parents.
    D. Communication with schools.
    E. Termination.
    F. Family therapy.
    G. Group therapy.
    H. Psychoanalysis and psychodynamic psychotherapy.
    I. Cognitive and behavioral therapies.
X. Psychopharmacological treatment—special considerations with adolescents.
XI. Hospitalization and alternative living arrangements.

REFERENCES

Aichhorn, A. 1935. *Wayward Youth*. New York: Viking.
American Medical Association. 1988. *1988–1989 Directory of Graduate Medical Education Programs Accredited by the Accreditation Council on Graduate Medical Education*. Chicago: American Medical Association.
American Society for Adolescent Psychiatry. 1971. Position statement on adolescent psychiatry. *Adolescent Psychiatry* 1:418–421.

American Society for Adolescent Psychiatry. 1986. *Report of the Future Directions Task Force*. Washington, D.C.: American Society for Adolescent Psychiatry.

Blos, P. 1967. The second individuation process of adolescence. *Psychoanalytic Study of the Child* 22:162–186.

Enzer, N.; Yager, J.; Bezek, P.; Kestenbaum, C.; and Hendron, R. 1986. Who is qualified to treat adolescents? Symposium presented at the annual meeting of the American Academy of Child and Adolescent Psychiatry, October 18, Los Angeles.

Erikson, E. 1950. *Childhood and Society*. New York: Norton.

Flaherty, L. 1986. Unpublished data.

Freud, A. 1958. Adolescence. *Psychoanalytic Study of the Child* 13:255–278.

Freud, S. (1905). Drei Abhandlungen zur Sexualtheorie. Vienna: Deuticke.

Hodgman, C. H. 1983. Current issues in adolescent psychiatry. *Hospital and Community Psychiatry* 34:514–521.

Keniston, K. 1971. Youth as a stage of life. *Adolescent Psychiatry* 1:161–175.

Kestenbaum, C. 1974. Child development: the early years and the middle years. From *The Electronic Textbook of Psychiatry*. New York: Columbia University, Departments of Psychiatry and Neurology, College of Physicians and Surgeons. Videorecording.

Kestenbaum, C. 1976. Child development: the adolescent boy. From *The Electronic Textbook of Psychiatry*. New York: Columbia University, Departments of Psychiatry and Neurology, College of Physicians and Surgeons. Videorecording.

Looney, J.; Ellis, W.; Benedek, E.; and Schowalter, J. 1985. Training in adolescent psychiatry for general psychiatry residents: elements of a model curriculum. *Adolescent Psychiatry* 12:94–103.

Masterson, J. 1971. To teach is to learn twice: teaching and learning the art of psychotherapy with adolescents. In D. Offer and J. Masterson, eds. *Teaching and Learning Adolescent Psychiatry*. Springfield, Ill.: Thomas.

Mead, M. 1928. *Coming of Age in Samoa*. New York: Morrow.

Meeks, J. 1980. *The Fragile Alliance*. 2d ed. Malibu, Fla.: Krieger.

Mental Health, United States: Suicide in the United States: 1958–1982. 1985. Publication (ADM) 85–1378. Washington, D.C.: Department of Health and Human Services.

Nadelson, C., and Robinowitz, C. 1987. Medical academics and economics: continued conflict or resolution. In C. Nadelson and C. Robinowitz, eds. *Training Psychiatrists for the '90s: Issues and Recommendations*. Washington, D.C.: American Psychiatric Press.

Offer, D., and Masterson, J., eds. 1971. *Teaching and Learning Adolescent Psychiatry*. Springfield, Ill.: Thomas.

Offer, D.; Ostrov, E.; and Howard, K. I. 1986. Self-image, delinquency, and help-seeking behavior among normal adolescents. *Adolescent Psychiatry* 13:121–138.

Offord, D. 1985. Child psychiatric disorders: prevalence and perspectives. *Psychiatric Clinics of North America* 8:637–652.

Parry-Jones, W. 1984. Adolescent psychiatry in Britain: a personal view of its development and present position. *Bulletin of the Royal College of Psychiatrists* 8:230–233.

Piaget, J. 1969. The intellectual development of the adolescent. In G. Caplan and S. Lebovici, eds. *Adolescence: Psychosocial Perspectives*. New York: Basic.

Reider, R. 1988. Subspecialization in psychiatry. *American Association of Directors of Psychiatric Residency Training Newsletter* 16:1–6.

Sharfstein, S.; Goldman, H.; and Stein, S. 1987. New reimbursement models and residency training: the changing clinical and educational future. In C. Nadelson and C. Robinowitz, eds. *Training Psychiatrists for the '90s: Issues and Recommendations*. Washington, D.C.: American Psychiatric Press.

Slaff, B. 1981. The history of adolescent psychiatry. *Adolescent Psychiatry* 9:7–21.

Tasman, A., and Kay, J. 1987. Setting the stage: residency training in 1986. In C. Nadelson and C. Robinowitz, eds. *Training Psychiatrists for the '90s: Issues and Recommendations*. Washington, D.C.: American Psychiatric Press.

Weithorn, L. 1988. Mental hospitalization of troublesome youth: an analysis of skyrocketing admission rates. *Stanford Law Review* 40:773–838.

Yager, J.; Langsley, D.; Peele, R.; McKegney, F.; and Fink, P. 1987. The future psychiatrist as subspecialist: there is no alternative. In C. Nadelson and C. Robinowitz, eds. *Training Psychiatrists for the '90s: Issues and Recommendations*. Washington, D.C.: American Psychiatric Press.

THE AUTHORS

ROBERT L. ARNSTEIN is Clinical Professor of Psychiatry, Yale University School of Medicine; and Chief Psychiatrist, Yale University Health Services, New Haven, Connecticut.

LEONA L. BACHRACH is Research Professor of Psychiatry, Maryland Psychiatric Research Center, University of Maryland School of Medicine, Catonsville, Maryland.

HOWARD S. BAKER is Clinical Associate Professor of Psychiatry, University of Pennsylvania; and Director, Student Mental Health Services, Drexel University, Philadelphia, Pennsylvania.

PETER BARGLOW is Associate Professor of Psychiatry, Pritzker School of Medicine, University of Chicago; and Director, Psychiatric Acute Care Unit, Michael Reese Hospital and Medical Center, Chicago, Illinois.

JULES BEMPORAD is Associate Professor in Psychiatry, Harvard Medical School; and Director of Training and Education, Massachusetts Mental Health Center, Boston, Massachusetts.

PETER BLOS is Supervisor of Adolescent Analysis, New York Psychoanalytic Institute; Faculty Member, Columbia University Center for Psychoanalytic Education and Research; and a recipient of the Distinguished Service Award of the American Society for Adolescent Psychiatry.

DAVID DEAN BROCKMAN is Clinical Professor of Psychiatry, University of Illinois College of Medicine; and Member, Psychoanalytic Education Council, Chicago Institute for Psychoanalysis.

ANDREW M. BOXER is Associate Director, Center for the Study of Adolescence, Michael Reese Hospital and Medical Center; and Faculty Member, Chicago Institute for Psychoanalysis, Chicago, Illinois.

EVAN BRAHM is Assistant Professor, Department of Psychiatry, McGill University; Faculty Member, Canadian Institute of Psychoanalysis; and Director, Youth Service, Sir Mortimer B. Davis–Jewish General Hospital, Montreal, Quebec, Canada.

ROBERT W. BUCHANAN is Clinical Assistant Professor of Psychiatry, Pritzker School of Medicine, University of Chicago.

REBECCA S. COHEN is Director, Clinical Social Work, Department of Psychiatry, Michael Reese Hospital and Medical Center, Chicago, Illinois.

BERTRAM J. COHLER is William Rainey Harper Professor of Social Sciences, Behavioral Sciences, Education, Psychiatry, and Divinity, the University of Chicago.

RHONDA DIMPERO is Associate Director of Nursing, Timberlawn Psychiatric Hospital, Dallas, Texas.

ANNETTE EHRLICH is Professor of Psychology, California State University at Los Angeles.

AARON H. ESMAN is Professor of Clinical Psychiatry, Cornell University Medical College, New York, New York.

ROSA LINDA ESPINOZA is a recent doctoral graduate, California Graduate Institute at Los Angeles. Her chapter is based, in part, on her doctoral dissertation.

SHERMAN C. FEINSTEIN is Clinical Professor of Psychiatry, Pritzker School of Medicine, University of Chicago; Senior Consultant in Adolescent Psychiatry, Michael Reese Hospital and Medical Center; and Editor-in-Chief of this volume.

LOIS T. FLAHERTY is Medical School Associate Professor and Director, Division of Child and Adolescent Psychiatry, University of Maryland School of Medicine, Baltimore, Maryland.

HOWARD H. GOLDMAN is Professor and Director, Mental Health Policy Studies Center, Department of Psychiatry, University of Maryland School of Medicine, Baltimore, Maryland.

ALEXANDER GRALNICK is Medical Director, High Point Hospital, Port Chester, New York.

EDWARD M. HALLOWELL is Instructor in Psychiatry, Harvard Medical School; and Associate Clinical Director, Massachusetts Mental Health Center, Boston, Massachusetts.

CHARLES JAFFE is Assistant Professor of Psychiatry, Rush Medical College; Attending Psychiatrist, Michael Reese Hospital and Medical Center; and Faculty Member, Chicago Institute for Psychoanalysis, Chicago, Illinois.

JAMES M. JONES is Associate Director, Clinical Social Work, Timberlawn Psychiatric Hospital, Dallas, Texas.

RUTHELLEN JOSSELSON is Associate Professor of Psychology, Towson State University, Towson, Maryland.

EUGENE H. KAPLAN is Professor, Department of Neuropsychiatry and Behavioral Science, University of South Carolina School of Medicine; and Training and Supervising Analyst, University of North Carolina–Duke University Psychoanalytic Training Program.

LEWIS A. KIRSHNER is Assistant Clinical Professor, Harvard Medical School; and Faculty Member, Boston Psychoanalytic Institute, Boston, Massachusetts.

CHARLES G. KRASNOW is Clinical Instructor in Psychiatry; and Acting Director, Pediatrics Consultation—Liaison Program, University of Michigan Medical School, Ann Arbor, Michigan.

JOHN G. LOONEY is Professor of Psychiatry and Director, Division of Child and Adolescent Psychiatry, Duke University Medical School; Director, Durham, North Carolina, Community Guidance Clinic for Children and Youth; and a Senior Editor of this volume.

CAROL C. NADELSON is Professor and Vice Chairman, Department of Psychiatry, Tufts University; and Director, Training and Education, Department of Psychiatry, New England Medical Center Hospitals, Boston, Massachusetts.

GLEN T. PEARSON is Clinical Associate Professor of Psychiatry, Southwestern Medical School; and Director, Adolescent Girls' Unit, Timberlawn Psychiatric Hospital, Dallas, Texas.

BERT PEPPER is Clinical Professor of Psychiatry, New York University School of Medicine; Lecturer, Department of Mental Hygiene, John Hopkins University, Baltimore, Maryland; and Director, Consultation Services, American Psychiatric Association, Washington, D.C.

VIVIAN M. RAKOFF is Professor and Chairman, Department of Psychiatry, University of Toronto; and Director and Psychiatrist-in-Chief, Clarke Institute of Psychiatry, Toronto, Ontario.

LEO RANGELL is Clinical Professor of Psychiatry, University of California, Los Angeles, School of Medicine; Clinical Professor of Psychiatry (Psychoanalysis), University of California, San Francisco; and Past President, American Psychoanalytic Association and International Psycho-Analytic Association.

JOHN J. RATEY is Assistant Professor in Psychiatry, Harvard Medical School; and Director of Research, Medfield State Hospital, Boston, Massachusetts.

M. SUSAN RIDGELY is Research Associate and Associate Director, Mental Health Policy Studies, Department of Psychiatry, University of Maryland School of Medicine, Baltimore, Maryland.

HILARY RYGLEWICZ is Clinical Assistant to the Commissioner and Co-ordinator of Family Services, Rockland County (New York) Department of Mental Health.

DEBRA SCHNALL was Supervising Social Worker, Adolescent Service, Bronx Children's Psychiatric Center. She is now in private practice.

BERTRAM SLAFF is Associate Clinical Professor of Psychiatry, Mt. Sinai School of Medicine, City University of New York; Historian, American Society for Adolescent Psychiatry; and Vice President, International Society for Adolescent Psychiatry.

S. DION SMITH is Director, Department of Adolescent Psychiatry, Kaiser Foundation, San Francisco, California; and President, American Society for Adolescent Psychiatry, 1988–1989.

MYRON STOCKING is Clinical Associate Professor, Division of Child and Adolescent Psychiatry, Department of Psychiatry, University of Minnesota; and a Training and Supervising Analyst, Institute for Psychoanalysis, Chicago, Illinois.

JOHN A. TALBOTT is Professor and Chairman, Department of Psychiatry, University of Maryland School of Medicine, Baltimore, Maryland.

SIDNEY H. WEISSMAN is Associate Professor of Psychiatry, Pritzker School of Medicine, University of Chicago; and Director of Training and Education, Department of Psychiatry, Michael Reese Hospital and Medical Center, Chicago, Illinois.

LLOYD A. WELLS is Associate Professor of Psychiatry, Mayo Medical School; and Head of Section on Child and Adolescent Psychiatry, Mayo Clinic, Rochester, Minnesota.

HELEN A. WIDEN is Psychotherapist, Mental Health Center, Northwestern University; Faculty, Child and Adolescent Psychotherapy Training Program, Chicago Institute for Psychoanalysis; and Faculty, Chicago Institute for Clinical Social Work, Chicago, Illinois.

JOSEPH YOUNGERMAN is Clinical Assistant Professor of Psychiatry, Albert Einstein College of Medicine; and Chief, Psychiatric Education, Bronx Children's Psychiatric Center, Bronx, New York.

525

CONTENTS OF VOLUMES 1–15

533

542

NAME INDEX

SUBJECT INDEX

Acting out, developmental function of,
    337–48
  case examples, 340–47
  ego-development theory and, 338–40
Adolescence, 372–85
  absence of, in earlier times, 375–77,
    387, 388
  age boundaries of, 54, 177, 374, 387,
    397
  as life-long expectation and opportu-
    nity, 383, 387, 390
  choice and, 377–78, 380, 388, 389, 391
  defining, 92–94, 176–77, 373–74, 397–
    98, 493–94
  developmental stages in, 400–402
  legal considerations and defining, 398
  leisure, and development of, 377
  postponement of, 177
  prolonged, 383, 397
  as recapitulation, 93
  self-determination and, 379–81
  selfobject issues and, 391. *See also*
    Object relations; Selfobject needs
    and functions
  social influences, 402–5
  sociocultural factors, 375–77, 383–84,
    398
  statistics on, 53
  suicide and, 380–81, 382, 389. *See also*
    Suicide
  tragedy and, 377, 388
  transition from, to young adulthood,
    127–38
  turmoil, 399–400
  twentieth century, 375
  value systems and, 400, 402–4
  see also Hospitalization; Seventeen; Tur-
    moil
Adolescent psychiatry
  defining, 493–96
  history of, 3–4, 31–49
  training in, 491–518

see also Training, for adolescent psy-
    chiatry
Adolescent tasks, 54–55, 130–35, 261
  identity formation, 142–54
  sexual identity, 6, 8–9, 11
  special set, for medical students, 235–
    36
  see also Career choices; Develop-
    mental tasks; Sexual identity; Iden-
    tity; Identity crisis; Intimacy
Adversarial selfobjects, 213
Affective illness, 57–61
  defining, 57–58
  statistics on, 58
  see also Depression
AIDS. *See* College students, risk of
    AIDS
Ainsworth Strange Situation, 351, 352,
    365, 366, 367
Al-Anon, 303
Alcoholics Anonymous, 293, 304–5
Alcohol use. *See* Substance abuse
Anomic suicide, 381–82, 384
Antabuse, 292, 301
Anxiety, in borderline personalities, 320
Assessment
  in adolescent psychiatry curriculum,
    506
  of adolescent surviving personal trag-
    edy, 417–18
  chronic mentally ill young adults, 298–
    300
  substance abuse, 299
  young adults with mental/emotional
    disorders, 285–86
Assessment, of young adults, 124, 246–
    56
  career choice and, 255
  case examples, 247–49, 254–55
  developmental tasks and, 246
  identification and, 251–52
  intimacy, capacity for, 252–55